Noninvasive Ventilation

Editors

LISA F. WOLFE
AMEN SERGEW

SLEEP MEDICINE CLINICS

www.sleep.theclinics.com

Consulting Editor
TEOFILO LEE-CHIONG Jr

December 2020 • Volume 15 • Number 4

ELSEVIER

1600 John F. Kennedy Boulevard • Suite 1800 • Philadelphia, Pennsylvania, 19103-2899

http://www.theclinics.com

SLEEP MEDICINE CLINICS Volume 15, Number 4
December 2020, ISSN 1556-407X, ISBN-13: 978-0-323-76476-6

Editor: Joanna Collett
Developmental Editor: Donald Mumford

Sleep Medicine Clinics (ISSN 1556-407X) is published quarterly by Elsevier Inc., 360 Park Avenue South, New York, NY 10010-1710. Months of issue are March, June, September and December. Business and Editorial Offices: 1600 John F. Kennedy Blvd., Ste. 1800, Philadelphia, PA 19103-2899. Customer Service Office: 3251 Riverport Lane, Maryland Heights, MO 63043. Periodicals postage paid at New York, NY and additional mailing offices. Subscription prices are $218.00 per year (US individuals), $100.00 (US and Canadian students), $518.00 (US institutions), $264.00 (Canadian individuals), $252.00 (international individuals) $135.00 (International students), $587.00 (Canadian and International institutions). Foreign air speed delivery is included in all *Clinics* subscription prices. All prices are subject to change without notice. **POSTMASTER:** Send change of address to *Sleep Medicine Clinics*, Elsevier Health Sciences Division, Subscription Customer Service, 3251 Riverport Lane, Maryland Heights, MO 63043. Customer Service: **Tel: 1-800-654-2452 (U.S. and Canada); 314-447-8871 (outside U.S. and Canada). Fax: 314-447-8029. E-mail: journalscustomerservice-usa@elsevier.com (for print support); journalsonline-support-usa@elsevier.com (for online support).**

Reprints. For copies of 100 or more of articles in this publication, please contact the Commercial Reprints Department, Elsevier Inc., 360 Park Avenue South, New York, NY 10010-1710. Tel.: 212-633-3874; Fax: 212-633-3820; E-mail: reprints@elsevier.com.

Sleep Medicine Clinics is covered in *MEDLINE/PubMed (Index Medicus).*

SLEEP MEDICINE CLINICS

SERIES OF RELATED INTEREST

Clinics in Chest Medicine
Available at: https://www.chestmed.theclinics.com/

THE CLINICS ARE AVAILABLE ONLINE!
Access your subscription at:
www.theclinics.com

Contributors

CONSULTING EDITOR

TEOFILO LEE-CHIONG, Jr, MD
Professor of Medicine, National Jewish Health,
Professor of Medicine, University of Colorado,
Denver, Colorado, USA; Chief Medical Liaison,
Philips Respironics, Pennsylvania, USA

EDITORS

LISA F. WOLFE, MD
Professor of Medicine, Division of Pulmonary
and Critical Care Medicine, Northwestern
University Feinberg School of Medicine,
Chicago, Illinois, USA

AMEN SERGEW, MD
Associate Professor, Division of Pulmonary,
Critical Care and Sleep Medicine, Section of
Critical Care Medicine, Department of
Medicine, National Jewish Health, Denver,
Colorado, USA

AUTHORS

VERONIQUE ADAM, RRT
Development Consultant, Programme National
d'assistance Ventilatoire à Domicile, McGill
University Health Center, Montreal, Quebec,
Canada

NAWAL AL-SHAMLI, MD
Division of Respiratory Medicine, Department
of Pediatrics, The Hospital for Sick Children,
University of Toronto, Toronto, Ontario,
Canada

RESHMA AMIN, MD, Msc
Division of Respiratory Medicine, Department
of Pediatrics, The Hospital for Sick Children,
University of Toronto, Toronto, Ontario,
Canada

ANA SANCHEZ AZOFRA, MD
Attending Pulmonologist, Hospital
Universitario de la Princesa, Madrid, Spain

JOSHUA O. BENDITT, MD
Medical Director, Respiratory Care Services
and General Pulmonary Clinic, Department of
Pulmonary, Critical Care, and Sleep Medicine,

University of Washington, UW Medical Center,
Seattle, Washington, USA

JEANETTE BROWN, MD, PhD
Assistant Professor, Division of Pulmonary
Medicine, University of Utah, Salt Lake City,
Utah, USA

MICHELLE CAO, DO
Clinical Associate Professor, Division of
Neuromuscular Medicine, Department of
Neurology, Division of Sleep Medicine,
Department of Psychiatry, Stanford University,
Palo Alto, California, USA

MAIDA L. CHEN, MD
Associate Professor, Department of Pediatrics,
University of Washington, Medical Director,
Sleep Disorders Program, Division of
Pulmonary and Sleep Medicine, Seattle
Children's Hospital, Seattle, Washington, USA

JACKIE CHIANG, MA, MD
Division of Respiratory Medicine, Department
of Pediatrics, The Hospital for Sick Children,
University of Toronto, Toronto, Ontario,
Canada

PHILIP CHOI, MD
Assistant Professor of Internal Medicine,
University of Michigan, Ann Arbor, Michigan,
USA

JOHN M. COLEMAN III, MD
Associate Professor of Medicine and
Neurology, Division of Pulmonary and Critical
Care Medicine, Department of Medicine,
Department of Neurology, Northwestern
University Feinberg School of Medicine,
Chicago, Illinois, USA

JESSICA A. COOKSEY, MD
Health System Clinician, Northwestern
University, Grayslake, Illinois, USA

DOM D'ANDREA, BS
Laboratory Technician in Regenerative
Neurorehabilitation Laboratory, Regenerative
Neurorehabilitation Laboratory (Biologics),
Shirley Ryan AbilityLab, Chicago, Illinois, USA

ASIL DAOUD, MD
Sleep Medicine Fellow, John D. Dingell VA
Medical Center, Department of Medicine,
Wayne State University, Detroit Medical
Center, Detroit, Michigan, USA

ELLEN FARR, MD
Resident Physician in Physical Medicine and
Rehabilitation, Regenerative
Neurorehabilitation Laboratory (Biologics),
Shirley Ryan AbilityLab, McGaw Medical
Center, Northwestern University, Chicago,
Illinois, USA

JUSTIN FIALA, MD
Pulmonary, Critical Care and Sleep Fellow,
Division of Pulmonary and Critical Care
Medicine, Department of Medicine,
Department of Neurology, Northwestern
University Feinberg School of Medicine,
Chicago, Illinois, USA

COLIN K. FRANZ, MD, PhD
Assistant Professor in Physical Medicine and
Rehabilitation, and Neurology, Director of the
Electrodiagnostic Laboratory, Regenerative
Neurorehabilitation Laboratory (Biologics),
Shirley Ryan AbilityLab, Northwestern
University Feinberg School of Medicine,
Chicago, Illinois, USA

SAMRAN HAIDER, MD
Pulmonary and Critical Care Medicine Fellow,
John D. Dingell VA Medical Center,
Department of Medicine, Wayne State
University, Detroit Medical Center, Detroit,
Michigan, USA

MARTA KAMINSKA, MD, MSc
Quebec National Program for Home Ventilatory
Assistance, Respiratory Division and Sleep
Laboratory, McGill University Health Centre,
Montreal, Quebec, Canada

ROOP KAW, MD
Departments of Hospital Medicine and
Anesthesiology Outcomes Research,
Cleveland Clinic, Cleveland, Ohio, USA

ERIN W. MACKINTOSH, MD
Acting Assistant Professor, Department of
Pediatrics, University of Washington, Division
of Pulmonary and Sleep Medicine, Seattle
Children's Hospital, Seattle, Washington, USA

KARA DUPUY-MCCAULEY, MD
Instructor of Medicine, Division of Pulmonary
and Critical Care Medicine, Center for Sleep
Medicine, Mayo Clinic, Rochester, Minnesota,
USA

JEREMY E. ORR, MD
Assistant Professor, Division of Pulmonary,
Critical Care, and Sleep Medicine, UC San
Diego School of Medicine, La Jolla, California,
USA

ASHIMA S. SAHNI, MD
Assistant Professor of Clinical Medicine,
Pulmonary, Critical Care, Sleep, and Allergy,
University of Illinois Hospital and Health
Sciences System, Chicago, Illinois, USA

ABDULGHANI SANKARI, MD, PhD
Director of Medical Education, John D. Dingell
VA Medical Center, Department of Internal
Medicine, Division of Pulmonary, Critical Care
and Sleep Medicine, Wayne State University,
Detroit, USA; Ascension Providence Hospital,
Southfield, Michigan, USA

BERNARDO SELIM, MD
Assistant Professor of Medicine, Director,
Respiratory Care Unit, Division of Pulmonary
and Critical Care Medicine, Center for Sleep

Medicine, Mayo Clinic, Rochester, Minnesota, USA

AMEN SERGEW, MD
Associate Professor, Division of Pulmonary, Critical Care and Sleep Medicine, Section of Critical Care Medicine, Department of Medicine, National Jewish Health, Denver, Colorado, USA

JENNY SHI, MD
Division of Respiratory Medicine, Department of Pediatrics, The Hospital for Sick Children, University of Toronto, Toronto, Ontario, Canada

GAURAV SINGH, MD, MPH
Staff Physician, Pulmonary, Critical Care, and Sleep Medicine Section, Department of Medicine, VA Palo Alto Health Care System, Clinical Assistant Professor, Division of Pulmonary, Allergy, and Critical Care Medicine, Department of Medicine, Stanford University, Palo Alto, California, USA

LAUREN A. TOBIAS, MD
Assistant Professor of Medicine, VA Connecticut Healthcare System, Yale School of Medicine, West Haven, Connecticut, USA

LIEN-KHUONG TRAN, MD
Attending Physician, Pulmonary, Critical Care and Sleep, Texas Pulmonary & Critical Care Consultants, Fort Worth, Texas, USA

LISA F. WOLFE, MD
Professor of Medicine, Division of Pulmonary and Critical Care Medicine, Northwestern University Feinberg School of Medicine, Chicago, Illinois, USA

DAVID ZIELINSKI, MD, FRCPC, FCCP
Associate Professor, Department of Pediatrics, McGill University, Montreal Children's Hospital, Research Institute of McGill University Health Centre, Montreal, Quebec, Canada

LAUREN A. TOBIAS, MD
Assistant Professor of Medicine, VA Connecticut Healthcare System, Yale School of Medicine, West Haven, Connecticut, USA

LISA ROUCHE TRAN, MD
Attending Physician, Pulmonary, Critical Care and Sleep, Texas Pulmonary & Critical Care Consultants, Fort Worth, Texas, USA

LISA F. WOLFE, MD
Professor of Medicine, Division of Pulmonary and Critical Care Medicine, Northwestern University Feinberg School of Medicine, Chicago, Illinois, USA

DAVID ZIELINSKI, MD, FRCPC, FCCP
Associate Professor, Department of Pediatrics, McGill University, Montreal Children's Hospital, Research Institute of McGill University Health Centre, Montreal, Quebec, Canada

Medicine, Mayo Clinic, Rochester, Minnesota, USA

AMEN SERGEW, MD
Associate Professor, Division of Pulmonary, Critical Care, and Sleep Medicine, Section of Chronic Care Medicine, Department of Medicine, National Jewish Health, Denver, Colorado, USA

JENNY SHI, MD
Internal Medicine/Respirology, Medicine Department, The Hospital for Sick Children, University of Toronto, Toronto, Ontario, Canada

GAURAV SINGH, MD, MPH
Staff Physician, Pulmonary, Critical Care, and Sleep Medicine Section, Department of Medicine, VA Palo Alto Health Care System, Clinical Assistant Professor, Division of Pulmonary, Allergy, and Critical Care Medicine, Department of Medicine, Stanford University, Palo Alto, California, USA

Contents

> Obesity hypoventilation syndrome is the most frequent cause of chronic hypoventilation and is increasingly more common with rising obesity rates. It leads to considerable morbidity and mortality, particularly when not recognized and treated adequately. Long-term nocturnal noninvasive ventilation is the mainstay of treatment but evidence suggests that CPAP may be effective in stable patients. Specific perioperative management is required to reduce complications. Some unique syndromes associated with obesity and hypoventilation include rapid-onset obesity with hypoventilation, hypothalamic, autonomic dysregulation (ROHHAD), and Prader-Willi syndrome. Congenital central hypoventilation syndrome (early or late-onset) is a genetic disorder resulting in hypoventilation. Several acquired causes of chronic central hypoventilation also exist. A high level of clinical suspicion is required to appropriately diagnose and manage affected patients.

> Individuals with spinal cord injury (SCI) are at increased risk of respiratory complications during wake and sleep. Sleep-disordered breathing (SDB) is commonly associated with SCI and requires an individualized approach to its management. Respiratory control plays a key role in the pathogenesis of SDB in cervical SCI. Noninvasive ventilation plays an important role in the management of respiratory complications in individuals with SCI acutely and in chronic phases. Positive airway pressure treatment may be effective in eliminating SDB and improving sleepiness symptoms, but adherence to treatment is poor and effect on long-term outcomes is questionable.

> Cumulative evidence supports the association of adverse postoperative outcomes with obstructive sleep apnea (OSA) and obesity hypoventilation syndrome (OHS). Although current guidelines recommend preoperative screening for OSA and OHS, the best perioperative management pathways remain unknown. Interventions attempting to prevent complications in the postoperative period largely are consensus based and focused on enhanced monitoring, conservative measures, and specific OSA therapies, such as positive airway pressure. Until further research is available to improve the quality and strength of these recommendations, patients with known or suspected OSA and OHS should be considered at higher risk for perioperative cardiopulmonary complications.

Individuals with Duchenne muscular dystrophy (DMD) have evolving sleep and res-piratory pathophysiology over their lifetimes. Across the lifespan of DMD, various sleep-related breathing disorders (SRBD) have been described, including obstruc-tive sleep apnea, central sleep apnea, and nocturnal hypoventilation. In addition to SRBD, individuals with DMD can be affected by insomnia, chronic pain and other factors interfering with sleep quality, and daytime somnolence. The natural progres-sion of DMD pathophysiology has changed with the introduction of therapies for downstream pathologic pathways and will continue to evolve with the development of therapies that target function and expression of dystrophin.

A significant body of literature supports the benefit of noninvasive ventilation (NIV) for acute hypercapnia in the setting of exacerbations of chronic obstructive pulmo-nary disease (COPD). In those with severe COPD with chronic hypercapnic respira-tory failure, however, the role of NIV has been more controversial. This article reviews the physiologic basis for considering NIV in patients with COPD, summa-rizes existing evidence supporting the role of NIV in COPD, highlights the patient population and ventilatory approach most likely to offer benefit, and suggests a po-tential clinical pathway for managing patients.

The need for long-term noninvasive positive pressure ventilation (NiPPV) in children with chronic respiratory failure is rapidly growing. This article reviews pediatric-specific considerations of NiPPV therapy. Indications for NiPPV therapy can be cate-gorized by the cause of the respiratory failure: (1) upper airway obstruction, (2) musculoskeletal and/or neuromuscular disease, (3) lower respiratory tract diseases, and (4) control of breathing abnormalities. The role of NiPPV therapy in select rare conditions (spinal muscular atrophy, congenital central hypoventilation syndrome, cerebral palsy, scoliosis, and Chiari malformations) is also reviewed.

Amyotrophic lateral sclerosis is a progressive neurodegenerative disease involving upper and lower motor neurons and has limited treatment options. The weakness progresses to involve the diaphragms, resulting in respiratory failure and death. Home noninvasive ventilation has been shown to improve survival and quality of life, especially in those with intact bulbar function. Once initiated, close monitoring with nocturnal oximetry, remote downloads from the home noninvasive ventilation machine, and measurement of serum bicarbonate should be conducted. Addition-ally, transcutaneous CO_2 monitoring can be considered if available. This article dis-cusses the indications, timing, initiation, and management of noninvasive ventilation in amyotrophic lateral sclerosis.

Weaning to noninvasive ventilation in intensive care unit and bridging the patients to home with respiratory support is evolving as the technology of noninvasive ventilation is improving. In patients with chronic obstructive pulmonary disease exacerbation, timing of initiation of noninvasive ventilation is the key, as persistently hypercapnic patients show benefits. High intensity pressure support seems to do better in comparison to low-intensity pressure support. In patients with obesity and hypercapnia, obesity hypoventilation cannot be ruled out especially in an inpatient setting, and it is crucial that these patients are discharged with noninvasive ventilation.

The number of patients experiencing prolonged mechanical ventilation is increasing over time. Patients who have a tracheostomy placed in a critical care setting have been described as having an average of 4 separate transitions between the acute care setting, long-term acute care (LTAC), and home. Transition points can be problematic if not addressed adequately; however, proactive planning can optimize patient care. Individual patient factors will determine if the patient will require long-term tracheostomy, transitioned to noninvasive positive pressure ventilation, or able to be decannulated. Patients and caregivers should be included in transition planning to optimize outcomes.

Preface

A Comprehensive View of Noninvasive Ventilation

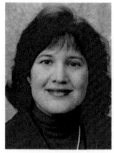 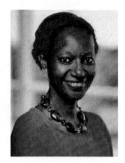

Lisa F. Wolfe, MD   Amen Sergew, MD

Editors

Noninvasive ventilation (NIV), often referred to interchangeably as noninvasive positive pressure ventilation, is the focus of the current issue. One of the earliest uses of the modern day NIV machines dates to the 1940s when a group from Columbia University at Bellevue Hospital devised an "automatic respirator" to provide intermittent positive pressure ventilation using a facemask for patients with acute respiratory failure.[1] NIV was used during the polio epidemic and was especially important for those with disabilities and chronic respiratory failure to be able to live independently in community-based living centers.[2] However, in the decades that followed, invasive ventilation become the mainstay for the management of acute respiratory failure while NIV fell out of favor. During the 1980s and 1990s, NIV came back into focus as convincing evidence was published to support the use of NIV for the hospital-based treatment of acute exacerbations of chronic obstructive pulmonary disease (COPD) and acute pulmonary edema.[3] NIV using a nasal mask (instead of a full facemask) was first reported in 1987 by Ellis and colleagues[4] in 5 patients with neuromuscular weakness, which provided more data and options for the use of long-term home NIV.

Over the years, the indications for NIV have expanded to include various disease states. In this issue, the authors discuss the key disease states in which long-term NIV is used: obesity hypoventilation (Kaw and Kaminska), spinal cord injury (Daoud and colleagues), Duchenne muscular dystrophy (MacKintosh and colleagues), COPD (Orr and colleagues), amyotrophic lateral sclerosis (Cooksey and Sergew), Neuralgic Amyotrophy (Farr and colleagues), and common uses of NIV in the pediatric population (Shi and colleagues). Over time, various modes and settings have been developed to improve synchrony and portability. These devices and modes are discussed (Singh and Cao) as well as the long-term follow up of NIV (Choi and colleagues). The use of NIV in the perioperative period (Dupuy-McCauley and Selim) and in the postacute phase, such as in long-term rehabilitation centers (Brown), is also discussed. NIV can be titrated in a sleep lab for optimal results when feasible and if outpatient titrations fail. Given the versatile patient population with vastly differing requirements, a thoughtfully designed and tailored sleep lab (Fiala and Coleman) provides more optimal and personalized results.

Our collection of articles provides a comprehensive review of the most pertinent issues in the use and management of NIV. We chose well-regarded experts in each topic, and we are immensely proud and grateful for their contributions. We are honored to have been a part of a series that will

Sleep Med Clin 15 (2020) xiii–xiv
https://doi.org/10.1016/j.jsmc.2020.09.001
1556-407X/20/© 2020 Published by Elsevier Inc.

highlight NIV to educate our colleagues on this fast-moving literature and are thankful to *Sleep Medicine Clinics* for this opportunity.

Lisa F. Wolfe, MD
Northwestern University
Feinberg School of Medicine
676 North St. Clair Street, Suite 1400
Chicago, IL 60611, USA

Amen Sergew, MD
National Jewish Health/University of Colorado
1400 Jackson St, B140
Denver, CO 80206, USA

E-mail addresses:
lwolfe@northwestern.edu (L.F. Wolfe)
sergewa@njhealth.org (A. Sergew)

REFERENCES

1. Motley HL, Werko L, Cournand A, et al. Observations on the clinical use of intermittent positive pressure. J Aviat Med 1947;18(5):417–35.
2. Headley J. Edward Verne Roberts. In: PolioPlace. 2011. Available at: http://www.polioplace.org/people/edward-verne-roberts. Accessed March 6, 2020.
3. Scala R, Pisani L. Noninvasive ventilation in acute respiratory failure: which recipe for success? Eur Respir Rev 2018;27(149).
4. Ellis ER, Bye PT, Bruderer JW, et al. Treatment of respiratory failure during sleep in patients with neuromuscular disease. Positive-pressure ventilation through a nose mask. Am Rev Respir Dis 1987; 135(1):148–52.

Obesity Hypoventilation
Traditional Versus Nontraditional Populations

Roop Kaw, MD[a,b,*], Marta Kaminska, MD, MSc[c]

KEYWORDS

- Hypoventilation • Obesity hypoventilation syndrome • Noninvasive ventilation • CCHS • ROHHAD

KEY POINTS

- Obesity hypoventilation syndrome should be suspected in obese patients with sleep-disordered breathing symptoms and otherwise unexplained increased serum bicarbonate levels, but confirmation requires arterial blood gas measurement.
- Continuous positive airway pressure is the preferred treatment of stable patients with OHS with severe OSA, but noninvasive ventilation is recommended for those without OSA and those presenting with acute hypercapnic respiratory failure.
- Unrecognized OHS increases the risk of postoperative complications. Considering the diagnosis preoperatively; avoiding general anesthesia over spinal/epidural, ensuring complete neuromuscular blockade reversal before awake extubation and avoiding high flow supplemental oxygen can minimize the risk.
- Sleep-related hypoventilation and progressive chronic respiratory failure can occur as a result of late-onset central congenital hypoventilation syndrome or other causes such that a high index of suspicion is necessary for diagnosis and appropriate management.

INTRODUCTION

Obesity hypoventilation syndrome (OHS) is characterized by a triad of chronic daytime hypercapnia ($Paco_2$ >45 mm Hg), sleep-disordered breathing (SDB), and obesity with a body mass index (BMI) >30 kg/m^2.[1] Its presumed prevalence in the general population, based on small clinical cohort studies, is 0.3% to 0.4%.[2] Among patients with known obstructive sleep apnea (OSA) the reported prevalence of OHS is between 10% and 20% and increases with obesity to as high as 50% as the BMI exceeds 50 kg/m^2. Compared with eucapnic patients with obesity, patients with OHS have higher odds of having heart failure, angina pectoris, cor pulmonale, pulmonary hypertension, higher mortality.[3,4]

Diagnosis

Typical signs and symptoms include dyspnea, nocturia, lower extremity edema, excessive daytime sleepiness, fatigue, loud disruptive snoring, witnessed apneas, and mild hypoxemia during wake but significant hypoxemia during sleep. A bicarbonate level less than 27 mmol/L effectively rules out hypercapnia. However, for obese patients with SDB who are strongly suspected of having OHS, the American Thoracic Society (ATS) recommends measuring $Paco_2$ directly to diagnose OHS, rather than bicarbonate or SpO_2 (**Fig. 1**). In contrast, for patients with low-moderate probability of OHS, $Paco_2$ only needs to be measured in patients with serum bicarbonate $\geq$27 mmol/L to confirm or rule out the diagnosis.

[a] Department of Hospital Medicine, Cleveland Clinic, 9500 Euclid Avenue, Suite M2-113, Cleveland, OH 44139, USA; [b] Department of Anesthesiology Outcomes Research, Cleveland Clinic, 9500 Euclid Avenue, Cleveland, OH 44139, USA; [c] Quebec National Program for Home Ventilatory Assistance, Respiratory Division and Sleep Laboratory, McGill University Health Centre, 1001 Decarie Boulevard, Montreal, Quebec H4A 3J1, Canada
* Corresponding author.
E-mail address: kawr@ccf.org

Sleep Med Clin 15 (2020) 449–459
https://doi.org/10.1016/j.jsmc.2020.08.001
1556-407X/20/© 2020 Elsevier Inc. All rights reserved.

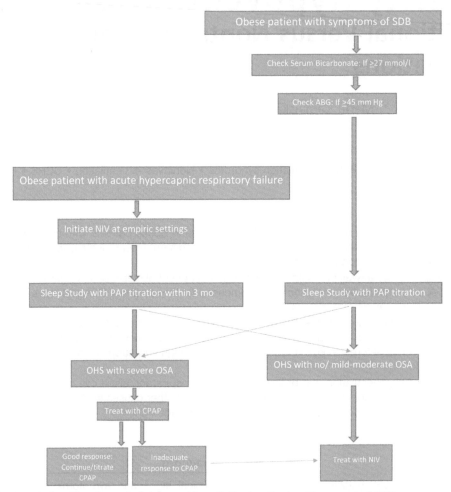

Fig. 1. Treatment algorithm for ambulatory and hospitalized patients with suspected OHS.

AMBULATORY MANAGEMENT OF OBESITY HYPOVENTILATION SYNDROME
Positive Airway Therapy

Positive airway therapy (PAP) is the primary treatment option for patients with OHS but accepted treatment targets and outcome measures are not determined yet. Patients with symptomatic OHS who also have cardiometabolic comorbidities (defined as stage IV OHS by the European Respiratory Society) and those with chronic respiratory failure after an episode of acute respiratory failure are more likely to benefit.[5] In patients with mild OHS (awake $Paco_2$: 45–50 mm Hg) or borderline OHS (stage I and II of obesity-associated sleep hypoventilation as defined by the European Respiratory Society) the treatment benefits are less certain.[5] Empirical settings for initial PAP in patients with OHS, without guidance of overnight respiratory monitoring, should be discouraged. Standardized education and training regarding

device and interface usage should be provided. Early follow-up (4–8 weeks) should be scheduled to assess clinical and physiologic response to PAP and should include monitoring objective adherence to therapy. Data show that higher rates of adherence to PAP are associated with superior control of respiratory failure in OHS.[6–8]

Continuous Positive Airway Pressure Versus BILEVEL Positive Airway Pressure

ATS recommends that, when effective, continuous positive airway pressure (CPAP) should be used over noninvasive ventilation (NIV) as the initial treatment of stable ambulatory adult patients with OHS and concurrent severe OSA (Apnea-Hypopnea Index $\geq$30 events per hour) presenting with chronic stable respiratory failure.[9] Reduction in Pco_2 levels is associated with improved prognosis.[10] Current data do not favor one form of PAP therapy over another in stable chronic OHS, in terms of short- and long-term mortality, composite cardiovascular events (including pulmonary hypertension and left ventricular diastolic dysfunction), resolution of hypercapnia, need for oxygen supplementation, and resolution of daytime sleepiness.[11] However, hypercapnia resolution may be slower with CPAP than with NIV. Patients presenting with more profound ventilatory failure, poorer lung function, advanced age, or less severe OSA may be less likely to respond to CPAP.[8,12,13] For these reasons, close monitoring is advised, especially during the first 2 months of treatment to ensure consistent improvement, with adjustment of therapy as required. NIV is more expensive than CPAP at baseline with additional resources needed for titration and training.[6] Adherence to CPAP and NIV are similar with reported use of 5 to 6 hours per night. Regardless of device, patient compliance predicts resolution of hypercapnia.

Obesity Hypoventilation Syndrome Without Severe Obstructive Sleep Apnea

OSA occurs in 90% of all OHS, with severe OSA in 73%.[14] In those without OSA, upper airway obstruction is unlikely to be the primary determinant of OHS. Pathophysiology in those cases is incompletely understood and may be heterogeneous. It likely involves unfavorable respiratory mechanics, altered central respiratory drive, and hormonal factors, including leptin abnormalities.[14,15] CPAP is believed to be ineffective in these cases, and NIV with backup rate has been successfully used. Although studies are mostly small or of limited duration, NIV in this context is more effective than lifestyle modification in improving P_{CO_2}, sleepiness, health-related quality of life, and polysomnographic parameters.[16] (see **Fig. 1**) Interestingly, improved CO_2 chemosensitivity was found to correlate with increasing leptin; this might reflect different pathophysiology from OHS with severe OSA where leptin is typically raised and decreases with NIV.[15,17] Further research is required to better characterize this population and determine optimal therapy.

Weight Loss as Management Strategy for Obesity Hypoventilation Syndrome

Limited data suggest, to achieve resolution of OHS, a long-term sustained weight loss of ≥25% to 30% of actual body weight is needed. The degree of weight loss necessary to mitigate cardiovascular and metabolic risk in patients with OHS is unknown. Intensive short- and long-term lifestyle interventions result in only about 2 to 12 kg weight loss.[18] Weight loss surgery, including laparoscopic sleeve gastrectomy, Roux-en-Y gastric bypass, or biliopancreatic diversion with duodenal switch but less likely laparoscopic gastric banding, is the only way to achieve sufficient weight loss. The choice of surgical procedure should be based on weighing potential risks of surgery against the maximum possible anticipated weight loss. Given that patients with OHS are at higher surgical risk, a balanced, patient-centered, risk-benefit discussion is important.[19]

INPATIENT MANAGEMENT OF SUSPECTED OBESITY HYPOVENTILATION SYNDROME

Up to 40% of patients with OHS first manifest with acute hypercapnic respiratory failure.[20] The underlying diagnosis of OHS may be overlooked, and appropriate treatment not initiated on discharge.[3] OHS should be considered in all obese patients presenting with hypercapnic respiratory failure. NIV should be initiated rapidly, if no contraindications exist, as it may help prevent intubation. Intubation is often difficult and the complications inherent to invasive mechanical ventilation are exacerbated in the obese.[21] NIV in the acute setting is at least as effective in OHS as in chronic obstructive pulmonary disease (COPD).[22]

Management at Hospital Discharge

Hospitalized patients suspected of having OHS who develop an acute-on-chronic hypercapnic respiratory failure have higher short-term (1–2 years) mortality than ambulatory patients with OHS.[23] An observational study reported a mortality of 23% at 18 months in patients discharged from the hospital without PAP.[3] In contrast, in another observational study in which all patients were discharged on NIV, the 2-year mortality was 8%.[10] ATS recommends that all hospitalized patients suspected of OHS be started on NIV before discharge and continued on such until outpatient workup and sleep laboratory titration after 3 months of therapy.[9,24]

PERIOPERATIVE CONSIDERATIONS IN OBESITY HYPOVENTILATION SYNDROME
Preoperative Assessment

In comparison with patients with OSA, patients with hypercapnia from definite or possible OHS or from overlap syndrome (OHS-COPD) are more likely to have postoperative respiratory failure, heart failure, prolonged intubation, postoperative intensive care unit (ICU) transfer, and longer ICU and hospital stays.[19] OHS should therefore be considered when postoperative respiratory failure occurs in an obese patient without other predispositions. Identifying those at risk helps to optimize management and prevent complications.

Patients with known or suspected OSA, who have a serum bicarbonate greater than 27 meq/L are likely to have OHS, which should be confirmed with measurement of $Paco_2$ (**Fig. 2**). A split-night (diagnostic and PAP titration) polysomnography is then recommended. The Society of Anesthesia and Sleep Medicine in its recent guideline recommends additional evaluation for preoperative cardiopulmonary optimization in patients with a partially treated OSA or suspected OSA when they have hypoventilation, pulmonary hypertension, and resting hypoxemia that are not attributable to other cardiopulmonary diseases.[25] If a split-night polysomnography is unavailable, the use of preoperative home sleep apnea testing combined with a secondary outpatient trial of auto-CPAP or NIV should be considered.

Intraoperative Considerations

Airway management
For laryngoscopy, sniffing position in general improves pharyngeal patency in anesthetized patients with OSA.[26] However, in morbidly obese patients, the head elevation laryngoscopy position, which horizontally aligns the auditory meatus and the sternal notch, with arms away from the chest, results in a better laryngeal view than the sniffing position.[27] If difficult mask ventilation is suspected, airway management in patients with OHS can be accomplished by awake fiber optic intubation under local anesthesia, instead of general anesthesia.

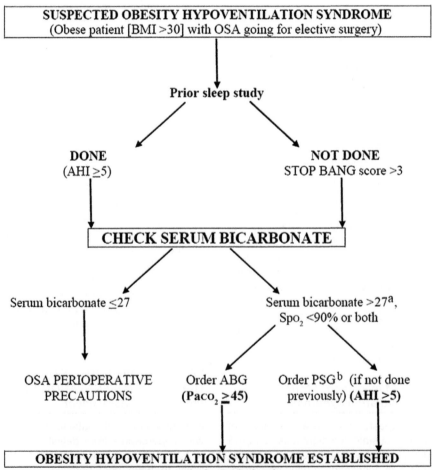

Fig. 2. Perioperative decision tree in patients with suspected OHS. [a] When metabolic alkalosis is not explained by causes other than chronic respiratory acidosis. [b] Whenever possible PSG should be arranged before surgery in this situation.

In patients with OHS, during periods of apnea the volume of oxygen absorbed from the lungs is more than the amount of carbon dioxide produced, creating a negative pressure, which assists in ventilation during the apnea period. Adding positive end-expiratory pressure (PEEP) up to 10 cm H_2O to oxygen for 5 minutes in a 25° head-up position during preintubation or apneic oxygenation during intubation using nasopharyngeal oxygenation or transnasal humidified rapid insufflation ventilator exchange prolongs nonhypoxic apnea because it ameliorates the drop in functional residual capacity (FRC) from position, paralysis, and absorptive atelectasis from high concentration oxygen.[28,29]

Choice of anesthesia technique

Central neuraxial anesthesia techniques (spinal and epidural anesthesia) can be problematic even if done with local anesthetics. Using fluoroscopic or ultrasound guidance to avoid airway instrumentation and limit the use of anesthetic agents can worsen an already blunted respiratory drive in patients with OHS.[30,31] Hypotension can be concerning in the obese patient during neuraxial anesthesia because they cannot tolerate supine or Trendelenburg positions. If pulmonary hypertension (PH) is suspected, epidural anesthesia is preferred over spinal anesthesia because of the latter's rapid onset and profound sympatholytic effect.[32]

Loading and maintenance doses of hydrophilic drugs, such as most neuromuscular blockers, should be based on lean body weight (LBW), whereas for lipophilic drugs, such as succinylcholine, the loading dose should be calculated based on total body weight (also because of higher plasma cholinesterase levels in the obese).[33] Rocuronium (dosed by LBW) is a good alternative for rapid induction when succinylcholine is contraindicated or unavailable.[34] Sugammadex and neostigmine reverse neuromuscular blockade. Their doses should be based on the total dose and half-time of neuromuscular blocking agents being reversed and should be titrated for the desired effect.[35,36] In patients with PH, etomidate is preferred for induction over propofol and sodium thiopental because of its minimal effect on myocardial contractility and systemic venous resistance, thereby avoiding right ventricular ischemia.[37] Nitrous oxide may increase pulmonary vascular resistance, and as such may be harmful to patients with right ventricular dysfunction.[38]

Intraoperative ventilation strategies

Intraoperative protective ventilation strategies (tidal volumes of 6–8 mL/kg of predicted body weight, PEEP of 6–8 cm H_2O, and lung recruitment in the form of 30 seconds of continuous positive airway pressure at 30 cm H_2O) have been used to reduce postoperative pulmonary complications.[21,39] However, recently, among obese patients (BMI ≥35) undergoing surgery lasting greater than 2 hours under general anesthesia, using high levels of PEEP (12 cm of H_2O) and alveolar recruitment maneuvers during intraoperative mechanical ventilation did not reduce postoperative pulmonary complications compared with low levels of PEEP (4 cm of H_2O).[40] This randomized controlled study did not specifically include patients with OHS or report its prevalence. Hypoxemia, however, was more frequent in the group randomized to lower levels of PEEP, resulting in higher need for rescue strategy for desaturation in this group.

Postoperative Considerations

Extubation and positive airway pressure after anesthesia

Awake extubation in a semisitting or sitting (beach chair) position avoids reduction in FRC and allows for rapid repositioning of the operating table for reintubation if extubation fails.

Subanesthetic residual concentrations of inhalational anesthetics impair hypoxic and hypercapnic drive and may contribute to hypoxemia/hypercapnia in patients with OHS.[41] The dose of volatile anesthetic and the time for its washout can be reduced with short-acting adjuvant medications, such as remifentanil, and by combining general and regional anesthetics.[42] Also, acute respiratory acidosis augments the activity of some neuromuscular blocking agents and interferes with their reversal. Adherence to extubation criteria and complete reversal of muscle relaxant effect is needed to prevent low tidal volumes, worsening respiratory acidosis and blunting of respiratory drive ultimately leading to CO_2 narcosis with hypoxemia despite oxygen therapy.[43] Use of PAP reduced postextubation respiratory failure in obese ICU patients.[44] Expiratory pressure at 1 to 2 cm higher than normal/optimal may be required to eliminate apneas. PAP therapy will also reduce postoperative atelectasis and avoid use of high Fio_2. Tidal volume on bilevel ventilation can be increased by increasing inspiratory pressure, shortening rise time, increasing inspiratory time, or lowering the expiratory sensitivity.[45] Backup respiratory rate can be set 2 to 3 breaths per minute below a patient's spontaneous rate. Volume assured pressure modes can adjust inspiratory PAP targeting a set tidal volume or alveolar ventilation. There is, however, no data currently to support their use perioperatively.[46]

Monitoring of opioid-induced ventilatory impairment and other clinical parameters

Obese patients have a higher central respiratory drive because they produce more carbon dioxide, and have a higher work of breathing and basal oxygen consumption in comparison with lean subjects. Opioids can shift the carbon dioxide response curve to the right and reduce the ventilatory response to $Paco_2$. Patients with OHS are particularly susceptible to opioid-induced ventilatory impairment (OIVI). Utilizing multimodal analgesic regimens, sedation scoring systems, such as the Ramsay Sedation Scale in postoperative patients, and implementing centralized continuous pulse oximetry monitoring, end-tidal or subcutaneous capnography monitors, or both, can help early detection and mitigation of OIVI.[47]

Postoperative supplemental oxygen

Up to 40% patients with OHS are prescribed nocturnal home oxygen in addition to adequately used PAP.[48] These patients may need higher amounts of oxygen postoperatively and pulse oximetry will not detect the onset or worsening of ventilatory depression.[49] Recent data advise extreme caution in administration of a high concentration (100%) of supplemental oxygen to this group of patients especially when they are sedated, asleep, or on intravenous opioids, because it suppresses ventilation and worsens hypercapnia.[50] In a recent trial of patients with OSA randomized to supplemental oxygen (max 3 L/min) or no oxygen postoperatively, 11% of the patients (mostly in the supplemental O_2 group) became significantly hypercapnic especially on the first postoperative night.[51] Hence, monitoring CO_2 is probably necessary in patients with OHS receiving supplemental oxygen after surgery.

SPECIFIC SYNDROMES WITH HYPOVENTILATION
Late-Onset Central Hypoventilation Syndrome

Congenital central hypoventilation syndrome (CCHS) results from mutations in the gene paired-like homeobox2B (*PHOX2B*) encoding the transcription factor responsible for regulating central and peripheral nervous system development. (See Shi and colleagues' article "Management of Rare Causes of Pediatric Chronic Respiratory Failure," in this issue.) Central chemoreception fails and patients have absent or diminished ventilatory response to CO_2, resulting in hypoventilation.[52] Most severe cases are detected in the neonatal period. However, the disease may first manifest after the neonatal period and into adulthood, then termed late-onset CCHS (LO-CCHS) (**Table 1**).

CCHS and LO-CCHS are characterized by hypoventilation in sleep and wakefulness, with absence of perception of hypercarbia/hypoxemia, and lack of arousal from sleep with development of physiologic compromise secondary to hypoventilation. There may be diffuse autonomic dysregulation, including cardiac arrhythmias that may require pacemaker insertion.[53]

Most CCHS cases result from a polyalanine repeat expansion mutation (PARM) in the PHOX2B gene, with a minority due to nonpolyalanine repeat mutation (NPARM), including frameshift, missense, and nonsense mutations. NPARMs typically occur de novo, whereas PARMs can be inherited (autosomal dominant) from apparently asymptomatic parents carrying either full PHOX2B gene mutation or mosaicism for this gene. The specific genotype is related to severity of the phenotype and helps predict severity of hypoventilation and risk of sudden cardiac death.[53] However, genotypes have incomplete penetrance and variable expressivity.[54] Families have been described with a mosaic mutation present in several family members, some of whom had minor or absent symptoms.[55]

LO-CCHS may be undetected until it is triggered by a physiologic disturbance, such as general anesthesia, respiratory infection, pregnancy, or administration of sedatives.[55,56] LO-CCHS should be suspected in cases of unexplained alveolar hypoventilation, increased serum bicarbonate, delayed recovery of spontaneous breathing after anesthesia or severe respiratory infection, and seizures or neurocognitive delay. Parents of known CCHS cases should be tested for the mutation.[57]

Ventilatory support management depends on the syndrome severity, with positive pressure ventilation by tracheostomy, bilevel NIV with backup rate, or negative pressure ventilators (although becoming rarer). Small children usually require tracheostomy ventilation, whereas older children and adults can often be managed with NIV. Continuous monitoring with pulse oximetry and end-tidal CO_2 is required in children. When LO-CCHS is diagnosed in adulthood, daytime support is generally not necessary. Nocturnal NIV is the mainstay of treatment and can be provided in volumetric or barometric mode, but a back-up rate is essential. To avoid complications, such as cognitive impairment and PH, periodic evaluation of adequacy of ventilation is required, using overnight pulse oximetry; overnight transcutaneous CO_2 recording can be useful when supplemental oxygen may mask hypoventilation.[58]

Table 1
Syndromes with hypoventilation

	Late-Onset CCHS	ROHHAD	Prader-Willi Syndrome
Cause of syndrome	*PHOX2B* mutations	Unknown, presumed dysfunction of neural crest-derived tissues; suggested: autoimmune, paraneoplastic, orexin system dysfunction	Genomic imprinting disorder with lack of expression of genes inherited from the paternal chromosome 15q11-q13 region
Cause of hypoventilation	Abnormal development of retrotrapezoid nucleus with reduced or absent CO_2 ventilatory response (also abnormal carotid bodies, cardiopulmonary afferents, and sympathetic ganglia)	Obesity and abnormal control of breathing	Obesity and abnormal control of breathing
Onset of syndrome	Any time after the neonatal period, including adulthood	Childhood, after initial normal development	Neonatal, different phases
Associated manifestations	Autonomic dysregulation (constipation, ophthalmologic abnormalities, arrhythmias), neural crest tumors	Rapidly progressing obesity, hypothalamic dysfunction (eg, growth hormone deficiency, diabetes insipidus, central precocious puberty), autonomic dysfunction, neurologic, and behavioral symptoms (eg, intellectual disability, seizures), neuroendocrine tumors	Obesity, hypothalamic, and autonomic dysfunction, intellectual disability, psychiatric disorders, short stature, hypogonadism, excessive daytime sleepiness, circadian rhythm disturbances, characteristic facial features

Abbreviations: CCHS, congenital central hypoventilation syndrome; ROHHAD, rapid-onset obesity with hypothalamic dysfunction, hypoventilation, and autonomic dysregulation.

Diaphragm pacers can be used for daytime support of ambulatory children and adults requiring full-time ventilatory support, with positive pressure ventilation at night. Pacers are also used in older patients during sleep only, to minimize the need for mechanical ventilation and potentially remove the tracheostomy.[59] Those relying on diaphragm pacing also require continuous monitoring with pulse oximetry and ideally end-tidal CO_2. OSA can complicate diaphragm pacing during sleep, but is correctable by adjusting pacer settings to lengthen inspiratory time and/or decrease inspiratory force.[60] CCHS does not resolve spontaneously and treatment is lifelong. Children with CCHS should be prohibited from competing in swimming and underwater sports as they will not perceive the hypercapnia/hypoxemia occurring with breath-holding and are at increased risk of drowning. The same risk likely exists in adults.

RAPID-ONSET OBESITY WITH HYPOVENTILATION, HYPOTHALAMIC, AUTONOMIC DYSREGULATION

Rapid-onset obesity with hypoventilation, hypothalamic, autonomic dysregulation (ROHHAD) syndrome is a rare disorder of respiratory failure presenting in a previously healthy child. A subset of patients with ROHHAD also develop neuroendocrine tumors (NET), then dubbed ROHHAD/NET. Rapidly progressing obesity and hypothalamic dysfunction are typically the presenting features. Autonomic dysregulation, and behavioral and neurologic symptoms can also occur. ROHHADNET is more frequent in girls, with a median age at diagnosis around 4 years.[31] Hypoventilation occurs early in the course and often requires ventilatory support. The origin of the ROHHAD phenotype is unknown.[61]

Mortality is high, often from cardiopulmonary arrest. Hypoventilation and respiratory failure are progressive, and presumed to relate to autonomic and central control of breathing abnormalities. However, ventilatory responses to hypoxia and hypercapnia were found to be only mildly abnormal.[62] OSA is common, often preceding evidence of hypoventilation.[63] Obesity likely plays a significant role, leading to upper airway obstruction, altered respiratory mechanics, hypoxemia, and hypoventilation. Clinically, patients lack perception of the physiologic disturbance and show no signs of respiratory distress.[62] Therefore, it is essential to obtain objective measures with pulse oximetry, and Pco_2 measurements using arterialized capillary blood, or end-tidal or transcutaneous CO_2 monitoring during both sleep and wakefulness.[33] Correction of SDB and chronic

hypoventilation using NIV is the mainstay of treatment. Timely initiation may prevent sudden death and neurocognitive impairment.[62] Upper airway obstruction in sleep, combined with lack of signs of respiratory distress, can lead to ventilatory failure despite NIV and complicate NIV management.[64] Ongoing monitoring with pulse oximetry seems essential in these patients. Compared with standard obesity hypoventilation seen in adults, ROHHAD is a much more fatal condition and requires more vigilance and close clinical monitoring.

Prader-Willi Syndrome

Prader-Willi syndrome (PWS) is a more common disorder, also presenting with hypothalamic and autonomic dysfunction, but manifesting first with neonatal hypotonia, poor feeding and growth, followed by rapid weight gain in early childhood and compulsive food-seeking behaviors in later childhood. The presentation of PWS is highly variable. OSA and sleep-related hypoventilation relate largely to obesity. However, reduced ventilatory responses to hypoxia and hypercapnia are present, and hypoxemia in sleep was more marked compared with matched controls in adults and adolescents with PWS, suggesting control of breathing abnormalities.[65,66] Chronic ventilatory failure is uncommon but occasional severe cases leading to death have been reported.[67,68] There is frequent use of testosterone replacement therapy, which can worsen SDB in PWS. Full polysomnography is recommended both before and after starting testosterone therapy.

Acquired central hypoventilation

Acquired causes of central hypoventilation include neurologic trauma, neurosurgical complications, ischemia (particularly lateral medullary strokes), mass, infection, demyelinating disease, anoxic-ischemic damage, and drugs (narcotics, sedatives, anesthetics).[52] Clinicians should be attentive to signs and symptoms of hypoventilation and SDB in disorders affecting the brainstem.

DISCLOSURE

investigator-initiated research support from Philips Respironics (In kind), VitalAire Inc (In kind), and Fisher Paykel (<15,000CAD); advisory board member for Biron Soins du Sommeil.

REFERENCES

1. Mokhlesi B, Tulaimat A, Faibussowitsch I, et al. Obesity hypoventilation syndrome: prevalence and

predictors in patients with obstructive sleep apnea. Sleep Breath 2007;11(2):117–24.

2. Kaw R, Hernandez AV, Walker E, et al. Determinants of hypercapnia in obese patients with obstructive sleep apnea. Chest 2009;136(3):787–96.

3. Nowbar S, Burkart KM, Gonzales R, et al. Obesity-associated hypoventilation in hospitalized patients: prevalence, effects, and outcome. Am J Med 2004;116(1):1–7.

4. Berg G, Delaive K, Manfreda J, et al. The use of health-care resources in obesity-hypoventilation syndrome. Chest 2001;120(2):377–83.

5. Randerath W, Verbraecken J, Andreas S, et al. Definition, discrimination, diagnosis and treatment of central breathing disturbances during sleep. Eur Respir J 2017;49(1):1600959.

6. Masa JF, Mokhlesi B, Benítez I, et al. Long-term clinical effectiveness of continuous positive airway pressure therapy versus non-invasive ventilation therapy in patients with obesity hypoventilation syndrome: a multicentre, open-label, randomised controlled trial. Lancet 2019;393(10182):1721–32.

7. Murphy PB, Davidson C, Hind MD, et al. Volume targeted versus pressure support non-invasive ventilation in patients with super obesity and chronic respiratory failure: a randomised controlled trial. Thorax 2012;67(8):727–34.

8. Mokhlesi B, Tulaimat A, Evans AT, et al. Impact of adherence with positive airway pressure therapy on hypercapnia in obstructive sleep apnea. J Clin Sleep Med 2006;2(1):57–62.

9. Mokhlesi B, Masa JF, Brozek JL, et al. Evaluation and management of obesity hypoventilation syndrome. An official American Thoracic Society clinical practice guideline. Am J Respir Crit Care Med 2019; 200(3):e6–24.

10. Budweiser S, Riedl SG, Jörres RA, et al. Mortality and prognostic factors in patients with obesity-hypoventilation syndrome undergoing noninvasive ventilation. J Intern Med 2007;261(4):375–83.

11. Masa JF, Mokhlesi B, Benítez I, et al. Echocardiographic changes with positive airway pressure therapy in obesity hypoventilation syndrome: long-term Pickwick randomized controlled trial. Am J Respir Crit Care Med 2019. https://doi.org/10.1164/rccm. 201906-1122OC. rccm.201906-1122OC.

12. Howard ME, Piper AJ, Stevens B, et al. A randomised controlled trial of CPAP versus non-invasive ventilation for initial treatment of obesity hypoventilation syndrome. Thorax 2017;72(5):437–44.

13. Pérez de Llano LA, Golpe R, Ortiz Piquer M, et al. Clinical heterogeneity among patients with obesity hypoventilation syndrome: therapeutic implications. Respiration 2008;75(1):34–9.

14. Piper AJ, Grunstein RR. Obesity hypoventilation syndrome: mechanisms and management. Am J Respir Crit Care Med 2011;183(3):292–8.

15. Redolfi S, Corda L, La Piana G, et al. Long-term non-invasive ventilation increases chemosensitivity and leptin in obesity-hypoventilation syndrome. Respir Med 2007;101(6):1191–5.

16. Masa JF, Corral J, Caballero C, et al. Non-invasive ventilation in obesity hypoventilation syndrome without severe obstructive sleep apnoea. Thorax 2016;71(10):899–906.

17. Yee BJ, Cheung J, Phipps P, et al. Treatment of obesity hypoventilation syndrome and serum leptin. Respiration 2006;73(2):209–12.

18. The Look AHEAD Research Group. Cardiovascular effects of intensive lifestyle intervention in type 2 diabetes. N Engl J Med 2013;369(2):145–54.

19. Kaw R, Bhateja P, Paz y Mar H, et al. Postoperative complications in patients with unrecognized obesity hypoventilation syndrome undergoing elective noncardiac surgery. Chest 2016;149(1):84–91.

20. Piper AJ, BaHammam AS, Javaheri S. Obesity hypoventilation syndrome. Sleep Med Clin 2017;12(4): 587–96.

21. Pépin JL, Timsit JF, Tamisier R, et al. Prevention and care of respiratory failure in obese patients. Lancet Respir Med 2016;4(5):407–18.

22. Carrillo A, Ferrer M, Gonzalez-Diaz G, et al. Noninvasive ventilation in acute hypercapnic respiratory failure caused by obesity hypoventilation syndrome and chronic obstructive pulmonary disease. Am J Respir Crit Care Med 2012;186(12):1279–85.

23. Marik PE, Chen C. The clinical characteristics and hospital and post-hospital survival of patients with the obesity hypoventilation syndrome: analysis of a large cohort. Obes Sci Pract 2016;2(1):40–7.

24. Mokhlesi B, Masa JF, Afshar M, et al. The effect of hospital discharge with empiric noninvasive ventilation on mortality in hospitalized patients with obesity hypoventilation syndrome: an individual patient data meta-analysis. Ann Am Thorac Soc 2020. https:// doi.org/10.1513/AnnalsATS.201912-887OC. AnnalsATS.201912-887OC.

25. Chung F, Memtsoudis SG, Ramachandran SK, et al. Society of Anesthesia and Sleep Medicine guidelines on preoperative screening and assessment of adult patients with obstructive sleep apnea. Anesth Analg 2016;123(2):452–73.

26. Isono S. Optimal combination of head, mandible and body positions for pharyngeal airway maintenance during perioperative period: lesson from pharyngeal closing pressures. Semin Anesth Perioper Med Pain 2007;26(2):83–93.

27. Collins JS, Lemmens HJM, Brodsky JB, et al. Laryngoscopy and morbid obesity: a comparison of the "Sniff" and "Ramped" positions. Obes Surg 2004;14(9):1171–5.

28. Patel A, Nouraei SAR. Transnasal humidified rapid-insufflation ventilatory exchange (THRIVE): a physiological method of increasing apnoea time in patients with difficult airways. Anaesthesia 2015;70(3):323–9.

29. Gander S, Frascarolo P, Suter M, et al. Positive end-expiratory pressure during induction of general anesthesia increases duration of nonhypoxic apnea in morbidly obese patients. Anesth Analg 2005; 100(2):580–4.

30. Zwillich CW, Sutton FD, Pierson DJ, et al. Decreased hypoxic ventilatory drive in the obesity-hypoventilation syndrome. Am J Med 1975;59(3): 343–8.

31. Shimura R, Tatsumi K, Nakamura A, et al. Fat accumulation, leptin, and hypercapnia in obstructive sleep apnea-hypopnea syndrome. Chest 2005; 127(2):543–9.

32. Minai OA, Yared J-P, Kaw R, et al. Perioperative risk and management in patients with pulmonary hypertension. Chest 2013;144(1):329–40.

33. Lemmens HJM, Brodsky JB. The dose of succinylcholine in morbid obesity. Anesth Analg 2006; 102(2):438–42.

34. Pösö T, Kesek D, Winsö O, et al. Volatile rapid sequence induction in morbidly obese patients. Eur J Anaesthesiol 2011;28(11):781–7.

35. Ingrande J, Lemmens HJM. Dose adjustment of anaesthetics in the morbidly obese. Br J Anaesth 2010; 105:i16–23.

36. Leykin Y, Miotto L, Pellis T. Pharmacokinetic considerations in the obese. Best Pract Res Clin Anaesthesiol 2011;25(1):27–36.

37. Ebert TJ, Muzi M, Berens R, et al. Sympathetic responses to induction of anesthesia in humans with propofol or etomidate. Anesthesiology 1992;76(5): 725–33.

38. McNulty SE, Weiss J, Azad SS, et al. The effect of the prone position on venous pressure and blood loss during lumbar laminectomy. J Clin Anesth 1992;4(3):220–5.

39. Futier E, Constantin J-M, Paugam-Burtz C, et al. A trial of intraoperative low-tidal-volume ventilation in abdominal surgery. N Engl J Med 2013;369(5): 428–37.

40. Writing Committee for the PROBESE Collaborative Group of the PROtective VEntilation Network (PRO-VEnet) for the Clinical Trial Network of the European Society of Anaesthesiology, Bluth T, Serpa Neto A, Schultz MJ, et al. Effect of intraoperative high positive end-expiratory pressure (PEEP) with recruitment maneuvers vs low PEEP on postoperative pulmonary complications in obese patients: a randomized clinical trial. JAMA 2019;321(23):2292.

41. Gupta A, Stierer T, Zuckerman R, et al. Comparison of recovery profile After ambulatory anesthesia with propofol, isoflurane, sevoflurane and desflurane: a systematic review. Anesth Analg 2004;632–41. https://doi.org/10.1213/01.ANE.0000103187.70627.57.

42. Seet E, Chung F. Management of sleep apnea in adults—functional algorithms for the perioperative period: continuing professional development. Can J Anesth 2010;57(9):849–64.

43. Kaw R, Argalious M, Aboussouan LS, et al. Obesity hypoventilation syndrome and anesthesia considerations. Sleep Med Clin 2014;9(3):399–407.

44. El Solh AA, Aquilina A, Pineda L, et al. Noninvasive ventilation for prevention of post-extubation respiratory failure in obese patients. Eur Respir J 2006; 28(3):588–95.

45. Squier SB, Patil SP, Schneider H, et al. Effect of end-expiratory lung volume on upper airway collapsibility in sleeping men and women. J Appl Physiol 2010; 109(4):977–85.

46. Selim BJ, Wolfe L, Coleman JM, et al. Initiation of noninvasive ventilation for sleep related hypoventilation disorders. Chest 2018;153(1):251–65.

47. Taenzer AH, Pyke JB, McGrath SP, et al. Impact of pulse oximetry surveillance on rescue events and intensive care unit transfers: a before-and-after concurrence study. Anesthesiology 2010;112(2): 282–7.

48. Banerjee D, Yee BJ, Piper AJ, et al. Obesity hypoventilation syndrome. Chest 2007;131(6):1678–84.

49. Fu ES, Downs JB, Schweiger JW, et al. Supplemental oxygen impairs detection of hypoventilation by pulse oximetry. Chest 2004;126(5):1552–8.

50. Wijesinghe M, Williams M, Perrin K, et al. The effect of supplemental oxygen on hypercapnia in subjects with obesity-associated hypoventilation. Chest 2011;139(5):1018–24.

51. Liao P, Wong J, Singh M, et al. Postoperative oxygen therapy in patients with OSA. Chest 2017;151(3): 597–611.

52. Zaidi S, Gandhi J, Vatsia S, et al. Congenital central hypoventilation syndrome: an overview of etiopathogenesis, associated pathologies, clinical presentation, and management. Auton Neurosci 2018;210: 1–9.

53. Weese-Mayer DE, Berry-Kravis EM, Ceccherini I, et al. An official ATS clinical policy statement: congenital central hypoventilation syndrome: genetic basis, diagnosis, and management. Am J Respir Crit Care Med 2010;181(6):626–44.

54. Amiel J, Laudier B, Attié-Bitach T, et al. Polyalanine expansion and frameshift mutations of the paired-like homeobox gene PHOX2B in congenital central hypoventilation syndrome. Nat Genet 2003;33(4): 459–61.

55. Klaskova E, Drabek J, Hobzova M, et al. Significant phenotype variability of congenital central hypoventilation syndrome in a family with polyalanine expansion mutation of the PHOX2B gene. Biomed Pap 2016;160(4):495–8.

56. Mahfouz AKM, Rashid M, Khan MS, et al. Late onset congenital central hypoventilation syndrome after exposure to general anesthesia. Can J Anesth 2011;58(12):1105–9.

57. Kasi AS, Kun SS, Keens TG, et al. Adult with *PHOX2B* mutation and late-onset congenital central hypoventilation syndrome. J Clin Sleep Med 2018; 14(12):2079–81.

58. Adam V, Zielinski D, Kaminska M. Feasibility of Overnight Transcutaneous CO2 Monitoring in the Home Setting. Presented at the 15th International Conference on Home Mechanical Ventilation. Lyon, March, 2018.

59. Diep B, Wang A, Kun S, et al. Diaphragm pacing without tracheostomy in congenital central hypoventilation syndrome patients. Respiration 2015;89(6): 534–8.

60. Wang A, Kun S, Diep B, et al. Obstructive sleep apnea in patients with congenital central hypoventilation syndrome ventilated by diaphragm pacing without tracheostomy. J Clin Sleep Med 2018; 14(02):261–4.

61. Barclay SF, Rand CM, Nguyen L, et al. ROHHAD and Prader-Willi syndrome (PWS): clinical and genetic comparison. Orphanet J Rare Dis 2018;13(1): 124.

62. Carroll MS, Patwari PP, Kenny AS, et al. Rapid-onset obesity with hypothalamic dysfunction, hypoventilation, and autonomic dysregulation (ROHHAD):

63. Reppucci D, Hamilton J, Yeh EA, et al. ROHHAD syndrome and evolution of sleep disordered breathing. Orphanet J Rare Dis 2016;11(1):106.

64. Graziani A, Casalini P, Mirici-Cappa F, et al. Hypoventilation improvement in an adult non-invasively ventilated patient with rapid-onset obesity with hypothalamic dysfunction hypoventilation and autonomic dysregulation (ROHHAD). Pneumol Buchar Rom 2016;65(4):222–4.

65. Nixon GM, Brouillette RT. Sleep and breathing in Prader-Willi syndrome. Pediatr Pulmonol 2002; 34(3):209–17.

66. Arens R, Gozal D, Burrell BC, et al. Arousal and cardiorespiratory responses to hypoxia in Prader-Willi syndrome. Am J Respir Crit Care Med 1996; 153(1):283–7.

67. Yee BJ, Buchanan PR, Mahadev S, et al. Assessment of sleep and breathing in adults with Prader-Willi syndrome: a case control series. J Clin Sleep Med 2007;3(7):713–8.

68. Schrander-Stumpel CTHRM, Curfs LMG, Sastrowijoto P, et al. Prader-Willi syndrome: causes of death in an international series of 27 cases. Am J Med Genet 2004;124A(4):333–8.

response to ventilatory challenges. Pediatr Pulmonol 2015;50(12):1336–45.

Noninvasive Ventilation and Spinal Cord Injury

Asil Daoud, MD[a,b,c], Samran Haider, MD[a,b,c], Abdulghani Sankari, MD, PhD[a,d,e],*

KEYWORDS

• Sleep • Sleep-disordered breathing • Spinal cord injury (SCI) • Noninvasive ventilation

KEY POINTS

• Spinal cord injury (SCI) is a common cause of paralysis and can lead to increased risk of respiratory complications acutely and for years after recovery.
• Sleep-disordered breathing (SDB) is common after SCI and contributes to poor sleep and quality of life.
• Positive airway pressure can improve sleepiness symptoms but evidence for its effect on neurocognitive outcome is lacking. In addition, there are several barriers to achieving effective management.
• Noninvasive ventilation is an effective therapeutic tool in the management of respiratory dysfunction in the setting of acute and chronic SCI; however, its role in treating SDB in this population is not well established.

INTRODUCTION

Spinal cord injury (SCI) is the second most common cause of paralysis after a stroke.[1] Traumatic injuries such as motor vehicle accidents are responsible for most SCIs, with more than half involving an injury to the cervical spine.[2] It is estimated that 1.9% of the US population, or 6 million people, live with paralysis.[2] The injury age distribution is bimodal: younger, predominantly men, involved in motor vehicle accidents; and older people injured during falls.[3]

Patients with SCI are at risk of respiratory complications secondary to neuromuscular respiratory weakness leading to ineffective cough, poor airway clearance, infections, and respiratory failure.[4] They are also at increased risk of sleep-disordered breathing (SDB), particularly obstructive sleep apnea (OSA), with ranges between 27% and 62%.[5] However, patients with SCI are also predisposed to central sleep apnea (CSA).[6]

The acute and chronic respiratory dysfunction depends on preexisting pulmonary status, level of SCI, and the quality of care provided in the management of impaired respiratory dysfunction.[7] The role of noninvasive ventilation (NIV) has been studied for decades in the management of respiratory dysfunction in the setting of acute and chronic SCI, and the evidence continues to grow in support of the role of NIV in the management of respiratory failure in SCI. However, it is considered a double-edged sword given the resulting complications, the burden on patients with SCI, and the limited evidence on the effect on overall survival, length of hospital stay, and quality of life.[8]

In this article, the focus is on the role of NIV in the management of acute and chronic respiratory failure in patients with SCI.

Funding: Dr A. Sankari is supported by VA for the research (in part) presented in this paper and his time as a PI.
[a] Department of Medicine, John D. Dingell VA Medical Center, Wayne State University, Detroit Medical Center, 3990 John R St, Detroit, MI 48201, USA; [b] Department of Medicine, Wayne State University, Detroit, MI, USA; [c] Detroit Medical Center, Detroit, MI, USA; [d] Department of Internal Medicine, Division of Pulmonary, Critical Care and Sleep Medicine, Wayne State University, 3990 John R, 3-Hudson, Detroit, MI 48201, USA; [e] Ascension Providence Hospital, Southfield, MI, USA
* Corresponding author. Division of Pulmonary, Critical Care and Sleep Medicine, Wayne State University, 3990 John R, 3-Hudson, Detroit, MI 48201.
E-mail address: asankari@wayne.edu

RESPIRATORY COMPLICATIONS AFTER ACUTE SPINAL CORD INJURY

Most patients with traumatic brain injury and SCI die because of respiratory muscle paralysis and apnea.[9,10] Those who survive are at risk of developing ventilatory failure during the first week of hospitalization.[9] Pulmonary complications are the leading cause of morbidity and death both in the short and long term after injury. It is estimated that up to 84% of patients with high cervical SCI (C1–C4) and 60% with low cervical (C5–C8) injuries experience respiratory compromise.[11]

Atelectasis is the most common respiratory complication overall, followed by pneumonia and respiratory failure, regardless of the level of injury. However, among patients with high cervical SCI (C1–C4), pneumonia is the most common complication and may occur in up to 63% of patients. Pleural effusions occur most frequently among patients with T1 to T12 level injuries, and the incidence may be as high as 38%.[12] Other pulmonary complications following SCI include pulmonary edema from excess fluid resuscitation in the acute phase and pulmonary embolism, which may occur in up to 4.5% patients in the first 3 months. The ability to cough is also severely impaired among patients with cervical or high thoracic injuries secondary to thoracic and abdominal muscle paralysis. This condition results in an inability to produce the forced expiration required for an effective cough.[13] In addition, in lesions above T6, there is impairment of the sympathetic nervous system with an unopposed parasympathetic activity, which results in bronchial reactivity. Such patients may benefit from inhaled anticholinergic agents. In addition to increased bronchial reactivity, a recent study showed an increase in nasal resistance, which may contribute to OSA among patients with high cervical injuries. Nasal resistance decreased with the use of phenylephrine.[14]

In the acute period of traumatic spinal injury, spinal shock may occur. This condition results in immediate flaccid paralysis of muscles below the level of the cord injury and can last for several months. As spinal shock resolves, spasticity of thoracic and abdominal muscles replaces the flaccid paralysis and this may improve lung volumes.[11,13] In the acute phase, spinal shock may be severe enough to require mechanical ventilatory assistance. Aggressive respiratory management has been recommended for the prevention and treatment of pulmonary complications among these patients.[11] Emesis and aspiration of gastric content is a risk, especially during the acute period of SCI when gastric emptying is slowed. If adequate monitoring and expertise are not available, it is best to intubate acutely injured patients.[15]

PATHOPHYSIOLOGY OF CHRONIC RESPIRATORY FAILURE IN SPINAL CORD INJURY
Mechanism of Chronic Respiratory Failure

Respiratory failure associated with SCI depends on the level of the injury, along with other factors such as age and preexisting medical illness. Following SCI, several respiratory muscles are affected, leading to impairment of respiratory and airway functions. The muscles that contribute to respiration can be divided into 3 groups: the intercostal and accessory muscles, the diaphragm, and the muscles of the abdomen.[7] The diaphragm, which is innervated by the phrenic nerve, originating from C3 to C5, is the most important muscle for inspiration, providing 65% of the tidal volume during normal breathing.[16,17] The intercostals, which are innervated by segmental spinal nerves arising from T1 through T11 and are lost in complete tetraplegia, and the accessory muscles help the diaphragm in the expansion of the chest wall in the process of inspiration.[17] Patients with injury above C5 have an impaired diaphragm and likely require a period of mechanical ventilation.[13]

Expiration is a passive process; however, abdominal muscles are important for augmentation of contractions and for the expulsive force needed for an effective cough and to clear secretions.[18] In complete tetraplegia, abdominal muscle function is absent, and, as the diaphragm relaxes during expiration, the flaccid chest wall moves outward, limiting the expiratory reserve volumes to less than 20% of normal.[17] Because abdominal musculature is also flaccid, forced expiration is even severely compromised during wakefulness and sleep.[19]

Several studies investigated the cause of pulmonary complications of SCI. De Vivo and colleagues[20] and Cotton and colleagues[4] suggested that injury to the cervical and upper thoracic cord disrupts the function of the diaphragm, intercostal muscles, accessory respiratory muscles, and abdominal muscles, which causes a reduction in lung volume parameters. This condition results in several chronic respiratory consequences, such as ineffective cough, difficulty clearing secretions, atelectasis, pulmonary infections, and hypoventilation and hypoxia episodes.

Vital capacity (VC), expiratory reserve volume, and maximum generated expiratory flow significantly decrease with cervical SCI. This decrease is worse among patients with cord injury above

C4. Close monitoring of VC and pulse oximetry among other clinical parameters is highly recommended in this population. VC should be measured every 8 hours and, if decreasing, mechanical ventilation should be started.[9]

Bach[21] described 3 categories of ventilatory failure complicating spinal injuries. The first category comprised patients with high spinal cord (C1–C4) injuries who are apneic at the time of injury. If these patients survive the initial injury, they require long-term ventilation. About 60% of patients in this category can be eventually weaned off but it may take up to 8 years. Patients in the second category have autonomous breathing at the time of presentation to the hospital regardless of the level of injury. These patients are at high risk of developing respiratory failure, which may occur 12 hours or more after injury. Ventilatory failure among these patients may last up to 5 weeks and most of these patients can be weaned off. The third category comprises patients who did not have ventilatory failure immediately after the injury or during the hospital admission but may have pulmonary complications, including respiratory failure many years later.

Patients with SCI may have an ineffective cough, which puts them at higher risk and aggressive mechanical airway clearance is recommended for these patients.[9,21,22] Ineffective cough may be caused by a weak inspiratory gasp secondary to weakness of the diaphragm or spinal deformity, weakness of bulbar muscles impairing glottis closure, or weakness of the expulsive phase of cough caused by weakness of intercostal and abdominal muscles. This condition may result in atelectasis, bacterial colonization, pneumonia, and respiratory failure.[23] Peak cough flow less than 160 L/min is considered ineffective for airway clearance. Values less than 270 L/min are considered low and put patients at higher risk of developing respiratory complications. Effective airway clearance with peak cough flow greater than 160 L/min has also been associated with successful extubation.[24] Large randomized controlled trials to assess the effectiveness of airway cough techniques among patients with SCI are lacking.[25]

Mechanism of Sleep-Disordered Breathing in Spinal Cord Injury

Several studies in the literature reported an increased incidence of SDB in individuals with SCI and a high level of injury.[26] Specifically, SDB was 5 times more common in patients with SCI than in the general population. Berlowitz and colleagues,[5] and Chiodo and colleagues[27] reported that more than 60% of people with tetraplegia have SDB. Sankari and colleagues[19] assessed the SDB and ventilation changes comparing 2 different levels of SCI: cervical and thoracic. This study revealed a higher prevalence of SDB in cervical SCI, 93% compared with 55% in thoracic SCI, which was similar to the prevalence reported in the literature. However, this study was unique because it showed, using in-laboratory polysomnography (PSG), that SDB in patients with thoracic SCI was mainly obstructive, whereas SDB in patients with cervical SCI seemed to be mixed and centrally mediated, with 1 in 4 patients having Cheyne-Stokes respiration pattern or CSA without evidence of heart failure.[19] Likewise, a subsequent case series using home sleep study combined with transcutaneous CO_2 monitoring showed that CSA was present in 23.8%.[28]

To identify therapeutic targets, researchers in recent years have attempted to understand the mechanisms responsible for the development of SDB in individuals with SCI, which is more complex than in the general population. Several pathophysiologic traits have been postulated, such as increased upper airway collapsibility (Pcrit),[29] a reduced dilator muscle responsiveness,[30] reduced arousal threshold,[31] and unstable ventilatory control[6] (**Fig. 1**).

Central SDB is a result of hypoventilation (hypercapnia) or a consequence of posthyperventilation (hypocapnia). This condition is thought to be caused by the loss of wakefulness drive to breath.[32] Adequate ventilation during sleep is critically dependent on levels of arterial CO_2 ($Paco_2$)[33]; thus, abnormal loop gain can cause CSA, which occurs when there is a fluctuation of $Paco_2$ below the apneic threshold. This condition is more likely when the $Paco_2$ level is close to the apneic threshold, called CO_2 reserve. Loop gain is an engineering term that refers to the propensity of a negative feedback control system to oscillate. Loop gain combines the response of the ventilatory system to changing $Paco_2$ (the controller or chemoreflex sensitivity), and the effectiveness of the lung/respiratory system in decreasing $Paco_2$ in response to hyperventilation (the plant)[34] (**Fig. 2**). Changes in either parameter change the requisite hypocapnia to reach central apnea, which is implied in patients with neuromuscular disease.[35,36] It seems that patients with cervical SCI are more susceptible to developing CSA mainly because of higher plant gain compared with individuals with thoracic SCI (**Fig. 3**). High plant gain can occur when a small change in ventilation results in a large change in CO_2. High plant gain can be found in individuals with cervical SCI because of small functional residual capacity and/or alveolar hypoventilation.[6]

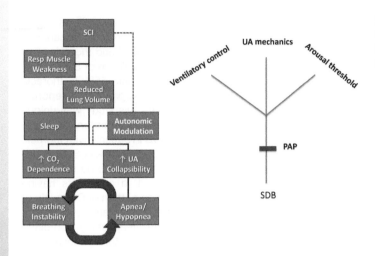

Fig. 1. The scope of the SDB and respiratory failure following SCI. PAP, positive airway pressure; UA, upper airway.

Central apnea may also influence the development of pharyngeal obstruction or narrowing when the ventilatory drive reaches a nadir during central apnea or hypopnea.[37] In contrast, pharyngeal collapses, combined with mucosal and gravitational factors, may impair pharyngeal opening and require a substantial increase in a drive that propagates breathing instability.

Hypoventilation in neuromuscular disease often first presents at night during sleep, particularly the rapid eye movement stage.[38] The weakness of muscles of inspiration and exhalation and the alteration of upper airway reflex leads to decreased respiratory efforts, which causes the failure of effective airflow during sleep.[30,39] Known risk factors of OSA in the general population, such as obesity, aging, and male gender, may also contribute to the incidence of SDB in people with SCI. In more recent studies, Wijesuriya and colleagues[40] reported that increased nasal resistance may contribute to SDB in people with tetraplegia.

In summary, the combination of sleep-related hypoventilation and increased peripheral chemoresponsiveness may explain why patients with cervical SCI show an increased propensity for CSA, whereas increased upper airway collapsibility (Pcrit) provides a physiologic explanation for increased risk of OSA in patients with cervical and thoracic SCI. Understanding the unique pathophysiologic mechanisms may inform the development of targeted therapies in this population.

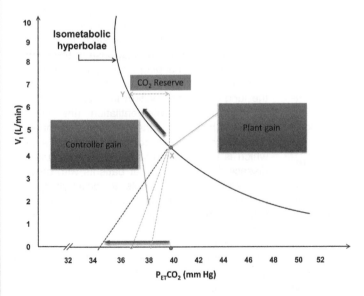

Fig. 2. The determinants of ventilatory instability (ie, hypocapnic central apnea). $P_{ET}CO_2$, end-tidal CO_2.

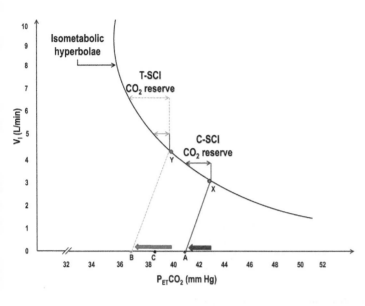

Fig. 3. The ventilatory responsiveness to CO_2 below eupnea in the cervical (C-SCI) and thoracic (T-SCI) patients for a given isometabolic hyperbolae. Two examples of SCI with similar chemoreflex sensitivity slopes. Note that in C-SCI (*solid lines*) a smaller change in $P_{ET}CO_2$ (from 42.8 mm Hg at baseline to 40.8 mm Hg) in response to hyperventilation is required to cross the apneic threshold (A) and results in apnea. In T-SCI (*dotted lines*), a larger change in $P_{ET}CO_2$ (from 40.0 mm Hg at baseline to 36.6 mm Hg) in response to hyperventilation is required to cross the apneic threshold (B) and develop an apnea. Note that the T-SCI is at a higher point (Y) on the isometabolic hyperbola than the C-SCI (X) despite a similar chemoreflex sensitivity. Slopes indicate the similar chemoreflex sensitivity below eupnea in the thoracic and cervical groups. The solid line and arrow in the T-SCI example indicate the estimated change in $P_{ET}CO_2$ (from 40.0 mm Hg at baseline to 38.5 mm Hg) for the same change in ventilation that is noted in C-SCI in response to hyperventilation reaching point C without crossing the apneic threshold (B). Example of decreasing plant gain by shifting the eupneic CO_2 to the steeper portion of the metabolic hyperbolae (X to Y). (*From* Sankari A, Bascom AT, Chowdhuri S, Badr MS. Tetraplegia is a risk factor for central sleep apnea. *J Appl Physiol (1985)*. 2014;116(3):345-353; with permission.)

Physiology and clinical manifestation of chronic respiratory failure and sleep-disordered breathing

A high prevalence of SDB among patients with SCI has been reported in multiple publications. As in the general population, SDB in individuals with SCI can manifest as daytime hypersomnolence, morning headaches, or unexplained nocturnal arousals.[30] The mechanism of SDB is likely secondary to the loss of the wakefulness drive to breathe. Bascom and colleagues[41] showed a decrease in tidal volume and minute ventilation with an increase in end-tidal CO_2 during the transition of wakefulness to the N1 stage among patients with SCI. Moreover, this effect was more pronounced among patients with cervical injuries compared with thoracic injuries. Therefore, PSG should be considered when symptoms of nocturnal hypoventilation are present.

At present, in the United States, the restrictive thoracic disorders for NIV are such that a low forced VC (<50%) is sufficient to initiate NIV in SCI; however, most physicians like PSG to support their diagnosis. In-laboratory sleep studies may require special accommodation and a personal attendant to accompany patients with SCI and debility. Thus, unattended home sleep studies or overnight oximetry and transcutaneous or end-tidal CO_2 level monitoring have been suggested to

substitute for in-laboratory studies. However, the sensitivity and specificity of these portable tests remain unclear for patients with SCI.[42]

ROLE OF NONINVASIVE VENTILATION
Role of Noninvasive Ventilation in the Management Following Acute Spinal Cord Injury

There is only a handful of observational studies published on the use of NIV for the management of acute SCI. Most patients with acute SCI also have other injuries, including facial trauma, brain injury, chest trauma, medical conditions, and opioid therapy for pain control, and hence pose a contraindication for use of NIV in this population.[9] In addition, NIV may cause emesis and aspiration. Therefore, clinical practice guidelines recommend the use of NIV among carefully selected patients with mild respiratory dysfunction and intact bulbar muscles who are medically stable, cooperative in the presence of experienced staff, and without any other contraindication in the acute period.[13]

In a study by Tromans and colleagues,[43] NIV was shown to be effective in 10 out of 17 patients (58%) for managing acute respiratory failure among patients with cervical SCI and decreased VC. Patients who failed NIV were noted to have a mean decrease of VC by approximately 50%

from their baseline at presentation. NIV was successfully used among patients with a decrease in VC of less than 20% from their respective baselines. In comparison, NIV was much more successfully used to wean patients off invasive ventilation, with 13 out of 15 (86%) patients successfully weaned. The investigators reduced inspiratory positive airway pressure (IPAP) by 2 cm H_2O at a time until the patient could tolerate a decrease by 2 cm H_2O for 24 hours. The cycle was repeated until the patient was completely weaned off.

Bach[9] also published a retrospective study comparing patients with neuromuscular weakness, including 19 patients with SCI. He assessed weaning from mechanical ventilation using NIV. He used the following criteria to assess the readiness of extubation: (1) fully alert and cooperative, receiving no sedative medications; (2) afebrile and normal white blood cell count; (3) $Paco_2$ less than or equal to 40 mm Hg at peak inspiratory pressures less than 30 cm H_2O on full ventilatory support and normal breathing rate; (4) Spo_2 greater than or equal to 95% for 12 hours or more in room air; (5) all oxyhemoglobin desaturations less than 95% reversed by suctioning via translaryngeal tube; (6) chest radiograph abnormalities cleared or clearing; and (7) air leakage via upper airway sufficient for vocalization on cuff deflation. Patients were extubated to NIV on assist/control mode with volume cycling targeting volumes of 800 to 1500 mL and respiratory rate 10 to 14 breaths/min provided by a 15-mm angled mouthpiece. Volume cycling was used to encourage air stacking to facilitate coughing and airway clearance. The mechanically assisted cough was provided to all patients to facilitate airway clearance and when Spo_2 decreased to less than 95%. All 19 patients were successfully weaned off invasive ventilation using this protocol without requiring reintubation during the hospitalization. Preextubation VC dictated the duration for weaning. Patients with VC of 250 mL or less required continuous NIV indefinitely, whereas those with VC of 250 mL or more were weaned off in 3 weeks, most of them continuing to need intermittent mouthpiece ventilation. Some patients continued to require NIV during sleep.[9]

Noninvasive Ventilation Management in Chronic Spinal Cord Injury

The benefits of long-term NIV in patients with nocturnal hypoventilation are well established in the literature and include improvement in gas exchange, normalizing tissue acidosis and hypoxia, in addition to improving the quality and physiology of sleep.[9] It has been also proposed that NIV has beneficial physiologic effects of pulmonary distension and improvement of sputum clearance, which could be of a great benefit for patients with SCI with nocturnal hypoventilation.[8,44] Patients with SCI who show symptoms suggesting the need for NIV, such as poor sleep quality, snoring, excessive daytime sleepiness, and unexplained comorbidities such as cardiovascular disease or pulmonary hypertension, should be referred to a specialized sleep center with skills to investigate the need for and implementation of NIV.[39] Indications for NIV in patients with SCI are similar to the indications in the general population with suspected wakeful or nocturnal hypoventilation. PSG, capnography, or nocturnal oximetry are usually the diagnostic tests of choice, in which findings of Spo_2 less than 88% for greater than 5 minutes, or Spo_2 less than 88% for greater than 10% of total sleep time (TST), or end-tidal CO_2 greater than 50 mm Hg for more than 50% of TST suggest hypoventilation.[45]

Nasal, oral-nasal, and nasal interfaces have been suggested for patients requiring chronic NIV. Nasal airway is preferred when the patients have weak facial musculature causing air leakage around the mouth. Custom-made molded mouthpieces may be required by some patients for more comfort. The intact bulbar function is a prerequisite for effective NIV.[46] Patients should also be motivated, cooperative, and medically stable.[9]

However, NIV is not adequate for the management of respiratory failure in all patients who require mechanical ventilation. Many patients with high cervical SCI (above C4 level) may require more advanced invasive ventilation via tracheostomy. Tracheostomy is associated with many complications, which include, but are not limited to, chronic bacterial colonization of the airway, nosocomial infections, tracheomalacia, tracheal perforation, stenosis, fistula formation, and impaired swallowing.[9,46] Several studies compared invasive positive pressure ventilation (IPPV) via tracheostomy with NIV, which suggested that NIV had higher patient satisfaction.[15,43,47,48] Bach[47] reported that NIV seemed to be more convenient; to have less untoward effect on speech, appearance, and comfort; and to be preferred overall to tracheostomy IPPV. Tracheostomy can also carry a great burden on the patient's family. Tracheostomy-dependent patients need frequent airway suctioning, which may require licensed personnel to be hired 24 hours or the patient to be staying in a 24-hour nursing facility. Among selected patients who are on chronic mechanic ventilation but have functional phrenic nerve motor neurons, diaphragmatic pacer may help wean off mechanical ventilation and tracheostomy. Weaning is more successful if the pacer is implanted within the first year of injury.[49] Thus, in the instance of wakeful hypoventilation and IPPV via tracheostomy and ventilator, the conversion to NIV should be considered whenever possible.[15,43,48]

Role of Airway Clearance

Airway clearance is a key component of rehabilitation among patients with SCI. Mucus secretions can build up secondary to ineffective clearance and cause atelectasis and pneumonia, which may be fatal for ventilator-dependent persons.[15] Chest physiotherapy and postural drainage, although helpful in certain able-bodied patients, may not be effectively used among patients with unstable spine or chest wall injuries. These therapies also require expertise and may have to be implemented multiple times a day for effective airway clearance.[24] There is a lack of clinical studies comparing various techniques of airway clearance among patients with SCI. Among the available studies, insufflation combined with manually assisted cough provided the most consistent, high-level evidence. Secretion removal techniques, including the use of expiratory pressure valve tracheal suctioning, and chest physiotherapy, shows benefit in small case series and case reports.[50]

In patients with cervical SCI (C4–C6 levels) and Association Impairment Scale injury with a functional glottis, breath stacking, with or without manually assisted cough, has been shown to increase peak cough flow. Torress-Castro and colleagues[51] published a study of 15 patients and showed near-normal peak cough flows among patients who had a combination approach with 2 to 3 stacked breaths with manual resuscitation bag followed by an assisted cough. Patients were asked to hold their breaths between the assisted breaths and cough forcefully while a therapist applied force on the patient's epigastrium, pushing the diaphragm up. This combined technique showed a higher mean peak cough flow compared with the individual technique.

Noninvasive Ventilation Titration in Patients with Spinal Cord Injury and Sleep-Disordered Breathing

Despite compelling evidence to support the use of NIV in chronic hypoventilation in patients with SCI, studies remain scarce on the best approach for NIV titration. The American Academy of Sleep Medicine (AASM) published recommendations and desired goals of NIV titration in the management of chronic hypoventilation in neuromuscular disease and obesity hypoventilation syndrome, which can be applied to patients with SCI because they manifest similar pathophysiology and end goals of the management of chronic hypoventilation. These goals are to eliminate obstructive events and improve ventilation such that the Spo_2 was greater than 90% and the transcutaneous Pco_2 was less than a set goal (such as 45–50 mm Hg) if sufficient pressure to achieve these goals was tolerated.[52]

Outpatient NIV treatment and titration have been an acknowledged practice in some sleep centers with considerable expertise in treating patients with neuromuscular disease after a period of daytime adaptation under direct supervision. If nocturnal noninvasive positive pressure ventilation is tolerated with low pressures, the settings are increased over weeks to months based on symptoms and/or daytime arterial Pco_2 measurement (or estimates of arterial Pco_2 such as end-tidal Pco_2). Gruis and colleagues[53] studied patients with amyotrophic lateral sclerosis (ALS) in whom NIV was titrated the aforementioned way; symptom relief was provided in 4 of 18 patients with the low initial settings, whereas most other patients required either 1 or 2 increases in pressure. Only 6 out of 19 required pressure support greater than 10 cm H_2O. Another study investigated the effects of bilevel positive airway pressure (PAP) in the spontaneous timed mode on survival and quality of life in patients with ALS, with average IPAP and expiratory PAP settings being 15 and 6 cm H_2O, respectively. All patients treated with NIV had an improvement in quality of life. However, patients with ALS and moderate to severe bulbar dysfunction tended to have more difficulty tolerating NIV and mask ventilation, and that group did not show improved survival.[53–55]

Autotitrating Positive Airway Pressure Versus Continuous Positive Airway Pressure

Patients with SCI have barriers to being diagnosed and treated for SDB, such as limited access to well-equipped sleep laboratories. Thus, home testing and initiating autotitrating PAP (APAP) for those diagnosed with SDB have been studied. Berlowtiz and colleagues[56] conducted a randomized clinical trial to test the effect of APAP use over 3 months in patients with acute cervical SCI. This study reported significant improvement in daytime sleepiness but no change in neurocognitive function over the follow-up of 3 months. Those findings were compatible with APPLES (Apnea Positive Pressure Long-Term Efficacy Study) trial,[57] in nondisabled patients, which showed improvement in daytime sleepiness in patients using PAP therapy, but no significant improvement in neurologic function. Note that these findings have limitations that were mentioned by Sankari and Badr.[58] Those limitations include low adherence rates; it only included patients with acute SCI, which may not be representative of the overall population of patients with SCI. Sankari and colleagues[58], in the same review, suggested a clinical approach for the application of APAP to individuals with SCI, which suggested that patients with OSA, with apnea-hypopnea index (AHI) between 5 and 50/h, can be placed on APAP, whereas patients with AHI greater than 50/h, central apneas, hypoxia, or nocturnal hypoventilation need in-laboratory PAP titration. However, limited evidence and trials have been conducted in this matter, and more investigation is needed.

Adherence to Positive Airway Pressure in Spinal Cord Injury

Despite the PAP benefits in SDB, efficacy remains limited because of poor adherence. PAP adherence is a complex process that remains inadequately explained, and range between 30% and 60% in patients with no known disabilities.[59] This finding has been attributed to many factors, including, but not exclusive to, lack of social/spousal support and limited access to treatment.[60] Reasons of nonadherence in patients with SCI are thought to be different from those in patients without disability because of additional physical and psychological burden, lack of social support, poor quality of sleep caused by spasm and pain, nasal congestion, and inability to adjust the mask because of mobility impairment.[61] There have been very few studies to investigate barriers to adherence to PAP in SCI. Graco and colleagues[62] followed 16 patients with SCI to assess the benefits and burden of PAP treatment caused by coexisting morbidities. The study reported that 25% of those patients were fully adherent (used >4 h/night) for 6 months to 1 year. Adherent patients showed significant improvement in their quality of sleep and less daytime sleepiness. Close follow-up with a sleep specialist had a significant effect on adherence.

SUMMARY

Respiratory complications from inadequate cough, infections, and respiratory failure to disordered breathing during sleep are common among individuals with SCI, particularly among those with cervical injury. The mechanisms for the SDB after surviving SCI are not clear, but evidence points to complex pathways that include increased susceptibility to central instability, nocturnal hypoventilation, and upper airway collapsibility. The current diagnostic and management approach of SDB in individuals with SCI is challenging because of complex pathophysiology, limited mobility, and high care needs. Mechanical intervention to assist ventilation and improve ineffective cough mechanically using NIV plays an important role in their management, but more studies are needed.

DISCLOSURE

This study was not industry supported. The authors have no financial conflicts of interest. The opinions expressed in this article reflect those of the authors and do not necessarily represent official views of Department of Veterans' Affairs (VA). Dr A. Sankari is supported by the Office of Research and Development from the VA award RX002885 and from the National Heart, Lung, and Blood Institute awards HL140447 and HL130552.

REFERENCES

1. Jackson AB, Dijkers M, Devivo MJ, et al. A demographic profile of new traumatic spinal cord injuries: change and stability over 30 years. Arch Phys Med Rehabil 2004;85(11):1740–8.
2. Spinal cord injury facts and figures at a glance. J Spinal Cord Med 2012;35(4):197–8.
3. Lee BB, Cripps RA, Fitzharris M, et al. The global map for traumatic spinal cord injury epidemiology: update 2011, global incidence rate. Spinal Cord 2014;52(2):110–6.
4. Cotton BA, Pryor JP, Chinwalla I, et al. Respiratory complications and mortality risk associated with thoracic spine injury. J Trauma 2005;59(6):1400–7 [discussion 1407–9].
5. Berlowitz DJ, Brown DJ, Campbell DA, et al. A longitudinal evaluation of sleep and breathing in the first year after cervical spinal cord injury. Arch Phys Med Rehabil 2005;86(6):1193–9.
6. Sankari A, Bascom AT, Chowdhuri S, et al. Tetraplegia is a risk factor for central sleep apnea. J Appl Phys (1985) 2014;116(3):345–53.
7. Galeiras Vazquez R, Rascado Sedes P, Mourelo Farina M, et al. Respiratory management in the patient with spinal cord injury. Biomed Res Int 2013; 2013:168757.
8. Clinical indications for noninvasive positive pressure ventilation in chronic respiratory failure due to restrictive lung disease, COPD, and nocturnal hypoventilation–a consensus conference report. Chest 1999;116(2):521–34.
9. Bach JR. Noninvasive respiratory management of high level spinal cord injury. J Spinal Cord Med 2012;35(2):72–80.

10. Hachen HJ. Idealized care of the acutely injured spinal cord in Switzerland. J Trauma 1977;17(12): 931–6.

11. Berney S, Bragge P, Granger C, et al. The acute respiratory management of cervical spinal cord injury in the first 6 weeks after injury: a systematic review. Spinal Cord 2011;49(1):17–29.

12. Jackson AB, Groomes TE. Incidence of respiratory complications following spinal cord injury. Arch Phys Med Rehabil 1994;75(3):270–5.

13. Berlowitz DJ, Wadsworth B, Ross J. Respiratory problems and management in people with spinal cord injury. Breathe (Sheff) 2016;12(4): 328–40.

14. Gainche L, Berlowitz DJ, LeGuen M, et al. Nasal resistance is elevated in people with tetraplegia and is reduced by topical sympathomimetic administration. J Clin Sleep Med 2016;12(11):1487–92.

15. Toki A, Tamura R, Sumida M. Long-term ventilation for high-level tetraplegia: a report of 2 cases of noninvasive positive-pressure ventilation. Arch Phys Med Rehabil 2008;89(4):779–83.

16. Winslow C, Rozovsky J. Effect of spinal cord injury on the respiratory system. Am J Phys Med Rehabil 2003;82(10):803–14.

17. Berlly M, Shem K. Respiratory management during the first five days after spinal cord injury. J Spinal Cord Med 2007;30(4):309–18.

18. Nockels RP. Nonoperative management of acute spinal cord injury. Spine (Phila Pa 1976) 2001; 26(24 Suppl):S31–7.

19. Sankari A, Bascom A, Oomman S, et al. Sleep disordered breathing in chronic spinal cord injury. J Clin Sleep Med 2014;10(1):65–72.

20. DeVivo MJ, Black KJ, Stover SL. Causes of death during the first 12 years after spinal cord injury. Arch Phys Med Rehabil 1993;74(3):248–54.

21. Bach JR. Alternative methods of ventilatory support for the patient with ventilatory failure due to spinal cord injury. J Am Paraplegia Soc 1991;14(4): 158–74.

22. Casha S, Christie S. A systematic review of intensive cardiopulmonary management after spinal cord injury. J Neurotrauma 2011;28(8):1479–95.

23. Jane M, Braverman PD. Airway clearance needs in spinal cord injury: an overview. Available at: https://pdfs.semanticscholar.org.pdf.

24. Bach JR, Saporito LR. Criteria for extubation and tracheostomy tube removal for patients with ventilatory failure. A different approach to weaning. Chest 1996;110(6):1566–71.

25. William A, Sheel P, Joseph F, et al. FRCPC. Respiratory management following spinal cord injury. Available at: https://scireproject.com/wp-content/uploads/FINAL-Resp-V6-Chapter-May-30-2018.pdf.

26. Tran K, Hukins C, Geraghty T, et al. Sleep-disordered breathing in spinal cord-injured patients: a short-term longitudinal study. Respirology 2010; 15(2):272–6.

27. Chiodo AE, Sitrin RG, Bauman KA. Sleep disordered breathing in spinal cord injury: a systematic review. J Spinal Cord Med 2016;39(4):374–82.

28. Bauman KA, Kurili A, Schotland HM, et al. Simplified approach to diagnosing sleep-disordered breathing and nocturnal hypercapnia in individuals with spinal cord injury. Arch Phys Med Rehabil 2016;97(3): 363–71.

29. Sankari A, Bascom AT, Badr MS. Upper airway mechanics in chronic spinal cord injury during sleep. J Appl Phys (1985) 2014;116(11):1390–5.

30. Wijesuriya NS, Gainche L, Jordan AS, et al. Genioglossus reflex responses to negative upper airway pressure are altered in people with tetraplegia and obstructive sleep apnoea. J Physiol 2018;596(14): 2853–64.

31. Rizwan A, Sankari A, Bascom AT, et al. Nocturnal swallowing and arousal threshold in individuals with chronic spinal cord injury. J Appl Phys 2018; 125(2):445–52.

32. Dempsey JA, Skatrud JB. A sleep-induced apneic threshold and its consequences. Am Rev Respir Dis 1986;133(6):1163–70.

33. Sullivan CE, Kozar LF, Murphy E, et al. Primary role of respiratory afferents in sustaining breathing rhythm. J Appl Phys 1978;45(1):11–7.

34. Dempsey JA, Smith CA, Przybylowski T, et al. The ventilatory responsiveness to CO(2) below eupnoea as a determinant of ventilatory stability in sleep. J Physiol 2004;560(Pt 1):1–11.

35. Khoo MC. Using loop gain to assess ventilatory control in obstructive sleep apnea. Am J Respir Crit Care Med 2001;163(5):1044–5.

36. Younes M, Ostrowski M, Thompson W, et al. Chemical control stability in patients with obstructive sleep apnea. Am J Respir Crit Care Med 2001;163(5): 1181–90.

37. Sankri-Tarbichi AG, Rowley JA, Badr MS. Expiratory pharyngeal narrowing during central hypocapnic hypopnea. Am J Respir Crit Care Med 2009; 179(4):313–9.

38. Culebras A, Kelly JJ. Sleep disorders and neuromuscular diseases. Rev Neurol Dis 2008;5(3):153–8.

39. <sleepapnea.pdf>. Available at: https://aasm.org/resources/factsheets/sleepapnea.pdf.

40. Wijesuriya NS, Lewis C, Butler JE, et al. High nasal resistance is stable over time but poorly perceived in people with tetraplegia and obstructive sleep apnoea. Respir Physiolo Neurobiol 2017;235:27–33.

41. Bascom AT, Sankari A, Goshgarian HG, et al. Sleep onset hypoventilation in chronic spinal cord injury. Phys Rep 2015;3(8):e12490.

42. Kirk VG, Flemons WW, Adams C, et al. Sleep-disordered breathing in Duchenne muscular dystrophy: a

preliminary study of the role of portable monitoring. Pediatr Pulmonol 2000;29(2):135–40.

43. Tromans AM, Mecci M, Barrett FH, et al. The use of the BiPAP biphasic positive airway pressure system in acute spinal cord injury. Spinal Cord 1998;36(7): 481–4.

44. Laffont I, Bensmail D, Lortat-Jacob S, et al. Intermittent positive-pressure breathing effects in patients with high spinal cord injury. Arch Phys Med Rehabil 2008;89(8):1575–9.

45. Robert D, Willig TN, Leger P, et al. Long-term nasal ventilation in neuromuscular disorders: report of a consensus conference. Eur Respir J 1993;6(4): 599–606.

46. Bach JR, Alba AS, Saporito LR. Intermittent positive pressure ventilation via the mouth as an alternative to tracheostomy for 257 ventilator users. Chest 1993;103(1):174–82.

47. Bach JR. A comparison of long-term ventilatory support alternatives from the perspective of the patient and care giver. Chest 1993;104(6):1702–6.

48. Bach JR, Alba AS. Noninvasive options for ventilatory support of the traumatic high level quadriplegic patient. Chest 1990;98(3):613–9.

49. Onders RP, Elmo M, Kaplan C, et al. Long-term experience with diaphragm pacing for traumatic spinal cord injury: early implantation should be considered. Surgery 2018;164(4):705–11.

50. Reid WD, Brown JA, Konnyu KJ, et al. Physiotherapy secretion removal techniques in people with spinal cord injury: a systematic review. J Spinal Cord Med 2010;33(4):353–70.

51. Torres-Castro R, Vilaro J, Vera-Uribe R, et al. Use of air stacking and abdominal compression for cough assistance in people with complete tetraplegia. Spinal Cord 2014;52(5):354–7.

52. Berry RB, Chediak A, Brown LK, et al. Best clinical practices for the sleep center adjustment of noninvasive positive pressure ventilation (NPPV) in stable chronic alveolar hypoventilation syndromes. J Clin Sleep Med 2010;6(5):491–509.

53. Gruis KL, Brown DL, Lisabeth LD, et al. Longitudinal assessment of noninvasive positive pressure ventilation adjustments in ALS patients. J Neurol Sci 2006; 247(1):59–63.

54. Bourke SC, Tomlinson M, Williams TL, et al. Effects of non-invasive ventilation on survival and quality of life in patients with amyotrophic lateral sclerosis: a randomised controlled trial. Lancet Neurol 2006; 5(2):140–7.

55. Benditt JO. Respiratory complications of amyotrophic lateral sclerosis. Semin Respir Crit Care Med 2002;23(3):239–47.

56. Berlowitz DJ, Ayas N, Barnes M, et al. Auto-titrating continuous positive airway pressure treatment for obstructive sleep apnoea after acute quadriplegia (COSAQ): study protocol for a randomized controlled trial. Trial 2013;14:181.

57. Kushida CA, Nichols DA, Holmes TH, et al. Effects of continuous positive airway pressure on neurocognitive function in obstructive sleep apnea patients: the apnea positive pressure long-term efficacy study (APPLES). Sleep 2012;35(12):1593–602.

58. Sankari A, Badr MS. Does auto-PAP work in patients with acute quadriplegia and sleep-disordered breathing? Thorax 2019;74(3):217–8.

59. Weaver TE, Sawyer AM. Adherence to continuous positive airway pressure treatment for obstructive sleep apnoea: implications for future interventions. Indian J Med Res 2010;131:245–58.

60. Ward K, Hoare KJ, Gott M. What is known about the experiences of using CPAP for OSA from the users' perspective? a systematic integrative literature review. Sleep Med Rev 2014;18(4):357–66.

61. Sankari A, Martin JL, Badr MS. Sleep disordered breathing and spinal cord injury: challenges and opportunities. Curr Sleep Med Rep 2017;3(4):272–8.

62. Graco M, Green SE, Tolson J, et al. Worth the effort? weighing up the benefit and burden of continuous positive airway pressure therapy for the treatment of obstructive sleep apnoea in chronic tetraplegia. Spinal Cord 2019;57(3):247–54.

Perioperative Care and Medication-related Hypoventilation

Kara Dupuy-McCauley, MD*, Bernardo Selim, MD

KEYWORDS

- Perioperative management • Obesity hypoventilation syndrome • Obstructive sleep apnea
- Medication related hypoventilation • Positive airway pressure • Postoperative complications

KEY POINTS

- Obstructive sleep apnea (OSA) and obesity hypoventilation syndrome (OHS) are common conditions. Prevalence is higher among obese individuals and in older age groups.
- OSA and OHS are associated with significant chronic comorbid conditions and increased risk of adverse cardiopulmonary events in the postoperative setting.
- During perioperative screening for OSA, increase in serum bicarbonate level ($\geq$27 mEq/L) may be a surrogate marker of hypercapnia and may increase detection of OHS in obese patients.
- Currently, recommended perioperative interventions largely are consensus based. Strategies may include enhanced monitoring, conservative measures, and positive airway pressure therapy for OSA and OHS during perioperative care.
- Further trials are required to better identify OSA and OHS patients at higher risk of perioperative cardiorespiratory complications and to test the impact of specific interventions on cardiopulmonary outcomes.

INTRODUCTION

Obstructive sleep apnea (OSA) and obesity hypoventilation syndrome (OHS) are prevalent chronic health conditions associated with a higher postoperative risk of adverse events.[1–3] Therefore, the identification of OHS and OSA prior to elective surgery has become an emerging topic in patient safety.

OSA is characterized by a cyclical alternating pattern between pharyngeal collapse or narrowing (apnea or hypopnea) and arousals during sleep. This pattern is associated with recurrent physiologic stressors (eg, nocturnal hypoxemia, hypercoagulability, and sympathetic surges)[4] and chronic comorbid conditions relevant to perioperative management (**Box 1**). Severity of OSA, a predictor of perioperative complication, is defined by the apnea-hypopnea index (AHI), with 5 to 14 events per hour being mild, 15 to 29 moderate, and greater than or equal to 30 severe.

OHS is defined by the American Academy of Sleep Medicine (AASM) as a triad of daytime hypercapnia ($Paco_2$ $\geq$45 mm Hg), obesity (body mass index [BMI] $\geq$30 kg/m^2) and the exclusion of other causes of hypercapnia, such as severe lung disease or neuromuscular disease. Although OSA often is present and severe in OHS patients (90%), a minority of them (10%) present with milder OSA but severe hypercapnia and typical rapid eye movement (REM) sleep hypoventilation secondary to decreased respiratory drive (sometimes referred as true pickwickian syndrome)[12] (see Roop Kaw and Marta Kaminska's article, "Obesity Hypoventilation: Traditional Versus Nontraditional Populations," in this issue).

Current perioperative guidelines from multiple anesthesia and sleep societies largely are

---

Mayo Clinic, 200 First Street Southwest, Rochester, MN 55905, USA
* Corresponding author.
E-mail address: Dupuy-McCauley.Kara@Mayo.edu

Sleep Med Clin 15 (2020) 471–483
https://doi.org/10.1016/j.jsmc.2020.08.008
1556-407X/20/© 2020 Elsevier Inc. All rights reserved.

Box 1
Comorbidities associated with obstructive sleep apnea and obesity hypoventilation syndrome

OSA	Arrhythmias, including atrial fibrillation
	Hypertension
	Fatal myocardial infarction
	Heart failure
	Cerebrovascular disease
	All-cause mortality
	Diabetes mellitus
OHS	Hypertension
	Pulmonary hypertension
	Diabetes mellitus
	COPD
	Stroke
	Renal failure
	Diabetes mellitus
	Atrial fibrillation/flutter
	Congestive heart failure
	Cor pulmonale

Data from Refs.[5–11]

Table 1
Prevalence of obstructive sleep apnea and obesity hypoventilation syndrome

	Men (%)	Women (%)	Both Genders (%)
Prevalence of OSA			
General US population, all OSA (AHI ≥5/h)	24	9	—
General US population, moderate–severe OSA (AHI ≥15/h)	9	4	—
Bariatric population (BMI 48.7 kg/m² ± [7.3])	—	—	73
Prevalence of OHS			
General US population	0.15–0.3		
BMI of 30–35 kg/m²	8–12		
BMI≥40 kg/m²	18–31		
OSA with BMI 30–40	9.8		
OSA with BMI >40	23.6		
Severe OSA	20–30		
Hospitalized patients with BMI >35 kg/m²	31		

Data from Refs.[19–24]

consensus based or have low-quality evidence. The impact of their recommendations on preventing acute complications in the postoperative period remains uncertain.[13–18] Based on the most updated literature, this review article addresses the perioperative care of patients with OSA and OHS.

EPIDEMIOLOGY OF OBSTRUCTIVE SLEEP APNEA AND OBESITY HYPOVENTILATION SYNDROME IN SURGICAL PATIENTS
Epidemiology of Obstructive Sleep Apnea

Overall prevalence of OSA in the US varies based on age and gender, with the disease most prevalent among obese individuals and older adults (Table 1).[19] More than 17 million ambulatory and inpatient surgery visits occurred in 2014.[25] In this population presenting for surgery, OSA is common and many (67%) are undiagnosed.[26]

Epidemiology of Obesity Hypoventilation Syndrome

Epidemiology of OHS in the referred surgical population is unknown. Among patients with OSA, an average of 17% (range of 4%–50%) have concomitant OHS.[27] Although OHS in the general population has not been measured directly, Mokhlesi[28] has inferred an estimated prevalence of 0.15% to 0.3% by extrapolating data from prevalence of obesity, OSA within the obese population, and OHS among those with OSA. Epidemiologic data on OHS are derived mostly from studies of patients referred for sleep evaluation (see Table 1), because 90% of patients with OHS also have OSA.[22] OHS also is common in the obese population, with a prevalence of 8% to 31% (see Table 1), and that number may be even higher when the BMI is greater than 40 kg/m².[20]

Rates of obesity in the United States continue to increase, but rates of severe obesity (BMI >40 kg/m²) are rising disproportionately to moderate obesity,[29] so an increasing incidence of surgical patients with OSA and OHS may be expected in the future.

PREOPERATIVE EVALUATION OF SLEEP-RELATED BREATHING DISORDERS

Preoperative Screening

Because most patients with sleep-related breathing disorders remain undiagnosed, it is not uncommon to recognize them for the first time in the perioperative setting due to anesthesia's close approximation to some aspects of the sleep state.[30,31] Therefore, evidence-based preoperative measures to screen for OSA and OHS and optimize prior to elective surgery have been proposed by several societies[13–18] (Box 2).

Pertinent obstructive sleep apnea history and physical

The American Society of Anesthesiologists (ASA) has recommended screening for OSA should begin with a focused history and physical examination directed at assessment of risk factors and symptoms of sleep apnea.[13] The history should take into account risk factors for OSA, including obesity, age, male gender, and female menopause. Questioning should focus on symptoms of OSA, including snoring, apneic episodes, frequent arousals during sleep, morning headaches, and daytime somnolence. The physical examination should include assessment of the oropharynx and neck circumference.[13] A neck circumference of greater than 17 in (43 cm) in men and greater than 16 in (40 cm) in women is a positive predictor for the presence of OSA.[13,17] Diagnosis and management of OSA should be attempted preoperatively but should not necessarily delay surgery.

Role of questionnaires in obstructive sleep apnea

The STOP-Bang questionnaire has been validated as a predictor of postoperative respiratory complications and is recommended for use during the presurgical outpatient visit.[14] This questionnaire has a sensitivity of 88% to 93% for detecting moderate OSA (AHI ≥15) and sensitivity of 97% for detecting severe OSA (AHI ≥30).[32] Chan and colleagues[26] found that an STOP-Bang of greater than or equal to 3 was associated with increased risk of a composite of myocardial injury, cardiac death, congestive heart failure, thromboembolism, new atrial fibrillation, and stroke within 30 days of surgery as well as myocardial injury, intensive care unit (ICU) readmission, and wound infection.

Specific screening for obesity hypoventilation syndrome

For complete recommendations from national societies, see Box 2. Because 90% of patients with OHS have concomitant OSA, the OSA-focused history and physical are applicable in most cases, but in obese patients (BMI ≥30 kg/m²), additional findings must be looked for that could suggest a diagnosis of OHS:

- Increase in serum bicarbonate greater than 27 mmol/L
- Persistent hypoxemia during polysomnography
- Pulmonary function testing showing a restrictive pattern[21,33]

The role of polysomnography

The utility of confirmatory testing in patients identified at high risk of OSA or OHS during preoperative screening is unclear. When feasible in the presurgical period, in-laboratory attended polysomnography is the gold standard diagnostic test for sleep-related breathing disorders. When time constraints exist, home sleep apnea testing using a portable type 3 device may be considered to determine the presence and severity of OSA.[34]

Preoperative Positive Airway Pressure Therapy

At time of preoperative evaluation, some patients with known OSA and OHS already may have started positive airway pressure (PAP) therapy. The mainstays of PAP therapy for sleep-related breathing disorders are continuous PAP (CPAP) for OSA and noninvasive ventilation (NIV) for disorders with predominant sleep-related hypoventilation. NIV most commonly is either bilevel PAP (BPAP) or volume-assured pressure support (VAPS).[18] Both CPAP and NIV act as pneumatic splints, eliminating airway occlusion, but NIV additionally supports and/or augments a patient's breath (tidal volume) and, hence, ventilation. NIV also may provide supplemental breaths should a patient's rate of breathing fall below the preset backup respiratory rate in order to better support ventilation. For a given patient, however, the tidal volume generated by NIV is not fixed, and it depends on the interaction between the preset pressure of the device, inspiratory time and effort, and the dynamic characteristics of the respiratory system during the perioperative period.

Airway obstruction and hypoventilation are common in the perioperative period and PAP can be administered as treatment of most patients at risk for OSA and OHS, provided there is no contraindication. These contradictions may include: cardiac or respiratory arrest; severe encephalopathy; severe upper gastrointestinal bleeding;

Box 2 Society recommendations on perioperative management of obstructive sleep apnea and obesity hypoventilation syndrome		
Screening	ASA	Evaluate for OSA long enough before surgery to allow for perioperative management plan.
		Preoperative evaluation should include review of medical records; history of difficult airway or anesthesia; comorbidities; physical examination, including oropharynx; and focused interview with patient/family directed at sleep complaints.
		Choice to proceed to surgery or diagnose and treat OSA prior to surgery
		Determine whether surgery should be inpatient/outpatient.
	SASM	OSA confers higher risk of postoperative complications.
		OSA should be identified before surgery.
		Screening tools like STOP-Bang can be used to identify OSA.
		Insufficient evidence to delay surgery with OSA alone
	AASM	Presence of OSA should be documented; patients at risk should be identified.
		A screening questionnaire might be useful.
Preoperative	ASA	Initiation of CPAP should be considered, especially if OSA is severe.
		NIV, if unresponsive to CPAP
		Weight loss or mandibular advancement device, if feasible and appropriate
		Patients with OSA should be assumed to have a "difficult airway."
	SASM	Care team should be aware of OSA diagnosis.
		Obtain sleep study and PAP settings prior to surgery if possible.
		PAP use preoperatively and postoperatively (home PAP vs hospital-provided PAP).
		Optimize comorbid conditions prior to surgery.
		People at high risk for OSA should proceed to surgery in same manner as patients with confirmed OSA.
	AASM	CPAP should be used in the perioperative period.
		Intubate with an oral or nasal airway when possible.
		There should be no unsupervised preoperative sedation.
		OSA should be handled as a high-risk intubation.
Intraoperative	ASA	Use local or regional anesthesia with moderate sedation when possible.
		Monitor ventilation continuously if using moderate sedation.
		Use CPAP or mandibular advancement device during sedation.
		General anesthesia with intubation is preferred over deep sedation without a secure airway.
		Extubate awake unless contraindicated.
		Fully reverse neuromuscular block before extubation.
		The patient should be in a nonsupine position during extubation and recovery.
	SASM	

		Known or suspected OSA should be considered an independent risk factor for difficult intubation, difficult mask ventilation, or a combination of both.
		Neuromuscular blockade may lead to increased risk of postoperative residual neuromuscular blockade, hypoxemia, or respiratory failure in patients with OSA.
		Opioids may cause increased risk of adverse respiratory events in patients with OSA.
		Propofol may put patients with OSA at increased risk for adverse respiratory events.
		Use intravenous benzodiazepines cautiously because patients with OSA may be at increased risk for adverse respiratory events as a result of sedation.
		Regional anesthesia is preferable over general anesthesia in patients with OSA.
	AASM	Use regional or local anesthesia, when possible.
		Wait to extubate until fully awake and upright.
		Use narcotics conservatively.
		Patients with mild OSA or tracheostomy may be candidates for outpatient procedures.
Postoperative	ASA	Avoid opioids, if possible, especially continuous infusions.
		Exercise caution with respiratory depressants like benzodiazepines and barbiturates.
		Use supplemental oxygen as needed but with caution due to potential of masking respiratory depression.
		Use CPAP or NIV continuously unless contraindicated for hypoxia and upper airway obstruction.
		Use continuous oxygen monitoring until no longer at risk for respiratory depression.
	AASM	Use CPAP even when the patient has not been using it at home: titrate pressures as needed.
		Use sedatives, hypnotics, and anxiolytics with caution.
		Continuous pulse oximetry and heart rate monitoring with alarms
	ATS	For high pretest probability of OHS, measure $Paco_2$ rather than serum bicarbonate or Spo_2 for diagnosis.
		For low to moderate probability: if serum bicarbonate <27 mmol/L, OHS is unlikely; if serum bicarbonate ≥27 mmol/L, measure $Paco_2$ to confirm or rule out OHS.
		Do not base decision to measure $Paco_2$ on awake Spo_2 if OHS suspected.
		For stable outpatients with OHS, treatment should be PAP during sleep.
		For stable outpatients with OHS and severe OSA, initiate CPAP rather than NIV.
		Hospitalized patients with respiratory failure and suspected OHS should be started on NIV before being discharged from the hospital.
		Weight loss should be attempted prior to surgery, if feasible.

Abbreviations: ATS, American Thoracic Society; SASM, Society of Anesthesia and Sleep Medicine.
   Data from Refs.[13,15,17,18]

hemodynamic instability; cardiac arrhythmia; upper airway obstruction; high risk for aspiration; recent facial trauma; inability to clear respiratory secretions, copious secretions; and uncooperative patient. In preparation for surgery, CPAP is a reliable means of treating obstructive apneas and hypopneas in OSA.[35] Autotitrating CPAP (APAP) also is an effective method of treatment whereby the pressure delivered to the patient is adjusted automatically in response to airflow limitation. APAP provides a reasonable alternative to CPAP in the perioperative period when night-to-night variability in pressure requirement is anticipated based on sleep position or opioid administration.[36] BPAP also may be used to control OSA, especially in patients who require high levels of PAP to eliminate obstruction of the upper airway or for those who have coexisting hypoventilation (eg, chronic obstructive pulmonary disease [COPD]).

For patients with OHS and severe OSA who are in stable respiratory condition, CPAP or APAP may be appropriate PAP modes to continue in the perioperative period. In those OHS patients with milder OSA but chronic hypercapnic respiratory failure (true pickwickian syndrome), however, NIV in the form of BPAP and VAPS may be considered better alternatives to CPAP to support ventilation during perisurgical respiratory management.[37]

THE INTRAOPERATIVE AND IMMEDIATE POSTOPERATIVE PERIODS
Perioperative Interactions Between Sleep-related Breathing Disorders and Medications

During surgery, anesthesia closely approximates the sleep state in several ways. Common to the anesthetized state and to sleep are decreased tone of the pharyngeal dilator muscles,[38] reduced hypoxic and hypercapnic respiratory drive, decreased activity of the respiratory muscles, increased dependence on the diaphragm, decreased respiratory stimulation, and reduced lung volume.[39] These physiologic changes may lead to increased severity of OSA and hypoventilation during the recovery period from the anesthetic.[40] Whereas during sleep one might arouse to an event, such as an obstructed airway, the deeply anesthetized state blunts the typical arousal mechanisms and the effect can linger until the offending medications have been metabolized.

Opioids commonly are used for postoperative analgesia and can cause sedation and respiratory depression.[41] Their effects in the intraoperative and immediate postoperative period often are potentiated by the presence of other central nervous system depressants, such as benzodiazepines and anesthetic agents, and also can be amplified by patient comorbidities, such as OSA, OHS, and neuromuscular disease. All opioids inhibit μ-opioid receptors distributed on respiratory neurons throughout the central and peripheral nervous system. Among the most important opioid-sensitive areas in respiratory centers are the pre–Bötzinger complex; glomus cells of the carotid body; bulbospinal inspiratory and expiratory premotor neurons that project to the phrenic, intercostal, and abdominal motoneurons; and the hypoglossal motor nucleus necessary for maintaining upper airway patency during sleep. Therefore, opioids have the potential to affect breathing frequency, tidal volume, rhythm, upper airway patency, and chemosensitivity to CO_2 and O_2 changes. Clinically, this may translate in the postoperative recovery period as changes of breathing pattern (ataxia or irregular vs regular), presence of sleep-related breathing disorders (central and/or obstructive apneas and hypopneas), gas exchange (hypoxia and hypercapnia), or a combination of them. Therefore, patients with OSA and OHS may be at a higher risk of respiratory arrest when they are given analgesics to treat postoperative pain, especially in an unmonitored environment.[42–44]

Intraoperative Use of Noninvasive Ventilation

NIV has been studied for use intraoperative use with anesthesia/analgesia in a variety of conditions, including neuromuscular disease, obesity, COPD, and others. In this setting, NIV may control hypoventilation and may be a feasible alternative to tracheal intubation and general anesthesia in selected situations. The existing literature, however, supporting the use of NIV intraoperatively is heterogeneous and consists mostly of smaller studies and, therefore, must be interpreted with caution.[45]

SLEEP-RELATED BREATHING DISORDERS IN THE POSTOPERATIVE PERIOD
Changes in Sleep in the Postoperative Period

Sleep architecture is altered significantly after surgery. On postoperative night 1, there is a significant reduction or elimination of REM sleep. This is thought to be a result of sleep fragmentation and anesthesia/analgesia administration in the immediate postoperative period. On night 3, there is a significant increase in the AHI in OSA and non-OSA patients. This increase may be explained by a rebound in REM sleep.[40] Furthermore, postoperative day 3 has been linked with increased risk of cardiovascular ischemia, which may be attributed to increased episodes of OSA-related hypoxemia.[46]

Postoperative Complications in Sleep-related Breathing Disorders

Most postoperative complications occur in the first 72 hours after surgery. The highest incidence of respiratory failure occurs during the first 24 hours, driven mainly by the residual effect of anesthetic, sedatives, and the use of narcotics for pain control.[47,48] Many studies demonstrate higher risk of postoperative complications in patients with untreated OSA and OHS.[1,3,26,49,50] OSA is directly linked with

- Longer length of stay
- More frequent ICU admission
- Higher admission costs
- Increased 30-day mortality[2,51]

Additionally, there are data on specific respiratory and cardiac outcomes related to sleep-related breathing disorders.

Postoperative Respiratory Complications in Obstructive Sleep Apnea

Risk factors for respiratory depression during acute recovery from surgery include sleep-related breathing disorders, increased doses of perioperative opioids, use of sedating medications, and use of more soluble anesthetic volatile agents, such as isoflurane.[41,48]

Patients with OSA are at higher risk for immediate postoperative respiratory complications:

- Hypoxia
- Acute respiratory distress syndrome
- Acute respiratory failure
- Pneumonia
- Intubation and mechanical ventilation[2,3,51–54]

Postoperative Cardiovascular Complications in Obstructive Sleep Apnea

Chan and colleagues[26] found that severe OSA was significantly associated with a higher rate of postoperative cardiovascular events even after a multivariable analysis controlling for perioperative factors known to affect outcomes adversely (adjusted hazard ratio [HR] 2.23 [95% CI, 1.49–3.34]; $P = .001$). This association was not seen, however, among patients with mild OSA (adjusted HR 1.36 [95% CI, 0.97–1.91]; $P = .08$) or moderate OSA (adjusted HR 1.47 [95% CI, 0.98–2.09]; $P = .07$).

In post hoc analysis of the data, severe OSA was associated with a higher risk of

- Postoperative cardiac death
- Myocardial injury
- Congestive heart failure
- New-onset atrial fibrillation
- Unplanned admission or readmission to the ICU
- Unplanned tracheal intubation or lung ventilation

Moderate OSA was associated with

- Cardiac death
- Unplanned ICU readmission
- Unplanned tracheal intubation
- Infections

Mild OSA was associated with

- Unplanned admission or readmission to the ICU
- Unplanned postoperative tracheal intubation of lung ventilation
- Pneumonia[26]

Postoperative Complications Specific to Obesity Hypoventilation Syndrome

By definition, OHS is characterized by hypercapnia, which is considered a stand-alone risk factor for perioperative complications.[11] Patients with hypercapnia from definite or possible OHS are at higher risk compared with those with OSA without hypercapnia independent from AHI and BMI:

- Postoperative respiratory failure
- Postoperative heart failure
- Prolonged intubation
- Postoperative ICU transfer
- Longer ICU and hospital lengths of stay
- Six-week posthospital mortality[55]

REDUCING POSTOPERATIVE COMPLICATIONS
Postoperative Monitoring for Respiratory Depression

There are no agreed-on strategies for stratifying and monitoring patients at risk for sleep-disordered breathing in the postoperative setting. In the postanesthesia care unit (PACU), Gali and colleagues assessed patients at 30 minutes, 60 minutes, and 90 minutes postoperatively and found that patients with high preoperative risk for OSA and recurrent immediate postoperative respiratory events (eg, recurrent bradypnea, apnea, desaturations, and pain-sedation mismatch) had the highest incidence of elevated oxygen desaturation index and postoperative respiratory complications. This strategy may help identify and stratify patients at higher risk for postoperative respiratory desaturations and respiratory complications who may benefit from a higher level of care and monitoring.[56] Pulse oximetry combined with arterial blood gases often are used to monitor extubated patients with or at risk for OSA or OHS in the PACU; however, extension of oximetry monitoring during subsequent days of surgical recovery has proved useful. Chan and colleagues[26] have shown that adult patients at risk for OSA with longer duration of postoperative oxygen desaturations less than 80% during the first 3 postoperative nights were at higher risk for postoperative cardiovascular events ($P<.001$). These findings suggest that it is important to continuously monitor oxygen saturations in postoperative patients. To date, however, there has been no consensus on the most suitable device for monitoring these patients while recovering on the wards. Current clinically available monitoring devices for respiration in suspected or confirmed OSA or OHS patients include continuous pulse oximetry and capnography monitors. Other less available monitoring tools in clinical practice are respiratory volume monitor, and photoplethysmography. According to the current literature, the continuous pulse oximetry, with its high sensitivity, still is the most widely used device due to its simplicity, short setup time, and short response time (seconds). Although cost effective, it has a low specificity, and, because it is not an instrument to measure ventilation, it lags as an indicator of respiratory failure. Capnography is the device used most widely for detection of hypoventilation. For extubated postanesthesia patients, the measurement of end-tidal CO_2 ($EtCO_2$) is done by placing a nasal cannula to obtain and analyze exhaled gas samples. $EtCO_2$ may detect apneic episodes and respiratory depression indicated by reduced rate of respiration per minute. In OSA patients, however, mouth breathing related to high nasal airway resistance or partial obstruction of the airway and mixing of exhaled air with ambient air may display a normal $EtCO_2$ value, even when $Paco_2$ detectable by blood gas analysis is high.[57]

The ASA and AASM have recommended close monitoring with pulse oximetry of those patients at risk for respiratory depression (eg, OSA and/or OHS) receiving intravenous or neuraxial opioids for adequacy of ventilation, oxygenation, and level of consciousness (see **Box 2**). The AASM does not mention the setting in which a patient should be monitored (eg, general care, step-down unit, or ICU) and the ASA states that evidence in the literature is insufficient in assessing the impact of monitoring patients for respiratory depression in different potential postoperative settings. The ASA acknowledges that the optimal duration for postoperative respiratory monitoring has not been established.[58]

Reducing Anesthesia-related Postoperative Complications

In patients with sleep-disordered breathing or hypoventilation, using a preventative strategy to avoid respiratory depression and/or worsening of OSA in the setting of opioid administration might be considered. This could involve limiting use of opioids by employing other methods of analgesia, such as regional blocks,[41] or titrating opioid dose carefully to the minimum amount required to achieve adequate pain control.[17] A close monitoring strategy also may be appropriate for postoperative patients receiving opioid pain medications. A recent meta-analysis suggested that continuous pulse oximetry used with capnography in patients who have received opioids in the postoperative period may aid in the detection of respiratory failure even before hypoxia is clinically evident.[59]

In OSA patients, most respiratory complications associated with opioid administration are related to relatively small doses of opioids (MEDD <10 mg) and they occur in the first 24 hours post-surgery, predominantly on the general hospital ward. In a recent published series of perioperative critical complications, including deaths in patients with OSA, morbid obesity, male sex, undiagnosed/untreated OSA, suboptimal use of postoperative CPAP, need for opioid analgesia, and lack of appropriate postoperative monitoring were the risk factors identified to predispose an OSA patient to critical complications.[60]

Because the effects of opioids on sleep-related breathing disorders are dose dependent, discontinuation or reduction of the dose of opioid as tolerated is considered first-line therapy to prevent opioid-related respiratory complications. Beyond dose, route of administration may influence respiratory status. Therefore, for patients with OSA/OHS, the ASA has recommended limiting general anesthesia by using regional pain control strategies when possible and CPAP whenever a patient is sedated.[13] CPAP has been studied in the setting of acute postoperative opioid use in a bariatric surgery cohort and shown to be effective in improving AHI, tidal volume, and minute ventilation.[61] For a complete list of postoperative recommendations, see **Box 2**.

Postoperative Positive Airway Pressure Therapy in Respiratory Stable Obstructive Sleep Apnea/Obesity Hypoventilation Syndrome Patients

CPAP and APAP are equally effective in the perioperative management of OSA in decreasing

AHI, improving oxygenation, and shortening length of stay, although their role in preventing other adverse postoperative outcomes remains unclear.[35]

In postoperative care, patients with a previous diagnosis of OSA or OHS with predominant OSA already may have CPAP at home and may know their pressure settings. In that situation, the home pressure setting may be a reasonable initial set-point, but the pressure may need to be adjusted to meet the acute needs of the patient during surgical recovery. For patients without a prior pressure setting, use of an APAP device or manual bedside titration with close monitoring may be required.[62]

When initiation of BPAP is selected for a stable chronic hypercapnic respiratory failure patient, expiratory PAP (EPAP) may be started at a low pressure level, except when either OSA or atelectasis related to morbid obesity is present (or suspected) for which a higher EPAP may be needed. The level of inspiratory PAP (IPAP) determines the pressure support (PS), which helps assist/augment inspiration (PS = IPAP − EPAP). Therefore, an initial setting of IPAP approximately 6 cm H_2O to 8 cm H_2O above the EPAP (PS) assists with ventilation. Further customization of PS may be needed, however, based on the level of respiratory support needed during a patient's surgical recovery. If a backup rate is desired in order to ensure a minimum minute ventilation (respiration rate × tidal volume), the BPAP device can be used in spontaneous timed mode, setting the initial respiratory rate at 2 breaths per minute to 3 breaths per minute below the patient's spontaneous respiratory frequency while in stable respiratory condition.[63] In some cases, a higher backup rate (increased proportion of mechanical breaths delivered by the NIV) may be associated with better control of nocturnal transcutaneous carbon dioxide ($PtCO_2$) and larger falls in daytime CO_2; however, patient-ventilator synchrony should be monitored closely.[64]

Alternatively to BPAP, VAPS also can be implemented in those patients with stable chronic hypercapnic respiratory failure. VAPS is a mode that tracks spontaneous respiratory rate, expiratory tidal volume, and ventilation, proportionally adjusting IPAP and/or the backup respiratory rate, with subsequent augmentation of breathing when needed to reach a respiratory target set by the provider. These respiratory targets could be either expiratory tidal volume or alveolar ventilation. In patients with inadequate ventilation due to a decrease in respiratory drive (eg, use of opioids), a backup respiratory rate from the VAPS supplies additional breaths to reach adequate minute ventilation. An auto-EPAP function also is available in more recent device models to self-adjust to upper airway resistance to maintain upper airway patency.[65] Like CPAP and BPAP, VAPS settings should be adjusted to meet the needs of the patient during surgical recovery (see Gaurav Singh and Michelle Cao's article, "Noninvasive Ventilator Devices and Modes," in this issue) NIV per se also might induce de novo undesirable respiratory events. Ventilation-induced hyperventilation might promote periodic breathing and glottic closure. Therefore, close monitoring is highly recommended to all patients initiated on NIV to assist/augment ventilation.

Postoperative Monitoring of Patients on Continuous Positive Airway Pressure and Noninvasive Ventilation

In the postoperative surgical period, OSA and OHS patients on CPAP or NIV may experience patient-ventilator asynchrony, increases in upper airway resistance (with or without increased respiratory drive), and pressure leak from the mask. Detection of these events is important in order to optimize appropriate ventilator settings and interface. While on PAP therapy, pulse oximetry is important to ensure that adequate oxygen saturation is provided and to detect either prolonged or short and recurrent desaturations. Like those patients on non-PAP therapy, however, the specificity of pulse oximetry tracings during NIV is low and should be interpreted cautiously. In PAP therapy, Spo_2 variations may reflect upper airway instability and residual obstructive events, decrease in respiratory drive, or repetitive pressure leaks from the mask interrupted by microarousals commonly seen during recovery.

Different from CPAP, in NIV $EtCO_2$ is a poor predictor of $Paco_2$. During bilevel PS therapy, variability in physiologic dead space and tidal volumes, and difficulties reaching an adequate plateau, make measuring $EtCO_2$ technically difficult in the setting of continuous flow through the mask. Different from $EtCO_2$, transcutaneous capnography ($PtcCO_2$) has a good agreement with $Paco_2$, and is preserved when patients are treated by CPAP or NIV. Transcutaneous capnography may help better discriminate between hypoxemia related to ventilation/perfusion mismatch and hypoventilation, document correction of nocturnal hypoventilation, and detect ventilator-induced hyperventilation, a possible cause for central apnea/hypopnea and glottic closure. The latest generation of PAP devices often is equipped with sophisticated built-in software capable of recording a wide range of respiratory parameters, thus offering information for clinicians to estimate ventilation, tidal volume, leaks, and the rate of inspiratory or expiratory triggering by the patient.[66]

Reduction of Postoperative Cardiac and Pulmonary Complications with PAP

There is contradictory evidence regarding the efficacy of PAP in postoperative cardiopulmonary risk reduction. A retrospective study found people who had been diagnosed with OSA and were using CPAP at home during the preoperative period were less likely to have postoperative complications.[52] Additionally, a meta-analysis found that postoperative use of PAP decreased respiratory complications not only in patients with OSA but also in patients without OSA.[67] In contrast, a meta-analysis by Nagappa and colleagues[68] did not find a difference in postoperative outcomes in surgical patients with OSA treated with CPAP versus no-CPAP. The investigators postulated that heterogeneity between the studies with regard to the definition of a postoperative event, and low CPAP compliance may have been responsible for these findings.[68] Poor PAP compliance is a real-world issue that must be taken into account when interpreting medical literature regarding PAP treatment outcomes and when considering PAP as a feasible means of postoperative risk reduction.

NIV has been studied for prophylactic perioperative use in patients undergoing bariatric surgery but has not been shown to be effective in reducing mortality, intubation, or length of hospital stay.[69]

SUMMARY

Sleep-related breathing disorders, including OSA and OHS, are common in adults presenting for surgery and are associated with increased risk of postoperative complications. Even when OSA/OHS is identified in the preoperative evaluation, the evidence regarding effective means of risk reduction is controversial and there is no clear recommendation for a universal postoperative management strategy.

Further clinical trials are required to better identify those OSA and OHS patients at higher risk of perioperative cardiorespiratory complications (phenotypes) and to test the impact of specific interventions on cardiovascular and pulmonary outcomes.

DISCLOSURE

Neither author has any relevant financial relationships to disclose.

REFERENCES

1. Kaw R, Chung F, Pasupuleti V, et al. Meta-analysis of the association between obstructive sleep apnoea and postoperative outcome. Br J Anaesth 2012; 109:897–906.
2. Memtsoudis SG, Stundner O, Rasul R, et al. The impact of sleep apnea on postoperative utilization of resources and adverse outcomes. Anesth Analg 2014;118:407–18.
3. Mutter TC, Chateau D, Moffatt M, et al. A matched cohort study of postoperative outcomes in obstructive sleep apnea: could preoperative diagnosis and treatment prevent complications? Anesthesiology 2014;121:707–18.
4. Abboud F, Kumar R. Obstructive sleep apnea and insight into mechanisms of sympathetic overactivity. J Clin Invest 2014;124:1454–7.
5. Mansukhani MP, Calvin AD, Kolla BP, et al. The association between atrial fibrillation and stroke in patients with obstructive sleep apnea: a population-based case-control study. Sleep Med 2013;14:243–6.
6. Young T, Peppard P, Palta M, et al. Population-based study of sleep-disordered breathing as a risk factor for hypertension. Arch Intern Med 1997;157: 1746–52.
7. Marin JM, Carrizo SJ, Vicente E, et al. Long-term cardiovascular outcomes in men with obstructive sleep apnoea-hypopnoea with or without treatment with continuous positive airway pressure: an observational study. Lancet 2005;365:1046–53.
8. Gottlieb DJ, Yenokyan G, Newman AB, et al. Prospective study of obstructive sleep apnea and incident coronary heart disease and heart failure: the sleep heart health study. Circulation 2010;122: 352–60.
9. Yaggi HK, Concato J, Kernan WN, et al. Obstructive sleep apnea as a risk factor for stroke and death. N Engl J Med 2005;353:2034–41.
10. Kessler R, Chaouat A, Schinkewitch P, et al. The obesity-hypoventilation syndrome revisited: a prospective study of 34 consecutive cases. Chest 2001;120:369–76.
11. Kaw R, Bhateja P, Paz YMH, et al. Postoperative Complications in patients with unrecognized obesity hypoventilation syndrome undergoing elective noncardiac surgery. Chest 2016;149:84–91.
12. Masa JF, Pepin JL, Borel JC, et al. Obesity hypoventilation syndrome. Eur Respir Rev 2019;28.
13. American society of anesthesiologists task force on perioperative management of patients with obstructive sleep a. practice guidelines for the perioperative management of patients with obstructive sleep apnea: an updated report by the American society of anesthesiologists task force on perioperative management of patients with obstructive sleep apnea. Anesthesiology 2014;120:268–86.

14. Ayas NT, Laratta CR, Coleman JM, et al, ATS Assembly on Sleep and Respiratory Neurobiology. Knowledge Gaps in the perioperative management of adults with obstructive sleep apnea and obesity hypoventilation syndrome. An official American thoracic society workshop report. Ann Am Thorac Soc 2018;15:117–26.

15. Chung F, Memtsoudis SG, Ramachandran SK, et al. Society of anesthesia and sleep medicine guidelines on preoperative screening and assessment of adult patients with obstructive sleep apnea. Anesth Analg 2016;123:452–73.

16. Memtsoudis SG, Cozowicz C, Nagappa M, et al. Society of anesthesia and sleep medicine guideline on intraoperative management of adult patients with obstructive sleep apnea. Anesth Analg 2018;127:967–87.

17. Meoli AL, Rosen CL, Kristo D, et al. Clinical practice review C, American academy of Sleep M. Upper airway management of the adult patient with obstructive sleep apnea in the perioperative period–avoiding complications. Sleep 2003;26:1060–5.

18. Mokhlesi B, Masa JF, Brozek JL, et al. Evaluation and management of obesity hypoventilation syndrome. an official american thoracic society clinical practice guideline. Am J Respir Crit Care Med 2019;200:e6–24.

19. Peppard PE, Young T, Barnet JH, et al. Increased prevalence of sleep-disordered breathing in adults. Am J Epidemiol 2013;177:1006–14.

20. Reed K, Pengo MF, Steier J. Screening for sleep-disordered breathing in a bariatric population. J Thorac Dis 2016;8:268–75.

21. Macavei VM, Spurling KJ, Loft J, et al. Diagnostic predictors of obesity-hypoventilation syndrome in patients suspected of having sleep disordered breathing. J Clin Sleep Med 2013;9:879–84.

22. Mokhlesi B, Tulaimat A, Faibussowitsch I, et al. Obesity hypoventilation syndrome: prevalence and predictors in patients with obstructive sleep apnea. Sleep Breath 2007;11:117–24.

23. Laaban JP, Chailleux E. Daytime hypercapnia in adult patients with obstructive sleep apnea syndrome in France, before initiating nocturnal nasal continuous positive airway pressure therapy. Chest 2005;127:710–5.

24. Young T, Palta M, Dempsey J, et al. Burden of sleep apnea: rationale, design, and major findings of the Wisconsin sleep cohort study. WMJ 2009;108:246–9.

25. Steiner CA (Institute for Health Research, Kaiser Permanente), Karaca Z (AHRQ), Moore BJ (IBM Watson Health), Imshaug MC (IBM Watson Health), Pickens G (IBM Watson Health). Surgeries in Hospital-Based Ambulatory Surgery and Hospital Inpatient Settings, 2014. HCUP Statistical Brief #223. May 2017. Rockville (MD): Agency for Healthcare Research and Quality. Available at www.hcup-us.ahrq.gov/reports/statbriefs/sb223-Ambulatory-Inpatient-Surgeries-2014.pdf.

26. Chan MTV, Wang CY, Seet E, et al. Postoperative vascular complications in unrecognized obstructive sleep apnea study i. association of unrecognized obstructive sleep apnea with postoperative cardiovascular events in patients undergoing major noncardiac surgery. JAMA 2019;321:1788–98.

27. Balachandran JS, Masa JF, Mokhlesi B. Obesity hypoventilation syndrome epidemiology and diagnosis. Sleep Med Clin 2014;9:341–7.

28. Mokhlesi B. Obesity hypoventilation syndrome: a state-of-the-art review. Respir Care 2010;55:1347–62 [discussion: 1363–5].

29. Sturm R, Hattori A. Morbid obesity rates continue to rise rapidly in the United States. Int J Obes (Lond) 2013;37:889–91.

30. Brown EN, Lydic R, Schiff ND. General anesthesia, sleep, and coma. N Engl J Med 2010;363:2638–50.

31. Chung F, Hillman D, Lydic R. Sleep medicine and anesthesia a new horizon for anesthesiologists. Anesthesiology 2011;114:1261–2.

32. Chung F, Yegneswaran B, Liao P, et al. STOP questionnaire: a tool to screen patients for obstructive sleep apnea. Anesthesiology 2008;108:812–21.

33. Boing S, Randerath WJ. Chronic hypoventilation syndromes and sleep-related hypoventilation. J Thorac Dis 2015;7:1273–85.

34. Kapur VK, Auckley DH, Chowdhuri S, et al. Clinical practice guideline for diagnostic testing for adult obstructive sleep apnea: an american academy of sleep medicine clinical practice guideline. J Clin Sleep Med 2017;13:479–504.

35. Liao P, Luo Q, Elsaid H, et al. Perioperative auto-titrated continuous positive airway pressure treatment in surgical patients with obstructive sleep apnea: a randomized controlled trial. Anesthesiology 2013;119:837–47.

36. Kushida CA, Berry RB, Blau A, et al. Positive airway pressure initiation: a randomized controlled trial to assess the impact of therapy mode and titration process on efficacy, adherence, and outcomes. Sleep 2011;34:1083–92.

37. Murphy PB, Davidson C, Hind MD, et al. Volume targeted versus pressure support non-invasive ventilation in patients with super obesity and chronic respiratory failure: a randomised controlled trial. Thorax 2012;67:727–34.

38. Eastwood PR, Szollosi I, Platt PR, et al. Comparison of upper airway collapse during general anaesthesia and sleep. Lancet 2002;359:1207–9.

39. Hillman DR, Chung F. Anaesthetic management of sleep-disordered breathing in adults. Respirology 2017;22:230–9.

40. Chung F, Liao P, Yegneswaran B, et al. Postoperative changes in sleep-disordered breathing and sleep architecture in patients with obstructive sleep apnea. Anesthesiology 2014;120:287–98.

41. Nagappa M, Weingarten TN, Montandon G, et al. Opioids, respiratory depression, and sleep-disordered breathing. Best Pract Res Clin Anaesthesiol 2017;31:469–85.

42. Macintyre PE, Loadsman JA, Scott DA. Opioids, ventilation and acute pain management. Anaesth Intensive Care 2011;39:545–58.

43. Ladd LA, Kam PC, Williams DB, et al. Ventilatory responses of healthy subjects to intravenous combinations of morphine and oxycodone under imposed hypercapnic and hypoxaemic conditions. Br J Clin Pharmacol 2005;59:524–35.

44. Hajiha M, DuBord MA, Liu H, et al. Opioid receptor mechanisms at the hypoglossal motor pool and effects on tongue muscle activity in vivo. J Physiol 2009;587:2677–92.

45. Cabrini L, Nobile L, Plumari VP, et al. Intraoperative prophylactic and therapeutic non-invasive ventilation: a systematic review. Br J Anaesth 2014;112:638–47.

46. Gogenur I, Rosenberg-Adamsen S, Lie C, et al. Relationship between nocturnal hypoxaemia, tachycardia and myocardial ischaemia after major abdominal surgery. Br J Anaesth 2004;93:333–8.

47. Thompson JS, Baxter BT, Allison JG, et al. Temporal patterns of postoperative complications. Arch Surg 2003;138:596–602 [discussion 602–3].

48. Lee LA, Caplan RA, Stephens LS, et al. Postoperative opioid-induced respiratory depression: a closed claims analysis. Anesthesiology 2015;122:659–65.

49. Mador MJ, Goplani S, Gottumukkala VA, et al. Postoperative complications in obstructive sleep apnea. Sleep Breath 2013;17:727–34.

50. Liao P, Yegneswaran B, Vairavanathan S, et al. Postoperative complications in patients with obstructive sleep apnea: a retrospective matched cohort study. Can J Anaesth 2009;56:819–28.

51. Kaw R, Pasupuleti V, Walker E, et al. Postoperative complications in patients with obstructive sleep apnea. Chest 2012;141:436–41.

52. Gupta RM, Parvizi J, Hanssen AD, et al. Postoperative complications in patients with obstructive sleep apnea syndrome undergoing hip or knee replacement: a case-control study. Mayo Clin Proc 2001;76:897–905.

53. Memtsoudis S, Liu SS, Ma Y, et al. Perioperative pulmonary outcomes in patients with sleep apnea after noncardiac surgery. Anesth Analg 2011;112:113–21.

54. Mokhlesi B, Hovda MD, Vekhter B, et al. Sleep-disordered breathing and postoperative outcomes after elective surgery: analysis of the nationwide inpatient sample. Chest 2013;144:903–14.

55. Nowbar S, Burkart KM, Gonzales R, et al. Obesity-associated hypoventilation in hospitalized patients: prevalence, effects, and outcome. Am J Med 2004;116:1–7.

56. Gali B, Whalen FX Jr, Gay PC, et al. Management plan to reduce risks in perioperative care of patients with presumed obstructive sleep apnea syndrome. J Clin Sleep Med 2007;3:582–8.

57. Zhang X, Kassem MA, Zhou Y, et al. A brief review of non-invasive monitoring of respiratory condition for extubated patients with or at risk for obstructive sleep apnea after surgery. Front Med (Lausanne) 2017;4:26.

58. Practice guidelines for the prevention, detection, and management of respiratory depression associated with neuraxial opioid administration: an updated report by the American society of anesthesiologists task force on neuraxial opioids and the American society of regional anesthesia and pain medicine. Anesthesiology 2016;124:535–52.

59. Lam T, Nagappa M, Wong J, et al. Continuous pulse oximetry and capnography monitoring for postoperative respiratory depression and adverse events: a systematic review and meta-analysis. Anesth Analg 2017;125:2019–29.

60. Subramani Y, Nagappa M, Wong J, et al. Death or near-death in patients with obstructive sleep apnoea: a compendium of case reports of critical complications. Br J Anaesth 2017;119:885–99.

61. Zaremba S, Shin CH, Hutter MM, et al. Continuous positive airway pressure mitigates opioid-induced worsening of sleep-disordered breathing early after bariatric surgery. Anesthesiology 2016;125:92–104.

62. Hillman DR, Jungquist CR, Auckley D. Perioperative implementation of noninvasive positive airway pressure therapies. Respir Care 2018;63:479–87.

63. Selim BJ, Wolfe L, Coleman JM 3rd, et al. Initiation of noninvasive ventilation for sleep related hypoventilation disorders: advanced modes and devices. Chest 2018;153:251–65.

64. Contal O, Adler D, Borel JC, et al. Impact of different backup respiratory rates on the efficacy of noninvasive positive pressure ventilation in obesity hypoventilation syndrome: a randomized trial. Chest 2013;143:37–46.

65. Selim B, Ramar K. Advanced positive airway pressure modes: adaptive servo ventilation and volume assured pressure support. Expert Rev Med Devices 2016;13:839–51.

66. Janssens JP, Borel JC, Pepin JL, et al. Nocturnal monitoring of home non-invasive ventilation: the contribution of simple tools such as pulse oximetry, capnography, built-in ventilator software and autonomic markers of sleep fragmentation. Thorax 2011;66:438–45.

67. Ferreyra GP, Baussano I, Squadrone V, et al. Continuous positive airway pressure for treatment of

respiratory complications after abdominal surgery: a systematic review and meta-analysis. Ann Surg 2008;247:617–26.

68. Nagappa M, Mokhlesi B, Wong J, et al. The effects of continuous positive airway pressure on postoperative outcomes in obstructive sleep apnea patients undergoing surgery: a systematic review and meta-analysis. Anesth Analg 2015;120:1013–23.

69. Stefan MS, Hill NS, Raghunathan K, et al. Outcomes associated with early postoperative noninvasive ventilation in bariatric surgical patients with sleep apnea. J Clin Sleep Med 2016;12:1507–16.

Lifetime Care of Duchenne Muscular Dystrophy

Erin W. MacKintosh, MD[a,b,*], Maida L. Chen, MD[a,b], Joshua O. Benditt, MD[c]

KEYWORDS

- Duchenne muscular dystrophy • Polysomnogram • Respiratory failure • Neuromuscular disease
- Noninvasive ventilation • Obstructive sleep apnea • Insomnia hypoventilation

KEY POINTS

- Although sleep-disordered breathing is one of the best recognized disorders of sleep in boys and men with Duchenne muscular dystrophy (DMD), disorders of initiation and maintenance of sleep are more common and can significantly impact quality of life.
- Changes in mobility status predict need for increasing respiratory support.
- Nighttime hypoventilation precedes daytime symptoms and may be identified only on polysomnogram.
- Nighttime respiratory support should generally begin with bilevel noninvasive positive-pressure ventilation (bipap) instead of continuous positive airway pressure, and oxygen should never be used alone, as this can obscure and worsen hypoventilation.
- The natural progression of DMD pathophysiology has changed with the introduction of therapies for downstream pathologic pathways and will continue to evolve with the development of therapies that target function and expression of dystrophin.

INTRODUCTION

Duchenne muscular dystrophy (DMD) is an X-linked recessive disorder, with a prevalence of 15.9 to 19.5 per 100,000 live male births,[1] that is caused by absence or deficiency of functional dystrophin protein. Dystrophin stabilizes skeletal and cardiac muscle by connecting actin in muscle fibers to the extracellular matrix; in the absence of dystrophin, recurrent muscle fiber injury leads to chronic inflammation, replacement of muscle with fibrotic and fatty tissue, and associated weakness.[2]

The progressive neuromuscular weakness is often first noted during the preschool years. Boys with DMD create accommodative patterns of movement, and independent ambulation has been prolonged with the widespread use of systemic steroids to minimize accumulation of chronic inflammation.[3,4] In the current era, ambulation continues until median age 12 years,[5] and adolescents typically begin noninvasive positive-pressure ventilation (NIPPV) for respiratory failure before age 18 to 20 years.[1,6] Historically, death was expected in the second or third decade, whereas boys born today have life expectancy beyond age 40[6] with ventilatory assistance. Rarely, female carriers can exhibit a milder phenotype.

The natural disease progression has been altered over past decades by the advent of therapies targeting the downstream pathways that lead to muscle destruction, and promising work is under way with genetic and molecular therapies to

[a] Department of Pediatrics, University of Washington, Box 359300, Seattle, WA 98195, USA; [b] Division of Pulmonary and Sleep Medicine, Seattle Children's Hospital, 4800 Sand Point Way Northeast, M/S OC.7.720, Seattle, WA 98115, USA; [c] Respiratory Care Services and General Pulmonary Clinic, Department of Pulmonary, Critical Care, and Sleep Medicine, University of Washington, UW Medical Center, 1959 Northeast Pacific Street, Seattle, WA 98195, USA
* Corresponding author. Division of Pulmonary and Sleep Medicine, Seattle Children's Hospital, 4800 Sand Point Way Northeast, M/S OC.7.720, Seattle, WA 98115.
E-mail address: erin.mackintosh@seattlechildrens.org

Sleep Med Clin 15 (2020) 485–495
https://doi.org/10.1016/j.jsmc.2020.08.011
1556-407X/20/© 2020 Elsevier Inc. All rights reserved.

restore function of partially functioning dystrophin protein.[2] Although the trajectory has changed over time, individuals with DMD continue to have progressive sleep and respiratory disturbances that are best addressed in an anticipatory fashion, before accumulation of morbidity.

SLEEP-RELATED BREATHING DISORDERS AND RESPIRATORY FAILURE

Respiratory sufficiency, which is dependent on adequate ventilatory muscle strength, decreases as muscle weakness progresses. The decline in respiratory function and eventual failure typically parallels ambulation, with emergence of respiratory insufficiency when independent ambulation is lost. The diaphragm is the largest and most active muscle involved in breathing and thus the first to become significantly damaged and weakened in DMD.

Given the natural decrease in muscle tone and ventilatory drive during sleep, respiratory abnormalities in those with DMD tend to manifest first during sleep. Across the lifespan of DMD, various sleep-related breathing disorders (SRBD) have been described, including obstructive sleep apnea (OSA), central sleep apnea (CSA),[7] and nocturnal hypoventilation (**Fig. 1**).

As respiratory complications are a major cause of morbidity and mortality in the individual with DMD,[8] the respiratory management of the Duchenne patient, particularly the adult, should be anticipatory and preventive. Monitoring of respiratory muscle function, diurnal and nocturnal ventilation, cough, and swallowing function are foundational.[8] Implementing a "package" of respiratory interventions at appropriate points is crucial for improvements in quality and length of life, and is discussed in detail as follows.[8,9]

Pathophysiology

Early ambulatory (0–10 years)
With the emergence of widespread newborn screening and genetic testing, many children are now diagnosed with DMD in infancy. Infants with DMD have normal or near-normal respiratory physiology for age. Early ambulatory children with DMD should have typical trajectories of respiratory illnesses when compared with healthy peers and should not require additional diagnostic or therapeutic measures.

The most common SRBD during toddlerhood/early school years is OSA associated with adenotonsillar hypertrophy. OSA has a prevalence of 1% to 5% in the general population[10]; specific rates of OSA in those with DMD during ambulatory years have not been studied. Manifestations of OSA in prepubertal childhood are different from those in older youth and adults. As opposed to overt sleepiness, younger children with OSA tend to have more difficulty with inattention and mood, manifestations of which can overlap with the comorbid attention-deficit hyperactivity disorder and/or autism present in DMD. Treatment of childhood OSA with adenotonsillectomy has been shown to help with behavior and quality of life.[11] Although this has not been studied specifically in children with DMD, there is no indication that treating OSA in a child with DMD would not provide at least some of the same benefits.

Late ambulatory (8–18 years)
The use of chronic systemic steroids is commonly acknowledged as a risk factor for OSA with presumptive mechanism being the association with obesity,[12,13] as well as increased fat deposits in the tongue and neck; this has not been well described.

Inhalation is an active process, whereas exhalation is passive. However, forced expiration maneuvers such as coughing are not passive, and are necessary to clear the airways of secretions or foreign matter. Although a strong, productive cough depends on muscles of expiration, it is just as dependent on first taking a large breath in: a cough with a low volume of air behind it will be less forceful.[14] As the muscles of a youth with DMD slowly weaken, the diaphragm will maintain the ability to take small, "tidal" breaths much longer than the ability to take a large-volume inhale needed to create a cough.

Thus, decreasing inspiratory muscle strength first presents clinically with diminishing cough strength and decreased ability to clear airway secretions, before affecting ventilation.[14] This becomes important in the setting of lower respiratory tract infections, with poor secretion clearance leading to atelectasis, VQ mismatch, hypoxemia, and increasing risk for secondary pneumonia and respiratory failure.

During times of health, late-ambulatory youth with DMD can maintain adequate minute ventilation when awake and upright, but ventilation can begin to be impaired during times of challenge (viral illnesses, sleep, supine positioning). Acute bone fractures can be associated with splinting of breathing, sedating pain medications, and changes to mobility status, which all increase the risk of hypoventilation.

Early nonambulatory (12–20 years)
Decreased mobility further limits airway clearance, again increasing risk of secondary pneumonia and respiratory failure with viral illnesses. Nonambulation is associated with development of scoliosis.

This typically begins as a thoracolumbar curve, and does not significantly affect respiratory status until later progression.

With progression of respiratory muscle weakness, the weakened diaphragm leaves the individual more dependent on muscles of the chest wall for respirations. This is first observed during rapid-eye movement (REM) sleep, when the diaphragm is unable to compensate for atonia of the chest wall, and hypoventilation develops. To compensate, individuals with DMD may show paradoxic breathing and tachypnea; this increased energy expenditure may prevent partial pressures of carbon dioxide ≥ 50 mm Hg from being captured on capnography, as required for American Academy of Sleep Medicine diagnosis of hypoventilation, at the cost of disrupted REM sleep and failure to thrive. In this group, $Pco_2 \geq 45$ mm Hg can be considered abnormal.

Late nonambulatory

Patients with DMD have significant reductions in both lung and chest wall compliance. Some of this decrease in compliance may be due to atelectasis that occurs at low lung volumes. The inability to hyperinflate the lung via sigh breaths, due to muscle weakness, likely contributes to this progressive loss of compliance.

In addition to respiratory muscle weakness, progressive pharyngeal weakness and prolonged steroid exposure lead to increased rates of OSA. Dysphagia is increasingly common,[15] and unlike in other disorders, occurs first with solid foods rather than liquids. Although clinically apparent choking can occur, it is often underrecognized and can lead to aspiration pneumonia.

Thoracolumbar scoliosis progresses to include compensatory thoracic curve with pelvic obliquity.[16] This leads to further restrictive lung disease, hypoventilation, and risk for progressive respiratory failure with acute illness. Hypoventilation progresses to non-REM sleep and wake states.

Assessments for Sleep-Related Breathing Disorders

Due to the evolving respiratory pathophysiology through the lifespan with DMD, focus should vary with age:

Physical examination and history

- Early ambulatory: evaluate for tonsillar hypertrophy, mouth breathing, history of snoring, restless sleep, and mood or attention concerns

- Late ambulatory: history of snoring, restless sleep, mood or attention concerns, prolonged cough with respiratory illnesses, history of pneumonia
- Nonambulatory: monitor for changes in chest wall shape and compliance, symmetry of chest auscultation, reports of poor sleep and daytime sleepiness, signs and symptoms of dysphagia

Pulmonary function testing

Simple spirometry should be performed annually in ambulatory individuals. More extensive testing should be performed twice annually in nonambulatory individuals.

Home pulse oximetry

A pulse oximeter should be considered in an individual who has been prescribed cough augmentation to identify early, mild hypoxemia with illness or mucus plugging.[17,18] A persistent value SpO2 of less than 95% suggests that cough therapy and lung volume recruitment (LVR) should be instituted aggressively. Oximetry used at night is not a sensitive method for detecting the hypoventilation that is a major issue during sleep for individuals with respiratory muscle weakness.

Polysomnography

Polysomnogram (PSG) with continuous carbon dioxide monitoring by end-tidal or transcutaneous monitoring should be performed as follows:

- For any symptomatic individual with DMD (snoring, morning headaches, daytime sleepiness, observed apneic pauses), or asymptomatic individuals with significant weight gain or adenotonsillar hypertrophy
- Annually for nonambulatory individuals not already using nocturnal ventilation
- Preoperative PSG, if no recent study

For adult men with DMD using nocturnal ventilation, ongoing management of device settings during sleep are managed by recorded downloads from their nocturnal ventilatory devices as well as monitoring symptoms and diurnal carbon dioxide levels.[8] A panel of clinical experts have suggested that yearly sleep studies should be performed in adults with DMD,[8] although many adult sleep laboratories are not equipped to handle individuals with significant mobility issues, nocturnal nursing, and caregiver needs (discussed in Justin A. Fiala and John M. Coleman III's article, "Tailoring the Sleep Laboratory for Chronic Respiratory Failure," in this issue).

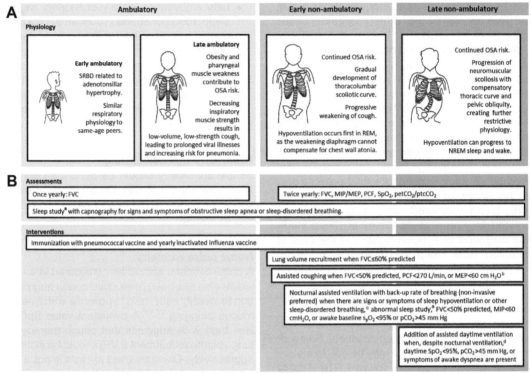

Fig. 1. Progression of respiratory pathophysiology and care by stage of disease. (*A*) Sleep-related respiratory pathophysiology in patients with DMD by stage of disease. (*B*) Assessments and interventions for respiratory care of patients with DMD by stage of disease. MEP, maximum expiratory pressure; MIP, maximum inspiratory pressure; PCF, peak cough flow; petCO$_2$, end-tidal partial pressure of CO$_2$; ptcCO$_2$, transcutaneous partial pressure of CO$_2$; SpO$_2$, blood oxygen saturation by pulse oximetry. [a] See text for definitions of sleep study results. [b] All specified threshold values of PCF, MEP, and MIP apply to older teenage and adult patients. [c] Fatigue, dyspnea, morning or continuous headaches, frequent nocturnal awakenings or difficult arousal, hypersomnolence, difficulty concentrating, awakenings with dyspnea and tachycardia, or frequent nightmares. [d] We strongly endorse the use of noninvasive methods of assisted ventilation instead of tracheostomy to optimize patient quality of life; indications for tracheostomy include patient preference, inability of patient to use noninvasive ventilation successfully, 3 failed extubation attempts during a critical illness despite optimum use of noninvasive ventilation and mechanically assisted coughing, or failure of noninvasive methods of cough assistance to prevent aspiration of secretions into the lungs due to weak bulbar muscles. ([*B*] *From* Birnkrant, DJ, Bush KM, Bann CM, et al., Diagnosis and management of Duchenne muscular dystrophy, part 2: respiratory, cardiac, bone health, and orthopaedic management., The Lancet Neurology, 2018; volume 17: 347–361; Reprinted with permission from Elsevier.)

Respiratory status during acute illness

Patients should be instructed to contact their medical care team with symptoms of respiratory tract infection. In addition to history and physical examination, chest radiograph, oximetry, and assessment of Pco$_2$ should be strongly considered. Patients and their families are often equipped to manage increased frequency of cough therapy and assisted ventilation; however, if adequate caregivers are unavailable at home or the trajectory of respiratory status is poor, admission to the hospital is appropriate for monitoring, augmented care, and family respite. Admission does not negate that family members often have better knowledge in assessment and treatment than some medical team members, as admissions overall for DMD are relatively uncommon. Use of oxygen without noninvasive ventilation (NIV) during hospitalization should be avoided given the risk of hypercarbia.

Respiratory Management During Childhood

Immunizations

- All infants/children with DMD should receive standard pediatric immunizations.
- All individuals with DMD should receive annual *inactivated* influenza vaccination.
- All individuals with DMD should receive pneumococcal vaccination per Centers for Disease

Control and Prevention (CDC)[19] guidelines for children with underlying medical conditions. At the time of this writing, recommendations are as follows:

○ PCV13 vaccine in a 4-part series before age 2 years
○ PPSV23 with first dose administered at age ≥2 years (at least 8 weeks after final indicated dose of PCV13), second dose 5 years after the first
○ See current guidelines for details

Adenotonsillectomy

Adenotonsillectomy should be considered in ambulatory children with OSA and in nonambulatory individuals with identified SRBD and adenotonsillar hypertrophy.

Cough augmentation

Diminishing percent-predicted forced vital capacity (FVC) or maximal inspiratory/expiratory pressures may correlate with decreasing efficacy of spontaneous airway clearance, as does prolonged cough or hypoxemia with viral illnesses. It benefits these patients to have equipment available at home before first severe respiratory exacerbation, so an anticipatory philosophy toward prescription of therapies is recommended. Cough augmentation is initiated when the patient's peak cough expiratory flow falls below 270 LPM.[20,21] There are 3 ways of increasing the cough peak flow.[22]

- Mechanical insufflator-exsufflator (MI-E): this device, colloquially referred to as "cough assist," is commonly prescribed in pediatric settings. It is an artificial cough generator used with a mask (or, later, tracheostomy adapter) that moves a volume of air into the subject's lungs via positive pressure, and then creates airflow out of the lung, "sucking" out secretions in the process, via rapid switch to a negative pressure. This is most effective with patients who can cooperate to keep the glottis and upper airway open to allow airflow out of the lung.
- Manually assisted cough (MAC): a trained assistant applies a thrust to the upper abdomen or lower ribcage to increase transpulmonary pressure during exhalation, thus increasing flow.
- LVR or "breath stacking": can be used either alone or in combination with MAC to increase flow. By increasing the volume of the lung before cough, there is a greater volume of air to exhale, as well as increased lung elastic recoil at greater lung volumes (see section on LVR in adult care).

Nighttime positive-pressure ventilation

Although the physiology of sleep-disordered breathing varies, it is generally recommended to begin nighttime respiratory support with bilevel pressure. Although continuous positive airway pressure (CPAP) may provide adequate initial support for OSA alone, CPAP may overpower respiratory muscle strength and worsen hypoventilation as weakness progresses. From a practical standpoint, initiation with bilevel support prevents the necessity of frequent follow-up polysomnograms as well as the need to upgrade the device. Oxygen should never be used in isolation to treat SRBD in DMD, as this can mask and worsen hypoventilation.[23]

Although there are times that NIPPV is started in the setting of an acute illness while hospitalized, NIPPV is best initiated in the outpatient setting. Ideally, NIPPV will have been discussed as part of anticipatory guidance before imminent need. Allowing youth with DMD to see, feel, and try different styles of mask interfaces before PSG may provide a better first-time positive airway pressure (PAP) experience, which may affect long-term adherence to prescribed PAP therapy. Mask selection depends on age, craniofacial structure including obesity, ability to self-adjust mask, but mostly patient preference and comfort. Nasal masks including pillows are often preferred for decreased risk of aerophagia. Split-night or titration PSG can be used to help initiate and/or fine tune settings, although this is not absolutely necessary. Once PAP treatment is begun, follow-up within 1 to 2 months is important to identify barriers to use as well as adequacy of treatment, both clinically and often for insurance coverage. Subsequent follow-up frequency is related to adherence, tolerance, subjective benefit, and overall clinical trajectory. Remote downloads and telemedicine can be useful adjuncts or even substitutes to in-person follow-ups, particularly with the explosion of telemedicine platforms related to the Coronavirus Disease 2019 pandemic.

Transition from Pediatric to Adult Care

Medical care for pediatric patients has become much more sophisticated over the past several decades, resulting in increased survival of high-technology needs individuals into adulthood. Transition has been defined by one investigator as "the purposeful, planned movement of adolescents with chronic medical conditions from child-centered to adult-oriented health care."[24] Transition usually occurs between the ages 17 and 21, depending on the health care system.

Components of transition programs necessary for a successful transition in other complex diseases have been identified.[25] These include the following:

- Disease-specific patient education including family self-management
- Creation of specific adolescent or joint pediatric/adult overlap clinics
- Creation of a transition-coordinator position with links to both programs

A list of important areas for consideration during transition specific to the young man with DMD is seen in **Fig. 2**.[26] Poorly planned transition can result in a deterioration of health status, a loss of confidence in the adult health care system due to perceived ignorance of pertinent diseases by adult providers, and a limited ability of some patients to direct their own health care in the adult environment.

Respiratory Management During Adulthood

Nighttime positive-pressure ventilation
Nearly all individuals with DMD will be on nocturnal ventilatory support before transition to adult care.

Cough augmentation
By the time the individual has transitioned to the adult clinic, cough augmentation strategies will have been in place already, as discussed previously.

Lung volume recruitment
Hyperinflation of the lung via LVR may reverse progressive loss of lung and chest wall compliance in the individual with DMD,[27–29] provide short-term and long-term improvements in lung compliance and vital capacity (VC),[28,30] and can enhance cough peak flow for secretion clearance.[31,32] LVR should be started when the FVC falls below 60% predicted and be performed 2 to 3 times per day.[8]

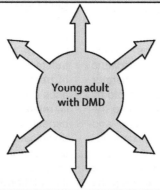

Relationships with others
- Develop skills to connect with others to manage own affairs (eg, social outings, appointments)
- Work towards desired level of autonomy and independence

Housing
- Examine where to live (family home vs elsewhere)
- Modify home for accessibility and safety
- Use assistive technology

Transportation
- Foster independent driving with vehicle modifications
- Modify family-owned vehicle
- Investigate accessible public transportation options

Young adult with DMD

Education or employment
- Plan early for future vocation
- Consider classes online vs on campus
- Contact campus programmes for students with disabilities
- Enlist employment or vocational planning resources

Activities of daily living
- Explore funding and benefits for care
- Learn to hire and train personal care attendants
- Ensure respite for family caregivers
- Consider need for guardianship or conservatorship

Health care
- Transition from paediatric to adult health care
- Move from family-centred to patient-centred provider interactions
- Discuss age-related changes in health-care benefits
- Assess the need for durable power of attorney for health care

Fig. 2. Social and medical considerations during transition to adulthood for young men with DMD. (*From* Birnkrant DJ, Bushby KM, Bann CM, et al., Diagnosis and management of Duchenne muscular dystrophy, part 3: primary care, emergency management, psychosocial care, and transitions of care across the lifespan., The Lancet Neurology, 2018; volume 17: 445-55; with permission.)

LVR, or "breath stacking," is an active assisted inhalation maneuver wherein the individual with DMD increases his lung volume above what he is able to achieve on his own by taking in extra positive-pressure breaths.[30] This larger, assisted lung volume has been referred to as the maximum inflation capacity or lung inflation capacity. The maneuver can be performed with a manual resuscitator bag attached to a mouthpiece, with an MI-E device, or with a mouthpiece ventilator in a volume mode, by taking multiple breaths without exhaling. The maneuver itself is relatively easily learned by the individual with DMD and is often very effective unless significant oral weakness leading to leak of volume is present.

Daytime noninvasive intermittent mechanical ventilation ("sip and puff")

Mouthpiece ventilation (MPV), also known as "sip and puff" ventilation, is a method using an open mouthpiece system that allows a breath to be delivered on demand when the patient "sips" from the mouthpiece interface[33] (**Fig. 3**). This requires a home ventilator that can deliver breaths in the volume mode. Modern ventilators can attach to the patient's wheelchair, and the mouthpiece interface is held in place by a flexible mechanical arm that can be adjusted to keep the mouthpiece stable in the proper position.

Patients who exhibit the need for ventilation during the daytime are candidates for MPV. Symptoms and signs that suggest that need include (1) dyspnea during the daytime, (2) elevated daytime CO_2 levels despite adequate treatment of sleep-disordered breathing, and (3) inadequate ability to phonate because of lack of breath volume. In addition, MPV allows for frequent user-controlled breath-stacking maneuvers that can be very helpful in increasing patient independence.

Tracheostomy/invasive mechanical ventilation

The need for and timing of tracheostomy is a debated topic,[34,35] but 24 hours per day noninvasive ventilation for individuals with DMD is entirely possible.[18,36] At our institution, we strongly support the use of NIPPV for 24 hours per day, via mask ventilation at night and MPV during the day. This avoids the tracheostomy procedure, the increased secretions caused by a tracheostomy tube, and allows the patient a greater ability for natural speech and swallowing.[37,38] Some have suggested that a patient requiring more than 16 hours per day of noninvasive ventilation should be considered for tracheostomy.[39]

A recent consensus statement suggested the following criteria for considering tracheostomy:[8]

- Three failed extubation attempts following intubation for a critical illness
- Patient preference
- Inability of the patient to use NIPPV successfully
- Presence of weak bulbar muscles causing failure of safe secretion management

OTHER SLEEP DISORDERS

In addition to direct benefits, treating these generalized sleep complaints is important in initiating and maintaining NIV in patients with DMD.

Insomnia

Prevalence

One cross-sectional study showed that insomnia is extremely common in boys and adolescents with DMD, with 30% of respondents screening positive for disorders of initiating or maintaining sleep.[40]

Etiology

Boys and men with DMD have multiple risk factors for insomnia, including the following:

- Medications: commonly prescribed medications that can disrupt sleep in this population include systemic steroids[41] and antidepressants.
- Psychological and socioeconomic stressors.

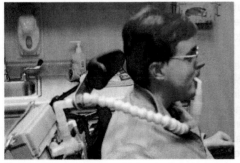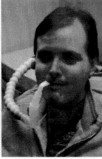

Fig. 3. Adult patient with DMD using MPV mounted to wheelchair.

- Sleep hygiene: Video games and online gaming are acknowledged by advocacy groups, such as Parent Project Muscular Dystrophy, as inclusive recreation that is popular for boys and men with DMD. While allowing for recreation and socializing, late-night and binged gaming sessions can contribute to poor sleep patterns if good sleep hygiene is not promoted.
- Pain: Most boys with DMD and their caregivers report chronic pain.[42] Pain is more common in nonambulatory individuals, possibly related to inability to independently shift body position requiring the caregiver to do so,[40] or associated with muscle contractures and positioning device (AFOs).[40]
- SRBD: unrecognized or undertreated SRBD can result in sleep onset and sleep maintenance insomnia.

Intervention

As with the general population, a detailed history of sleep patterns and environment will often yield potential areas for intervention. Promoting good sleep hygiene is important regardless of the presence of an organic etiology for sleep disturbance; in particular, regular sleep-wake cycles and limits to nighttime screen usage are important to recommend. Ensuring that the sleep environment that is conducive to restfulness includes addressing chronic pain and nighttime caregiver availability.

Treating SRBD may promote more continuous and restful sleep. For medication-related sleep disturbances, consider alternatives to prescribed medications that can cause insomnia and recommend dosing systemic steroids in the morning.

For more challenging or multifactorial cases of insomnia, melatonin may help promote regular sleep cycles when combined with sleep hygiene practices; due to the potential to suppress respiratory drive, hypnotics/medications with sedative effects should be avoided when possible. Cognitive Behavioral Therapy for Insomnia can also be a useful therapy and may benefit those with DMD as well as their caregivers.

Abnormal Autonomic Regulation

Symptoms of excess sympathetic tone, including tachycardia, reduced heart rate variability, and hyperhidrosis, are commonly seen in individuals with DMD.[43] In addition to physical discomfort that may interfere with sleep, abnormal autonomic tone may potentially contribute to psychological symptoms, such as depression.[44]

Restless Leg Syndrome

Immobility, muscle contractures, and postural equipment (orthotics) can be associated with extremity pain and discomfort. In this setting, symptoms of restless leg syndrome (RLS) may be overlooked. An individual with underlying propensity for RLS may have symptoms exacerbated by other medications prescribed for neuromuscular pains or depression (tricyclic antidepressants, selective serotonin reuptake inhibitor, serotonin-norepinephrine reuptake inhibitors).[45,46]

PALLIATIVE/END-OF-LIFE CARE

With the advent of noninvasive ventilation and advances in medications for the treatment of cardiomyopathy, individuals with DMD are currently living into their fourth and fifth decades. This is new territory for individuals with DMD and has been termed "unexpected adulthood." As men with DMD age into their 40s and even 50s, the issue of losing parental or other family caregivers due to death arises. Therefore, advanced planning for both advanced care and end-of-life (EOL) issues is crucial. Unfortunately, it is difficult to determine when EOL is near in individuals with DMD.[47]

One group has proposed the following indicators as indicating the approach of EOL in patients with neuromuscular diseases[48]: a marked decline in pulmonary function, particularly FVC and peak cough flow, marked weight loss, recurrent infections (typically pulmonary or urinary), inability to heal wounds/pressure ulcers, swallowing problems, and cognitive decline. These predictors have not been studied in DMD and may be more appropriate for other diseases, such as amyotrophic lateral sclerosis. Ventilatory failure can generally be well controlled in patients with DMD, and therefore end-stage cardiomyopathy may be an important marker of EOL in DMD.[49]

EOL issues and questions are best addressed through regular and open communication among the patient, their family/caregivers, and members of the health care team in advance of emergency situations. Patients and/or substitute decision-makers should be informed of the changes in respiratory function that can be expected over time, and the potential options available to address these changes. Rather than asking them to simply choose from a menu of options, a shared decision-making model is advocated when the right course is uncertain; health care providers should make recommendations after eliciting the values and preferences of decision-makers. Unfortunately, these discussions rarely happen. In a recent qualitative interview study of 15 young men with DMD in Britain, none of the men could recall any discussion about EOL with any clinician while on pediatric or adult services.[50] Too often, health care providers and caregivers of patients with DMD are unprepared for EOL, preventing death from happening in the location and manner desired by the patient or the patient's family. It may be helpful to engage a hospital-based or clinic-based palliative care service if providers are uncomfortable approaching these subjects with their patients.

Dyspnea is a common and distressing symptom at the EOL, and NIV can play a substantial role in palliation of dyspnea for patients with DMD and others with advanced ventilatory failure.[51] Most individuals with DMD will already have been using NIV before this point in their disease trajectory and so it is natural, and very appropriate, to continue during EOL care with the purpose of relieving dyspnea as opposed to prolonging care. Clear communication with hospice or home nursing services is important to make sure that NIV is not stopped abruptly and that transition to using dyspnea-relieving medications is gradual and with input from the patient and their caregivers.

SUMMARY

The natural progression of DMD pathophysiology has changed with the introduction of therapies for downstream pathologic pathways and will continue to evolve with the development of therapies that target function and expression of dystrophin. However, the respiratory and sleep needs in this population are largely predictable over the lifespan, and are best handled in an anticipatory manner. The profile of SRBD changes through childhood and adolescence due to progressive respiratory pathology. Boys treated with systemic steroids develop increased rates of OSA, and progression of chest wall weakness leads to hypoventilation during sleep before daytime symptoms and may only be identified on polysomnogram. Nighttime respiratory support should generally begin with bilevel NIPPV instead of CPAP, and oxygen should never be used alone, as this can obscure and worsen hypoventilation. Although less commonly recognized than SRBD, boys and men with DMD are at increased risk for disorders of initiation and maintenance of sleep, caused by SRBD, anxiety/depression, autonomic dysregulation, and as a side effect from commonly prescribed medications.

CLINICS CARE POINTS

- Decline in respiratory function typically parallels decline in ambulation.

- Intermittent nighttime hypoventilation precedes daytime symptoms and may be identified only on polysomnogram.
- Oxygen should never be used alone for acute illness or sleep disordered breathing, as this can mask or worsen hypoventilation.
- Boys and men with DMD benefit from anticipatory guidance with regard to respiratory disturbances and support, transition from pediatric to adult care, and transition to end-of-life care.

DISCLOSURE

Dr E.W. MacKintosh has no relevant disclosures.

REFERENCES

1. Ryder S, Leadley RM, Armstrong N, et al. The burden, epidemiology, costs and treatment for Duchenne muscular dystrophy: an evidence review. Orphanet J Rare Dis 2017;12:79.
2. Verhaart IEC, Aartsma-Rus A. Therapeutic developments for Duchenne muscular dystrophy. Nat Rev Neurol 2019;15:373–86.
3. Griggs RC, Miller JP, Greenberg CR, et al. Efficacy and safety of deflazacort vs prednisone and placebo for Duchenne muscular dystrophy. Neurology 2016;87:2123–31.
4. Guglieri M, Bushby K, Mcdermott MP, et al. Developing standardized corticosteroid treatment for Duchenne muscular dystrophy. Contemp Clin Trials 2017;58:34–9.
5. Janssen MMHP, Bergsma A, Geurts ACH, et al. Patterns of decline in upper limb function of boys and men with DMD: an international survey. J Neurol 2014;261:1269–88.
6. Kieny P, Chollet S, Delalande P, et al. Evolution of life expectancy of patients with Duchenne muscular dystrophy at AFM Yolaine de Kepper centre between 1981 and 2011. Ann Phys Rehabil Med 2013;56:443–54.
7. Barbe F, Quera-Salva MA, Mccann C, et al. Sleep-related respiratory disturbances in patients with Duchenne muscular dystrophy. Eur Respir J 1994; 7:1403–8.
8. Birnkrant DJ, Bushby K, Bann CM, et al. Diagnosis and management of Duchenne muscular dystrophy, part 2: respiratory, cardiac, bone health, and orthopaedic management. Lancet Neurol 2018;17:347–61.
9. Birnkrant DJ, Bushby KM, Amin RS, et al. The respiratory management of patients with duchenne muscular dystrophy: a DMD care considerations working group specialty article. Pediatr Pulmonol 2010;45:739–48.

10. Marcus CL, Brooks LJ, Draper KA, et al. Diagnosis and management of childhood obstructive sleep apnea syndrome. Pediatrics 2012;130:e714–55.

11. Marcus CL, Moore RH, Rosen CL, et al. A randomized trial of adenotonsillectomy for childhood sleep apnea. N Engl J Med 2013;368: 2366–76.

12. Mcdonough AK, Curtis JR, Saag KG. The epidemiology of glucocorticoid-associated adverse events. Curr Opin Rheumatol 2008;20:131–7.

13. Peckett AJ, Wright DC, Riddell MC. The effects of glucocorticoids on adipose tissue lipid metabolism. Metabolism 2011;60:1500–10.

14. Lomauro A, Romei M, D'angelo MG, et al. Determinants of cough efficiency in Duchenne muscular dystrophy. Pediatr Pulmonol 2014;49:357–65.

15. Toussaint M, Davidson Z, Bouvoie V, et al. Dysphagia in Duchenne muscular dystrophy: practical recommendations to guide management. Disabil Rehabil 2016;38:2052–62.

16. Archer JE, Gardner AC, Roper HP, et al. Duchenne muscular dystrophy: the management of scoliosis. J Spine Surg 2016;2:185–94.

17. Bach JR, Ishikawa Y, Kim H. Prevention of pulmonary morbidity for patients with Duchenne muscular dystrophy. Chest 1997;112:1024–8.

18. Bach JR, Martinez D. Duchenne muscular dystrophy: continuous noninvasive ventilatory support prolongs survival. Respir Care 2011;56:744–50.

19. Centers for Disease Control and Prevention. Available at: https://www.cdc.gov/vaccines/hcp/acip-recs/vacc-specific/mmr.html. Accessed February 26, 2020.

20. Basser PJ, Mcmahon TA, Griffith P. The mechanism of mucus clearance in cough. J Biomech Eng 1989; 111:288–97.

21. Bianchi C, Baiardi P. Cough peak flows: standard values for children and adolescents. Am J Phys Med Rehabil 2008;87:461–7.

22. Tzeng AC, Bach JR. Prevention of pulmonary morbidity for patients with neuromuscular disease. Chest 2000;118:1390–6.

23. Wagner MH, Berry RB. Disturbed sleep in a patient with Duchenne muscular dystrophy. J Clin Sleep Med 2008;4:173–5.

24. Blum RW. Introduction. Improving transition for adolescents with special health care needs from pediatric to adult-centered health care. Pediatrics 2002; 110:1301–3.

25. Peters A, Laffel L, American Diabetes Association Transitions Working, Group. Diabetes care for emerging adults: recommendations for transition from pediatric to adult diabetes care systems: a position statement of the American Diabetes Association, with representation by the American College of Osteopathic Family Physicians, the American Academy of Pediatrics, the American Association of Clinical Endocrinologists, the American Osteopathic Association, the Centers for Disease Control and Prevention, Children With Diabetes, the Endocrine Society, the International Society for Pediatric and Adolescent Diabetes, Juvenile Diabetes Research Foundation International, the National Diabetes Education Program, and the Pediatric Endocrine Society (formerly Lawson Wilkins Pediatric Endocrine Society). Diabetes Care 2011;34: 2477–85.

26. Birnkrant DJ, Bushby K, Bann CM, et al. Diagnosis and management of Duchenne muscular dystrophy, part 3: primary care, emergency management, psychosocial care, and transitions of care across the lifespan. Lancet Neurol 2018;17:445–55.

27. Katz SL, Barrowman N, Monsour A, et al. Long-term effects of lung volume recruitment on maximal inspiratory capacity and vital capacity in Duchenne muscular dystrophy. Ann Am Thorac Soc 2016;13: 217–22.

28. Mckim DA, Katz SL, Barrowman N, et al. Lung volume recruitment slows pulmonary function decline in Duchenne muscular dystrophy. Arch Phys Med Rehabil 2012;93:1117–22.

29. Molgat-Seon Y, Hannan LM, Dominelli PB, et al. Lung volume recruitment acutely increases respiratory system compliance in individuals with severe respiratory muscle weakness. ERJ Open Res 2017; 3. 00135-2016.

30. Kaminska M, Browman F, Trojan DA, et al. Feasibility of lung volume recruitment in early neuromuscular weakness: a comparison between amyotrophic lateral sclerosis, myotonic dystrophy, and postpolio syndrome. PM R 2015;7:677–84.

31. Kang SW, Kang YS, Moon JH, et al. Assisted cough and pulmonary compliance in patients with Duchenne muscular dystrophy. Yonsei Med J 2005;46:233–8.

32. Sancho J, Servera E, Diaz J, et al. Efficacy of mechanical insufflation-exsufflation in medically stable patients with amyotrophic lateral sclerosis. Chest 2004;125:1400–5.

33. Carilho R, De Carvalho M, Kuehl U, et al. Erythropoietin and amyotrophic lateral sclerosis: plasma level determination. Amyotroph Lateral Scler 2011;12: 439–43.

34. Katz SL, Mckim D, Hoey L, et al. Respiratory management strategies for Duchenne muscular dystrophy: practice variation amongst Canadian sub-specialists. Pediatr Pulmonol 2013;48: 59–66.

35. Rodger S, Woods KL, Bladen CL, et al. Adult care for Duchenne muscular dystrophy in the UK. J Neurol 2015;262:629–41.

36. Bach JR, Goncalves MR, Hon A, et al. Changing trends in the management of end-stage neuromuscular respiratory muscle failure: recommendations

of an international consensus. Am J Phys Med Rehabil 2013;92:267–77.

37. Britton D, Hoit JD, Benditt JO, et al. Swallowing with noninvasive positive-pressure ventilation (NPPV) in individuals with muscular dystrophy: a qualitative analysis. Dysphagia 2020;35:32–41.

38. Britton D, Hoit JD, Pullen E, et al. Experiences of speaking with noninvasive positive pressure ventilation: a qualitative investigation. Am J Speech Lang Pathol 2019;28:784–92.

39. Jeppesen J, Green A, Steffensen BF, et al. The Duchenne muscular dystrophy population in Denmark, 1977-2001: prevalence, incidence and survival in relation to the introduction of ventilator use. Neuromuscul Disord 2003;13:804–12.

40. Bloetzer C, Jeannet P-Y, Lynch B, et al. Sleep disorders in boys with Duchenne muscular dystrophy. Acta Paediatr 2012;101:1265–9.

41. Chrousos GP, Kino T. Glucocorticoid action networks and complex psychiatric and/or somatic disorders. Stress 2007;10:213–9.

42. Zebracki K, Drotar D. Pain and activity limitations in children with Duchenne or Becker muscular dystrophy. Dev Med Child Neurol 2008;50:546–52.

43. Angelini C, Di Leo R, Cudia P. Autonomic regulation in muscular dystrophy. Front Physiol 2013;4:257.

44. Sabharwal R. Autonomic regulation in muscular dystrophy. Front Physiol 2014;5:61.

45. Akamine RT, Grossklauss LF, Nozoe KT, et al. Restless leg syndrome exacerbated by amytriptiline in a patient with Duchenne Muscular Dystrophy. Sleep Sci 2014;7:178–80.

46. Kolla BP, Mansukhani MP, Bostwick JM. The influence of antidepressants on restless legs syndrome and periodic limb movements: a systematic review. Sleep Med Rev 2018;38:131–40.

47. Edwards JD, Kun SS, Graham RJ, et al. End-of-life discussions and advance care planning for children on long-term assisted ventilation with life-limiting conditions. J Palliat Care 2012;28:21–7.

48. Carter GT, Joyce NC, Abresch AL, et al. Using palliative care in progressive neuromuscular disease to maximize quality of life. Phys Med Rehabil Clin N Am 2012;23:903–9.

49. Tripodoro VA, De Vito EL. What does end stage in neuromuscular diseases mean? Key approach-based transitions. Curr Opin Support Palliat Care 2015;9:361–8.

50. Abbott D, Prescott H, Forbes K, et al. Men with Duchenne muscular dystrophy and end of life planning. Neuromuscul Disord 2017;27:38–44.

51. Curtis JR, Cook DJ, Sinuff T, et al. Noninvasive positive pressure ventilation in critical and palliative care settings: understanding the goals of therapy. Crit Care Med 2007;35:932–9.

Management of Chronic Respiratory Failure in Chronic Obstructive Pulmonary Disease: High-Intensity and Low-Intensity Ventilation

Jeremy E. Orr, MD[a],*, Ana Sanchez Azofra, MD[b], Lauren A. Tobias, MD[c]

KEYWORDS

- Chronic obstructive pulmonary disease (COPD) • High-intensity noninvasive ventilation (HI-NIV)
- Home mechanical ventilation • Hypercapnia • Low-intensity NIV (LI-NIV)
- Noninvasive ventilation (NIV) • Positive airway pressure (PAP) • Chronic respiratory failure

KEY POINTS

- Chronic obstructive pulmonary disease (COPD) is associated with several alterations in respiratory physiology resulting hypercapnia, which is most prominent during sleep.
- Although the use of bilevel noninvasive positive pressure ventilation (NIV) has been shown to improve outcomes in acute hypercapnic respiratory failure in COPD, the use of long-term NIV for chronic hypercapnia failed to show benefit in early studies.
- An emerging literature suggests that the use of "high-intensity" NIV (ie, inspiratory positive airway pressure [IPAP] >18 cmH2O) aimed at normalizing or maximally reducing $Paco_2$ may improve mortality and reduce rehospitalization in patients with severe COPD associated with chronic hypercapnia.
- The use of "low-intensity" NIV (ie, IPAP <18 cmH2O) may be considered when obstructive sleep apnea or obesity may be driving hypercapnia. In these settings, improvement in $Paco_2$ likely remains important.
- To effectively deploy NIV in clinical practice, dedicated pathways are needed to identify hypercapnic COPD, initiate and titrate NIV, and maintain appropriate follow-up. Specific strategies will depend on local expertise, institutional resources, and payor considerations.

INTRODUCTION

Chronic obstructive pulmonary disease (COPD) is a highly prevalent disease characterized by incompletely reversible airflow limitation and is the third leading cause of death worldwide.[1] In addition, COPD leads to substantial impairments in quality of life, function limitation, and frequent hospitalizations. Nocturnal noninvasive ventilation (NIV) is a strategy to attempt to correct COPD-related impairments in work of breathing, diaphragm effectiveness, and ventilation/gas exchange. Among patients with hypercapnia, emerging evidence suggests that NIV, particularly when paired with a "high-intensity" strategy aimed at reducing $Paco_2$, may improve quality of life, hospitalization rates, and mortality. However, effective utilization of NIV in clinical practice

^a Division of Pulmonary, Critical Care, and Sleep Medicine, UC San Diego School of Medicine, 9300 Campus Point Drive, MC 7381, La Jolla, CA 92130, USA; ^b Hospital Universitario de la Princesa, Calle Diego de León 62, Madrid 28006, Spain; ^c Veterans Affairs Connecticut Healthcare System, Yale University School of Medicine, 950 Campbell Avenue, West Haven, CT 06516, USA
* Corresponding author.
E-mail address: j1orr@health.ucsd.edu

Sleep Med Clin 15 (2020) 497–509
https://doi.org/10.1016/j.jsmc.2020.08.007
1556-407X/20/© 2020 Elsevier Inc. All rights reserved.

requires an understanding of patient, mode, and device selection, as well as titration and follow-up. In addition, health care systems issues in the United States present challenges to optimal deployment.

PHYSIOLOGY OF BREATHING IN CHRONIC OBSTRUCTIVE PULMONARY DISEASE AND DURING SLEEP

Chronic obstructive pulmonary disease (COPD) is associated with high mortality and morbidity.[2] Characterized by small airway inflammation (chronic bronchitis) and parenchymal destruction (emphysema), COPD is often considered a disease resulting in expiratory impairment: narrowing and pruning of small airways along with a loss of elastic recoil leads to expiratory flow limitation. However, inspiratory challenges are clearly also important. Air trapping leading to intrinsic positive end-expiratory pressure places a threshold load on initiation of inspiration, lung hyperinflation leads to malpositioning of the diaphragm (and potentially other muscles), and prolonged exhalation time limits available time for inspiration. Other changes that limit effective ventilation include systemic myopathy, ventilation-perfusion mismatch and dead space, pulmonary hypertension and left ventricular impairment, and comorbidities such as obstructive sleep apnea (OSA). These physiologic changes place a challenge on maintaining carbon dioxide (CO_2) homeostasis. Indeed, in some individuals, control of breathing maintains the CO_2 set point, despite the high energy costs of breathing, classically conceptualized as the "pink puffer." In other individuals, the CO_2 set point is lost or otherwise changed, resulting in hypercapnia and classically conceptualized as the "blue bloater." It should be noted that there appears to be a spectrum of phenotypes rather than a dichotomization.

During sleep, several physiologic changes may result in alterations in breathing for patients with COPD (Fig. 1). In healthy individuals, sleep is associated with a reduced responsiveness to both hypoxemia and hypercapnia, along with worsened ventilation-perfusion matching,[3,4] effects that may be exaggerated in patients with pulmonary disease.[5] Resulting alveolar hypoventilation during sleep leads to elevations in the partial pressure of carbon dioxide ($Paco_2$), which may be pronounced in those with COPD.[6] These changes are particularly prominent during rapid eye movement (REM) sleep, when ventilatory responses are most blunted and skeletal muscle atonia shifts work of breathing toward the diaphragm, which may be ineffective in those with COPD.[7] An

example of sleep-related hypoventilation in a patient with advanced COPD is shown in Fig. 2. Sleep is also associated with decreased tone of the upper airway dilator muscles, which may result in limitation to inspiratory airflow.[8] Of note, overnight increases in $Paco_2$ may drive up daytime $Paco_2$ likely via increases in bicarbonate retention or changes in cerebrospinal fluid.[9] These sleep-related physiologic alterations may be ameliorated by the use of nocturnal ventilatory support, which is the focus of this article.

POTENTIAL IMPORTANCE OF HYPERCAPNIA IN CHRONIC OBSTRUCTIVE PULMONARY DISEASE

Patients with COPD who develop chronic hypercapnic respiratory failure have an elevated risk of developing exacerbations, reduced health-related quality of life, and higher risk of mortality than those who are normocapnic.[10–15] Given the substantial impact of disease-related hospitalizations on both the patient and the health care system, a major goal in chronic management of patients with COPD is minimizing such episodes. Thus, exploring interventions that could prevent episodes of acute hypercapnic respiratory failure has generated significant interest.

In addition, the loss of CO_2 homeostasis suggests a failure of the ventilatory system, the correction of which may improve outcomes. Other potential explanations for why hypercapnia may result in poor outcomes include apparent contributions to pulmonary hypertension, central nervous system consequences, immunologic effects, and a higher risk of developing decompensated respiratory failure in the setting of respiratory illness or even during supplemental oxygen administration.[16]

PHYSIOLOGY OF NONINVASIVE VENTILATION

NIV refers to a ventilatory support strategy whereby bilevel positive airway pressure (PAP) is delivered through a nasal or oronasal mask. Ventilation is often delivered in a pressure-targeted mode, although volume-targeted modes are also sometimes used. In either case, the physiologic rationale for NIV in patients with COPD is based on the concept that offloading the respiratory muscles and allowing the ventilatory system to "rest" may preserve or promote awake ventilatory muscle strength, while improving the drive to breathe and blood gases. In the setting of air trapping and hyperinflation, the use of positive end-expiratory pressure (PEEP) can increase respiratory system compliance via alveolar recruitment

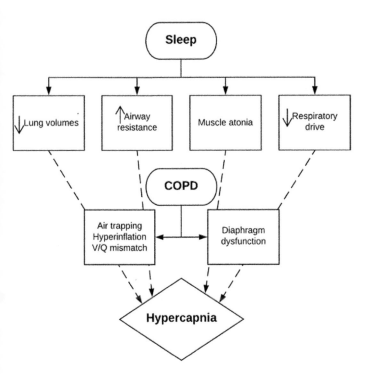

Fig. 1. Pathophysiology of sleep-related respiratory changes in COPD. Sleep has negative effects on various aspects of respiration resulting in worsening hypercapnia and hypoxemia. FRC, functional residual capacity; V/Q, ventilation/perfusion ratio. (*Adapted from* McNicholas, W.T., J. Verbraecken, and J.M. Marin, *Sleep disorders in COPD: the forgotten dimension.* European Respiratory Review, 2013. **22**(129): p. 365-375; with permission.)

and overcome intrinsic PEEP, reducing respiratory muscle load. Incorporation of a "backup rate" to reduce or eliminate the need for patient-triggered breaths may further reduce diaphragmatic effort and augment ventilation. The rationale for applying such therapy during sleep relates to both the potentially adverse physiologic changes during sleep (discussed previously), as well as the practical need to provide a meaningful duration of therapy.

In patients with COPD, empiric data confirm the ability of NIV to effectively increase the tidal volume (TV) and the alveolar ventilation, with resulting improvements in gas exchange.[17] These blood gas changes can be seen both during NIV use during sleep but also extend after NIV is removed into the daytime. NIV has also been confirmed to decrease work of breathing.[18] In general, nocturnal NIV does not appear to have consistent sustained impacts on daytime lung function as measured by the forced expiratory volume in 1 second (FEV1),[19] but some studies have suggested a reduction in air trapping and hyperinflation.[20,21] In addition, imaging data suggest that NIV results in clinically significant improvements in ventilation-perfusion matching.[22,23] Whether a reduction in $Paco_2$ itself has important effects (ie, beyond being a marker of effective ventilation) is unclear and difficult to isolate; in one study, however, a reduction in $Paco_2$ was associated with

reduction in cardiac biomarkers (eg, pro brain natriuretic peptide).[24] Hypercapnia itself has been found to increase the risk of pneumonia and infection, and reducing $Paco_2$ may help to reduce infection by improving immune function.[25]

It is important to note the possible adverse effects of NIV, including the potential for pulmonary hyperinflation resulting in increased risk of barotrauma, the potential for diaphragmatic atrophy due to minimizing inspiratory muscle activity, and disruption of sleep due to leaks and patient-ventilator asynchrony. Others have cited concerns that the application of very high inspiratory pressures could reduce cardiac output,[26] but in one 6-week study, cardiac output was not affected.[27] The latter may limit the application of NIV in patients with preexisting cardiac disease, discussed more discussed more later.[28]

EARLY TRIALS OF NONINVASIVE VENTILATION IN STABLE CHRONIC OBSTRUCTIVE PULMONARY DISEASE

For patients with an *acute* respiratory acidosis associated with exacerbations of COPD, the benefit of NIV is well established, with studies showing lower rates of intubation and improved survival when compared with standard care.[29–32]

Investigation about the possible role for NIV as *chronic* domiciliary therapy for COPD began in

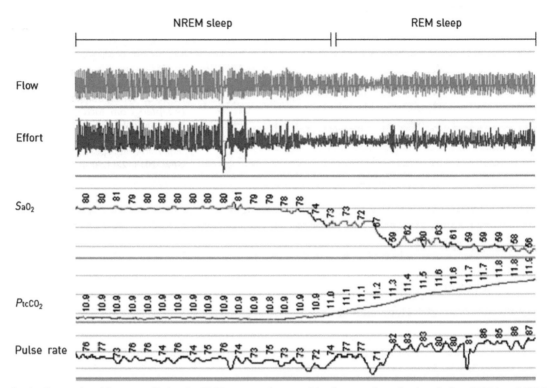

Fig. 2. Sleep-related hypoventilation in COPD. Image shows ∼30 minutes of respiration during NREM and REM sleep in a patient with stable, advanced COPD. The level of arterial oxygen saturation (SaO2) and transcutaneous carbon dioxide tension (PtcCO2) is already reduced during NREM stage 2 sleep compared with values during wakefulness (SaO2 90%). No repetitive apnea/hypopnea occurred. In the transition to REM sleep, a physiologic reduction in respiratory efforts (reduced amplitude in the thoracic effort signal) with a corresponding decrease in airflow amplitude occurred. A further reduction in SaO2 and a significant increase in PtcCO2 is the consequence of REM-related sleep hypoventilation. Heart rate increases as an indirect sign of increased sympathetic activity. (*From* McNicholas, W.T., et al., Sleep in chronic respiratory disease: COPD and hypoventilation disorders. Eur Respir Rev, 2019. **28**(153); with permission.)

the 1990s. The results of these smaller trials suggested some improvement in symptoms and quality of life, but "hard" outcomes such as reductions in hospitalizations or mortality were overall negative.[33–35] At the time, a systematic review including these studies of noninvasive ventilation failed to find any improvement in gas exchange with NIV.[36]

Subsequently, an Australian study randomized 144 patients with severe hypercapnic COPD to long-term oxygen therapy (LTOT) versus LTOT plus NIV. Chronic hypercapnia in this study was defined as a $Paco_2$ greater than 46 mm Hg at least twice in the prior 6 months (although participants' actual $Paco_2$ was ∼53 mm Hg at baseline). NIV was initiated in a resource-intensive 3-day to 4-day hospital stay during which NIV was titrated during nightly polysomnography (PSG) delivered via auto-adjusting, bilevel device with a target inspiratory positive airway pressure (IPAP) – expiratory positive airway pressure (EPAP) difference

of 10 cmH2O or greater (though observed mean IPAP was 12.9 and EPAP was 5.1). They found that although NIV improved sleep quality and sleep-related hypercapnia acutely, there was no long-term effect on gas exchange and some evidence for worsened quality of life. After adjustment for baseline variables, NIV did appear to have a mortality benefit.[37]

Thereafter, a 2013 Cochrane systematic review concluded that in patients with hypercapnic COPD, nocturnal NIV at home for at least 3 months failed to show a consistent clinically or statistically significant benefit on gas exchange, exercise tolerance, health-related quality of life, lung function, respiratory muscle strength, or sleep efficiency, but noted that the small sample sizes of included studies precluded a definitive conclusion regarding the effects of noninvasive positive pressure ventilation in COPD.[38]

Similarly, the RESCUE trial (REspiratory Support in COPD after acUte Exacerbation) published in 2014 failed to show a positive effect on patient-oriented outcomes. The study enrolled 201 patients with COPD admitted for acute hypercapnic respiratory failure who had persistently elevated levels of $Paco_2$ more than 48 hours after ventilatory support was discontinued. Patients were randomized to either NIV or standard treatment.[39] Although diurnal $Paco_2$ improved significantly only in the NIV group, the investigators failed to find a difference in either readmission or survival between groups at 1 year. However, it is likely that any treatment effect was diluted by inclusion of patients without truly chronic hypercapnia, because more than a quarter of the control group had normalized their $Paco_2$ levels within 3 months.

HIGH-INTENSITY NONINVASIVE VENTILATION

Since these early largely negative results, it has been argued that IPAP used in these studies, which ranged from 0 to 18 cmH2O, was insufficient as evidenced by its inability to reduce levels of arterial carbon dioxide tension ($Paco_2$). Accordingly, a growing body of evidence has suggested that NIV may in fact be beneficial only when ventilation is sufficient to lower $Paco_2$ as much as possible, with a goal of achieving normocapnia.[40] This approach, termed "high-intensity" NIV (HI-NIV), uses relatively high levels of IPAP (defined typically as >18 cm H_2O) and pressure support (PS) adjusted to augment alveolar ventilation, and a backup rate to achieve maximal control of a patient's breathing, with the goal of minimizing $Paco_2$ and causing near-abolition of diaphragmatic activity.[41]

The potential superiority of HI-NIV was first put forth by Dreher and colleagues,[42] who performed a 6-week study of 17 patients comparing HI-NIV (using mean inspiratory pressures of 29 cmH2O) with low-intensity NIV (LI-NIV; mean inspiratory pressures of 15). HI-NIV resulted in higher measured expiratory volumes and a significantly greater reduction in nocturnal $Paco_2$ than in the low-intensity group.[42] The study also called into question the common notion that HI-NIV might be poorly tolerated by patients, because patients on HI-NIV were no less likely to drop out of the trial and in fact demonstrated higher nightly usage (mean difference of 3.6 h/d, $P = .024$). Other favorable effects of HI-NIV included significant improvements in exercise-related dyspnea, daytime $Paco_2$, and FEV1. Others have suggested that the high levels of PS used during HI-NIV have the potential to disrupt sleep, but evidence has not borne out this concern. In a randomized controlled crossover trial comparing sleep quality during HI-NIV versus LI-NIV (mean IPAPs of 29 and 14 cmH2O, respectively), no significant difference was seen in sleep quality, as captured by several including arousal index, percentage of sleep time spent in non-rapid and rapid eye movement (NREM and REM, respectively) stage 3 sleep or sleep efficiency.[43]

Subsequently, 2 large randomized trials have been performed to evaluate the use of HI-NIV in 2 distinct populations: (1) stable hypercapnic COPD, and (2) persistent hypercapnia post-acute hypercapnic respiratory failure:

- In those with stable hypercapnic COPD, Kohnlein and colleagues[44] showed that in patients with severe COPD, HI-NIV (targeted to reduce the baseline $Paco_2$ by at least 20% or to achieve $Paco_2$ <48 mm Hg) was associated with a reduction in 1-year mortality from 33% in the control group to 12% in the intervention group. This was the first trial demonstrating a significant reduction in mortality from NIV compared with conventional treatment. In contrast to the prior outcomes-based clinical trials, a clear effect on $Paco_2$ was achieved, with mean $Paco_2$ of 48.8 mm Hg in the intervention group versus 55.5 in the control group at 12 months. NIV settings reflected an HI-NIV strategy, with a mean IPAP of 21.6 cmH2O, EPAP of 4.8 cmH2O, and backup rate of 16.1, with mean use of 5.9 h/d.
- In those with a recent severe COPD exacerbation, the Home Oxygen Therapy-Home Mechanical Ventilation (HOT-HMV) trial[45] recruited 116 patients from across the United Kingdom who had both persistent hypercapnia as defined by a $Paco_2$ more than 53 mm Hg 2 to 4 weeks after resolution of a decompensated respiratory acidemia requiring hospitalization. Participants were randomized to treatment with either home oxygen therapy (HOT) plus HMV or HOT alone. Importantly, they used median home ventilator settings using a much higher PS than is typically used in clinical practice along with a backup rate; the median IPAP was 24 cmH2O, EPAP was 4 cmH2O, and backup rate was 14 breaths per minute. They found a significant reduction in their composite endpoint of readmission or death at 12 months: 63% in the home oxygen plus home NIV group as compared with 80% in the home oxygen alone group (**Fig. 3**), representing an absolute risk reduction of 17% or a number needed to treat of 5.8. In other words, fewer than 6 patients needed to be treated with home NIV for a year to prevent 1 readmission or

Forest plot 13: PCO2 subgroup analysis - targeted PCO2 vs. non-targeted PCO2

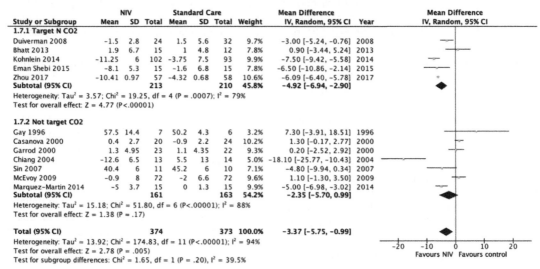

Fig. 3. Forest plot demonstrating the effect of long-term NIV on partial pressure of carbon dioxide. (Reproduced with permission of the © ERS 2020: European Respiratory Journal 2019 54: 1901003; 10.1183/13993003.01003-2019.)

death. Also notable was their high rates of adherence to NIV, with a mean 4.7 hours of nightly usage at 6 weeks and an increase to 7.6 hours at 12 months. No mortality difference was observed between the 2 groups. Other recent observational studies have specifically focused on use of NIV to prevent hospital readmissions, with supportive results.[46,47]

Putting this, as well as other, available randomized trial evidence[48] together, a meta-analysis of NIV for patients with hypercapnic COPD (both stable and postexacerbation) was performed as part of both the recent European Respiratory Society Guidelines and the American Thoracic Society guidelines.[49] These documents found several benefits to home NIV including improved symptoms and quality of life, and a possible benefit in terms of mortality. When examining studies using a high intensity strategy to reduce $PaCO_2$, there was a signal towards more symptomatic and functional benefit, and a clear improvement in $PaCO_2$ (**Fig. 4**). Overall, this body of evidence suggests that use of "high-intensity" NIV may be superior to that of LI-NIV for patients with severe hypercapnic COPD, reflected in the trend toward more recent trials using higher levels of IPAP.[50]

HIGH VERSUS LOW INTENSITY: DOES ONE SIZE FIT ALL?

Based on available clinical trial data, ATS and ERS guidelines suggest the use of NIV for the treatment of hypercapnic COPD in the long-term home setting, including among patients with stable hypercapnic respiratory failure and those with a recent episode of acute hypercapnic respiratory failure[19,49]. The recommendations further suggest that settings should be titrated to normalize or significantly reduce the $Paco_2$. Notably, the guidelines did not address specific pressure targets, but do make note that high pressure strategies were used in positive clinical trials. Similarly, the newest 2020 report from the Global Initiative for Chronic Obstructive Lung Disease (GOLD) group states that NIV "may improve hospitalization-free survival in selected patients after recent hospitalization, particularly in those with pronounced daytime persistent hypercapnia ($Paco_2 \geq 52$ mm Hg) (Evidence B)."

On the other hand, whether all patients with hypercapnic COPD require *high-intensity* ventilation has been called into question. Although there no comparative effectiveness data regarding high-intensity versus low-intensity treatment for long-term outcomes, there are several observations to be considered:

1. High-intensity NIV has been associated with a reduction in cardiac output compared with LI-NIV. Presumably this is due to larger positive intrathoracic pressure swings leading to decreases in right heart preload, increase in right ventricular afterload (increased pulmonary vascular resistance), and potential increases/swings in left heart preload.

2. Adherence to HI-NIV may be difficult to achieve in some individuals, particularly in "real-world" populations rather than those enrolled in clinical trials. Whether increased use at lower pressures might be comparable to lower use at high pressures is unclear.
3. Individual-level goals for reduction in Pa_{CO_2} remain unclear, and accordingly the amount of inspiratory pressure required is not known. For example, a patient may have substantial reduction in Pa_{CO_2} with pressures that do not meet the definition of HI-NIV.
4. Patients with COPD-OSA overlap syndrome were likely excluded from these trials, as patients with a body mass index greater than 35 were excluded. Such patients may develop hypercapnia (particularly with obesity) despite less severe lung function and may be a particularly high-risk group.[51,52] Although data are limited, these patients may represent a large proportion of hypercapnic COPD based on the high general population prevalence of OSA. Similarly, some patients may overlap with obesity hypoventilation syndrome. Although such patients may benefit from continuous positive airway pressure (CPAP), hypercapnia also appears to be a risk factor for CPAP failure.[53] In this case, NIV could be considered but an LI-NIV strategy may be sufficient to treat OSA and reduce Pa_{CO_2}.

A previously proposed clinical pathway to use in determining whether a patient with severe COPD may benefit from NIV.[54]

PRACTICAL CONSIDERATIONS FOR USE OF NONINVASIVE VENTILATION IN CHRONIC OBSTRUCTIVE PULMONARY DISEASE
Timing and Testing

The first consideration is when to initiation NIV. In the intensive care unit, patients are often placed on empiric IPAP and EPAP settings titrated to reduction of hypercapnia. Unfortunately, the inpatient setting during acute illness is not an optimal environment for a patient to first experience NIV for several reasons: (1) critically ill patients experience NIV in the setting of severe dyspnea and anxiety associated with acute illness, (2) the number of available interfaces in most inpatient settings is limited, (3) inpatient respiratory therapists may have less expertise with home ventilation and limited time to devote to helping patients acclimate, and (4) not all patients with acute respiratory failure need long-term NIV. Many will resolve their hypercapnia as they return to baseline.

Accordingly, it has been difficult to demonstrate that patients in whom home NIV is started immediately following an episode of acute respiratory failure have improvement in survival.[39]

It is recommended to wait 2 to 4 weeks following a COPD exacerbation before obtaining an arterial blood gas for the purposes of determining whether to initiate NIV,[19] although a clear prior history of sustained hypercapnia may warrant earlier initiation particularly among patients at high risk for recurrent decompensation.[55]

There exist differing viewpoints about whether diagnostic PSG is needed before initiation of NIV, but in general would be performed only if there was concern for coexisting OSA (ie, "overlap syndrome").[56] In the United States, obesity is present in more than a third of patients with COPD[57] and studies suggest that most patients with COPD also have OSA.[58] Undiagnosed OSA in patients with COPD is associated with adverse outcomes including worse quality of life.[59] If performed, PSG testing ideally should include PSG with use of capnometry, either by end-tidal or transcutaneous CO_2 (PtcCO2). PtcCO2 allows noninvasive and continuous measurements of Pa_{CO_2} and is generally preferable in patients with COPD because of its greater sensitivity for hypoventilation.[60,61]

Modes, Devices, and Interfaces

NIV is most often provided using a bilevel (ie, PS) mode, without a backup rate ("Bilevel-S") or with a backup rate ("Bilevel ST"). Of note, these modes are sometimes referred to as "BIPAP," but this is a brand name and is often conflated with the type of device used, so we suggest this term be avoided. Time-cycled pressure assist control ("PAC") is used less often due to potentially increased issues related to patient-ventilator cycling asynchrony. In contrast, bilevel modes usually allow for an inspiratory window ("Ti min" and "Ti max"), which can help to ensure that breath duration is appropriate. Volume assist control ("ACV") is rarely used; however, volume-assured PS modes ("VAPS") are effectively bilevel ST modes that use an algorithm to adjust PS to meet a set TV ("AVAPS") or ventilation target ("iVAPS"). It should be noted that adaptive servo-ventilation ("ASV") is a form of NIV to stabilize breathing in central sleep apnea, and should under no circumstances be used in the setting of hypercapnic COPD. Other potentially relevant settings include trigger and cycle sensitivity; details regarding modes are available in other publications.

Devices are either bedside machines (Medicare terms "Respiratory Assist Devices" or RAD) or ventilators. With technological convergence, RAD devices can typically provide the same level of support as a ventilator, along with built-in humidifiers and a smaller form factor. Importantly, ventilators have batteries and alarms, higher pressure capabilities, and are engineered as life support devices. The appropriate device therefore depends more on patient severity than mode or settings considerations.

Recommendations for specific modes and settings are not well established. One major controversy is the role of the backup rate; whereas the Dreher and Kohnlein studies have used relatively high rates (such that many breaths are likely timed, rather than spontaneous), other studies have used lower rates, with similar changes in $Paco_2$.[62] Whether fully spontaneous modes could achieve adequate support is not clear, but may depend on the individual. With regard to breath type, most studies have focused on the use of pressure-targeted forms of NIV rather than volume-targeted NIV (ie, VAPS). Two small studies have shown that patients with stable hypercapnic COPD treated with VAPS had equivalent physiologic benefits, including on reductions in PtcCO2, as those treated with HI-NIV,[63,64] and may reduce the amount of time and effort needed to initiate NIV. In addition, auto-titrating EPAP has been evaluated in single night studies including individuals with COPD.[65,66] Future technological improvements to the design of NIV equipment and software will be aimed at facilitating setup, improving patient tolerance, promoting effective

ventilation, and minimizing patient-ventilator dyssynchrony.

Several types of nasal and oronasal interfaces are available and the choice is largely based on patient comfort and preference. It should be noted that nasal masks are generally preferred over oronasal masks based on data in OSA indicating fewer issues with leak, lower pressure requirements, and better adherence.[67] Regardless, ensuring a good fit is paramount, as leaks may lead to disrupted sleep, ineffective ventilation, and patient-ventilator asynchrony. A good fit is particularly important during use of HI-NIV, given the high chance of leaks with high pressure.

Initial Titration

Titration of NIV may be performed in one of several settings. Traditionally, NIV titration has been performed in a monitored environment (either a hospitalized setting after the patient has medically stabilized, or sleep laboratory) under the supervision of trained health care providers using a systematic approach.[68] PSG or more limited respiratory monitoring may be used during titration. When sleep-disordered breathing is present, the first goal of a titration is to determine the optimal EPAP to facilitate airway patency. Next, an IPAP is chosen, typically beginning 6 to 8 cmH2O of PS above the EPAP. The resulting tidal volumes are monitored and the IPAP level is titrated toward goals of increasing minute ventilation and reducing hypercapnia. One example of a protocol that may be used to guide NIV titration

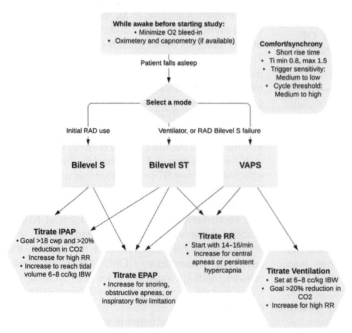

Fig. 4. Suggested protocol for in-laboratory titration of noninvasive positive pressure ventilation in patients with COPD in the United States. Bilevel-S, no back up rate; Bilevel-S/T, backup rate; cwp, centimeters of water pressure; IBW, ideal body weight; RR, respiratory rate; Ti, inspiratory time. (*Adapted from* van der Leest, S. and M.L. Duiverman, *High-intensity non-invasive ventilation in stable hypercapnic COPD: Evidence of efficacy and practical advice.* Respirology, 2019. **24**(4): p. 318-328; and Coleman, J.M., 3rd, L.F. Wolfe, and R. Kalhan, *Noninvasive Ventilation in Chronic Obstructive Pulmonary Disease.* Ann Am Thorac Soc, 2019. **16**(9): p. 1091-1098; with permission.)

in patients with COPD and chronic respiratory failure is shown in **Fig. 4**. Nonetheless, most sleep laboratories/technicians do not have extensive experience with such potentially complex titrations. Issues that arise include appropriate response to various patient-ventilator dyssynchronies (eg, ineffective triggering, glottic closure), uncertainty regarding appropriate use of supplemental oxygen, and an individual's goal $Paco_2$ reduction during the first night titration. Evidence regarding the utility of in-laboratory titrations is limited, and in the authors' experience the success rates for such titrations can be low.

Although all the European studies were conducted in the setting of prolonged hospital stays for titrations, this is not feasible in the United States. Many advocate for initiation of NIV at home, on the basis of convenience to the patient to allow time for desensitization, decreased need for specialized ancillary services, and cost considerations. This process may include an introduction to the device in the clinic, with a mask fitting and subsequently having the patient lie supine while the device is applied, and initial settings are determined based on observed breathing and patient comfort. Alternatively, setup may be carried out by an external durable medical equipment (DME) provider at the patient's home. Regardless, initially prescribed settings typically mirror those used as a starting point for the sleep laboratory starting with relatively low settings (see **Fig. 4**). Because many patients will obtain equipment via external DME companies, the clinician should be aware of the DME's service limitations and anticipate potential issues (eg, prescription being lost, requested device not available, remote monitoring not connected). Titration toward the target pressures is then performed over the course of several weeks, using in-clinic evaluations and often telemedicine/remote monitoring tools, discussed later in this article. "Intelligent" modes such as auto-EPAP and VAPS may be particularly useful for home titration.

Studies suggest that starting NIV in the home is a feasible and effective option for patients with neuromuscular disease,[69] and recent data have indicated success in those with COPD.[70] If the decision is made to initiate NIV empirically in a patient's home, and adjust settings based on clinical response, it is crucial to have a plan in place for close-clinical follow-up, ideally with the ability to retrieve data remotely and change settings as needed. Serial data downloads should be reviewed to ensure settings are effective and to make adjustments when needed. Other factors that might add to success include visits from specialized nurses early in the process to assist

with NIV setup, provide education, and facilitate practice using the device.[70] Overall, the method used for titration will depend on local expertise, institutional resources, patient preference, and urgency.

Monitoring and Follow-up

Follow-up at 2-week to 4-week intervals is initially needed to ensure adequate titration and adherence. Once settings appear optimized, many clinicians obtain arterial blood gas testing to ensure that the $Paco_2$ has been adequately controlled. If the patient is having difficulty, or data are not suggesting optimal titration, considerations include evaluating the patient while wearing the device in clinic during the day, or an in-laboratory evaluation under PSG. Once the patient is stable on NIV, visits can be every few months.

Frequent in-person follow-up may be challenging in the multimorbid and often frail population of patients with hypercapnic COPD. Telemonitoring offers the theoretic benefits of rapid intervention for suboptimal adherence, monitoring for signs of clinical deterioration or the need to alter ventilator settings, and cost savings.[71] One study in the Netherlands showed a 33% cost reduction with telemonitoring of patients on home NIV for COPD with chronic hypercapnic respiratory failure.[72] However, other studies have failed to show benefit; a study in the United Kingdom showed no benefit of telemonitoring for altering time to next hospitalization or quality of life and rather an increased number of hospital admissions and home visits overall.[73]

Payor/Policy Issues

To qualify patients with COPD for the use of home NIV in the United States, certain criteria must be met. **Fig. 5** outlines the Centers for Medicare and Medicaid Services (CMS) guidelines for qualifying patients for NIV. The term "respiratory assist device (RAD)" refers to NIV without a backup rate (EO470 devices, eg, Bilevel-S) or with a backup rate (E0471 devices, eg, Bilevel ST, VAPS). Clinicians may encounter several practical challenges when attempting to qualify patients for an RAD device. For inpatients, many institutions lack the ability to perform sleep studies or overnight oximetry on inpatients, and clinicians may be hesitant to down-titrate supplemental oxygen. For outpatients, barriers to sleep studies include insurance approval and patient ability, whereas overnight oximetry is not performed by many DME companies. In addition, a major question surrounding the prescription for NIV involves the issue of use of a backup rate. The aforementioned studies supporting the benefit of NIV on major outcomes used ventilator settings including a backup rate and thereby allowing for maximal unloading of respiratory muscles. Currently there exists no pathway for initial prescription of an RAD device with a backup rate; however, failure of an RAD without a backup rate must be documented after a minimum of 2 months of usage. A ventilator can be used to provide a backup rate, although whether this represents appropriate use of this level of therapy is not established.

Issues for Future Study

Further research is needed to clarify the best setting and strategic approach to initiation of NIV, whether in the hospital or at home and with what type of device.[19] Beyond the presence of chronic hypercapnia, we know little about the specific clinical phenotypes of COPD that may derive the greatest benefit from NIV initiation, and further study will be helpful in defining this patient population. COPD is a disorder with systemic manifestations including cardiovascular disease and mental health among others, and it remains to be seen how NIV impacts clinical outcomes beyond the respiratory system. Although studies to date have focused on respiratory-specific outcomes, rehospitalizations, mortality, and quality of life, future work should explore whether NIV affects other patient-centered outcomes, including cognitive function, pulmonary hypertension, and immune function. Significant effort has been devoted to identifying predictors of adherence to PAP therapy in OSA, but further work should attempt to delineate predictors and mediators of adherence in the typically frailer population of patients with hypercapnic COPD. Cost-effectiveness data also will be crucial to moving the discussion about NIV in COPD going forward, as it may provide the tools necessary to implement change on both an institutional level as well as potentially impact national policy regarding coverage of these devices. Along these lines, telemedicine (including remote monitoring) clearly has a role in optimizing therapy but requires more systemic study to determine best practices. From an implementation standpoint, there is a need to develop effective education for clinicians caring for those with COPD regarding the role and management of NIV in patients with hypercapnic COPD. Finally, the likely negative effects of burdensome insurance requirements limiting the availability of RAD devices should be evaluated.

| Diagnosis of COPD |

| **ABG** (while awake & on prescribed FiO2) PaCO2≥ 52 mm Hg |

| **Sleep oximetry** with SaO2 ≤88% for ≥5 min, <u>mininum</u> 2 h recording time (on 2L/min or prescribed FiO2, whichever is higher) |

| OSA & CPAP treatment has been considered and ruled out (no formal PSG is needed) |

| **E0470*** (bilevel device without a backup rate) |

| **For continued E0470 coverage:** |
| - Device must be re-evaluated no sooner than 61 d after initiating therapy |
| - Must document progress of relevant symptoms |
| - Signed/dated statement by treating |

Fig. 5. RAD Qualifying Guidelines as per the Centers for Medicare and Medicaid Services (CMS), revised 2014. *For patients with COPD to qualify for a RAD with backup rate (E0471), either of the following must occur: (1) after period of initial use of an E0470; ABG (done while awake and on prescribed Fio₂) shows Paco₂ worsens ≥7 mm Hg compared with original ABG result; facility-based PSG demonstrates oxygen saturation ≤88% for ≥ a cumulative 5 minutes with minimum 2 hours nocturnal recording time while on an E0470 and not caused by obstructive upper airway events (ie, apnea hypopnea index [AHI] <5). 2. No sooner than 61 days after initial issue of E0470, an ABG (done while awake and on prescribed Fio₂) shows Paco₂ ≥52 mm Hg OR sleep oximetry on an E0470 demonstrates oxygen saturation ≤88% for ≥ a cumulative 5 minutes with minimum 2 hrs nocturnal recording time, on 2 L/min O₂ or patient's prescribed Fio₂, whichever is higher). ABG, arterial blood gas. (*Courtesy of* the Centers for Medicare and Medicaid Services, Baltimore, MD.)

SUMMARY

Patients with advanced COPD with persistent hypercapnia should be strongly considered for long-term home NIV. An emerging literature suggests that in general, HI-NIV is more effective than LI-NIV, but low-intensity may be considered in certain circumstances. For NIV in general, the goal is normalizing, or at least significantly reducing, $Paco_2$. Recent studies suggest that this approach may reduce hospital readmissions and decrease mortality.[45]

CLINICS CARE POINTS

- Home non-invasive ventilation may be helpful in patients with chronic hypercapnic COPD.
- Reducing $PaCO_2$, usually via high inspiratory pressure settings, appears to be an important target of therapy.
- Titration and close clinical follow up are key to effective treatment.

REFERENCES

1. Organization, W.H. Source: global health estimates 2016: death by cause, age, sex, by country and by region, 2000–2016. Geneva (Switzerland): World Health Organization; 2018.
2. Vogelmeier CF, Criner GJ, Martinez FJ, et al. Global strategy for the diagnosis, management, and prevention of chronic obstructive lung disease 2017 Report: GOLD executive summary. Eur Respir J 2017;49(3):1700214.
3. Douglas NJ, White DP, Weil JV, et al. Hypoxic ventilatory response decreases during sleep in normal men. Am Rev Respir Dis 1982;125(3):286–9.
4. Douglas NJ, White DP, Weil JV, et al. Hypercapnic ventilatory response in sleeping adults. Am Rev Respir Dis 1982;126(5):758–62.
5. McNicholas WT, Verbraecken J, Marin JM. Sleep disorders in COPD: the forgotten dimension. Eur Respir Rev 2013;22(129):365–75.
6. O'Donoghue FJ, Catcheside PG, Ellis EE, et al. Sleep hypoventilation in hypercapnic chronic obstructive pulmonary disease: prevalence and associated factors. Eur Respir J 2003;21(6):977–84.
7. Becker HF, Piper AJ, Flynn WE, et al. Breathing during sleep in patients with nocturnal desaturation. Am J Respir Crit Care Med 1999;159(1):112–8.
8. O'Donoghue FJ, Catcheside PG, Eckert DJ, et al. Changes in respiration in NREM sleep in hypercapnic chronic obstructive pulmonary disease. J Physiol (Lond) 2004;559(Pt 2):663–73.
9. Norman RG, Goldring RM, Clain JM, et al. Transition from acute to chronic hypercapnia in patients with periodic breathing: predictions from a computer model. J Appl Physiol (1985) 2006;100(5):1733–41.
10. Yang H, Xiang P, Zhang E, et al. Is hypercapnia associated with poor prognosis in chronic obstructive pulmonary disease? A long-term follow-up cohort study. BMJ Open 2015;5(12):e008909.
11. Budweiser S, Hitzl AP, Jörres RA, et al. Health-related quality of life and long-term prognosis in chronic hypercapnic respiratory failure: a prospective survival analysis. Respir Res 2007;8:92.
12. Aida A, Miyamoto K, Nishimura M, et al. Prognostic value of hypercapnia in patients with chronic respiratory failure during long-term oxygen therapy. Am J Respir Crit Care Med 1998;158(1):188–93.
13. Foucher P, Baudouin N, Merati M, et al. Relative survival analysis of 252 patients with COPD receiving long-term oxygen therapy. Chest 1998;113(6):1580–7.
14. Almagro P, Barreiro B, Ochoa de Echaguen A, et al. Risk factors for hospital readmission in patients with chronic obstructive pulmonary disease. Respiration 2006;73(3):311–7.
15. Costello R, Deegan P, Fitzpatrick M, et al. Reversible hypercapnia in chronic obstructive pulmonary disease: a distinct pattern of respiratory failure with a favorable prognosis. Am J Med 1997;102(3):239–44.
16. Abdo WF, Heunks LM. Oxygen-induced hypercapnia in COPD: myths and facts. Crit Care 2012;16(5):323.
17. Nickol AH, Hart N, Hopkinson NS, et al. Mechanisms of improvement of respiratory failure in patients with restrictive thoracic disease treated with non-invasive ventilation. Thorax 2005;60(9):754–60.
18. Nava S, Ambrosino N, Rubini F, et al. Effect of nasal pressure support ventilation and external PEEP on diaphragmatic activity in patients with severe stable COPD. Chest 1993;103(1):143–50.
19. Ergan B, Oczkowski S, Rochwerg B, et al. European Respiratory Society guidelines on long-term home non-invasive ventilation for management of COPD. Eur Respir J 2019;54(3):1901003.
20. Budweiser S, Heinemann F, Fischer W, et al. Long-term reduction of hyperinflation in stable COPD by non-invasive nocturnal home ventilation. Respir Med 2005;99(8):976–84.
21. Díaz O, Bégin P, Torrealba B, et al. Effects of noninvasive ventilation on lung hyperinflation in stable hypercapnic COPD. Eur Respir J 2002;20(6):1490–8.
22. De Backer L, Vos W, Dieriks B, et al. The effects of long-term noninvasive ventilation in hypercapnic COPD patients: a randomized controlled pilot study. Int J Chron Obstruct Pulmon Dis 2011;6:615–24.
23. Hajian B, De Backer J, Sneyers C, et al. Pathophysiological mechanism of long-term noninvasive ventilation in stable hypercapnic patients with COPD using functional respiratory imaging. Int J Chron Obstruct Pulmon Dis 2017;12:2197–205.
24. Dreher M, Schulte L, Müller T, et al. Influence of effective noninvasive positive pressure ventilation on inflammatory and cardiovascular biomarkers in

stable hypercapnic COPD patients. Respir Med 2015;109(10):1300–4.

25. Gates KL, Howell HA, Nair A, et al. Hypercapnia impairs lung neutrophil function and increases mortality in murine pseudomonas pneumonia. Am J Respir Cell Mol Biol 2013;49(5):821–8.

26. Lukacsovits J, Carlucci A, Hill N, et al. Physiological changes during low- and high-intensity noninvasive ventilation. Eur Respir J 2012;39(4):869–75.

27. Duiverman ML, Maagh P, Magnet FS, et al. Impact of High-Intensity-NIV on the heart in stable COPD: a randomised cross-over pilot study. Respir Res 2017;18(1):76.

28. Duiverman ML. Noninvasive ventilation in stable hypercapnic COPD: what is the evidence? ERJ Open Res 2018;4(2). 00012-2018.

29. Brochard L, Mancebo J, Wysocki M, et al. Noninvasive ventilation for acute exacerbations of chronic obstructive pulmonary disease. N Engl J Med 1995;333(13):817–22.

30. Bott J, Carroll MP, Conway JH, et al. Randomised controlled trial of nasal ventilation in acute ventilatory failure due to chronic obstructive airways disease. Lancet 1993;341(8860):1555–7.

31. Ram FS, Picot J, Lightowler J, et al. Non-invasive positive pressure ventilation for treatment of respiratory failure due to exacerbations of chronic obstructive pulmonary disease. Cochrane Database Syst Rev 2004;(1):CD004104.

32. Plant PK, Owen JL, Elliott MW. Early use of non-invasive ventilation for acute exacerbations of chronic obstructive pulmonary disease on general respiratory wards: a multicentre randomised controlled trial. Lancet 2000;355(9219):1931–5.

33. Clini E, Sturani C, Rossi A, et al. The Italian multicentre study on noninvasive ventilation in chronic obstructive pulmonary disease patients. Eur Respir J 2002;20(3):529–38.

34. Tsolaki V, Pastaka C, Karetsi E, et al. One-year non-invasive ventilation in chronic hypercapnic COPD: effect on quality of life. Respir Med 2008;102(6):904–11.

35. Casanova C, Celli BR, Tost L, et al. Long-term controlled trial of nocturnal nasal positive pressure ventilation in patients with severe COPD. Chest 2000;118(6):1582–90.

36. Kolodziej MA, Jensen L, Rowe B, et al. Systematic review of noninvasive positive pressure ventilation in severe stable COPD. Eur Respir J 2007;30(2):293–306.

37. McEvoy RD, Pierce RJ, Hillman D, et al. Nocturnal non-invasive nasal ventilation in stable hypercapnic COPD: a randomised controlled trial. Thorax 2009;64(7):561–6.

38. Struik FM, Lacasse Y, Goldstein R, et al. Nocturnal non-invasive positive pressure ventilation for stable chronic obstructive pulmonary disease. Cochrane Database Syst Rev 2013;(6):CD002878.

39. Struik FM, Sprooten RT, Kerstjens HA, et al. Nocturnal non-invasive ventilation in COPD patients with prolonged hypercapnia after ventilatory support for acute respiratory failure: a randomised, controlled, parallel-group study. Thorax 2014;69(9):826–34.

40. Windisch W, Vogel M, Sorichter S, et al. Normocapnia during nIPPV in chronic hypercapnic COPD reduces subsequent spontaneous PaCO2. Respir Med 2002;96(8):572–9.

41. van der Leest S, Duiverman ML. High-intensity non-invasive ventilation in stable hypercapnic COPD: evidence of efficacy and practical advice. Respirology 2019;24(4):318–28.

42. Dreher M, Storre JH, Schmoor C, et al. High-intensity versus low-intensity non-invasive ventilation in patients with stable hypercapnic COPD: a randomised crossover trial. Thorax 2010;65(4):303–8.

43. Dreher M, Ekkernkamp E, Walterspacher S, et al. Noninvasive ventilation in COPD: impact of inspiratory pressure levels on sleep quality. Chest 2011;140(4):939–45.

44. Kohnlein T, Windisch W, Köhler D, et al. Non-invasive positive pressure ventilation for the treatment of severe stable chronic obstructive pulmonary disease: a prospective, multicentre, randomised, controlled clinical trial. Lancet Respir Med 2014;2(9):698–705.

45. Murphy PB, Rehal S, Arbane G, et al. Effect of home noninvasive ventilation with oxygen therapy vs oxygen therapy alone on hospital readmission or death after an acute COPD exacerbation: a randomized clinical trial. JAMA 2017;317(21):2177–86.

46. Galli JA, Krahnke JS, James Mamary A, et al. Home non-invasive ventilation use following acute hypercapnic respiratory failure in COPD. Respir Med 2014;108(5):722–8.

47. Coughlin S, Liang WE, Parthasarathy S. Retrospective assessment of home ventilation to reduce rehospitalization in chronic obstructive pulmonary disease. J Clin Sleep Med 2015;11(6):663–70.

48. Zhou L, Li X, Guan L, et al. Home noninvasive positive pressure ventilation with built-in software in stable hypercapnic COPD: a short-term prospective, multicenter, randomized, controlled trial. Int J Chron Obstruct Pulmon Dis 2017;12:1279–86.

49. Macrea M, Oczkowski S, Rochwerg B, et al. Long-Term Noninvasive Ventilation in Chronic Stable Hypercapnic Chronic Obstructive Pulmonary Disease. An Official American Thoracic Society Clinical Practice Guideline. Am J Respir Crit Care Med 2020;202(4):e74–87.

50. Storre JH, Callegari J, Magnet FS, et al. Home noninvasive ventilatory support for patients with chronic

obstructive pulmonary disease: patient selection and perspectives. Int J Chron Obstruct Pulmon Dis 2018;13:753–60.

51. Resta O, Foschino Barbaro MP, Brindicci C, et al. Hypercapnia in overlap syndrome: possible determinant factors. Sleep Breath 2002;6(1):11–8.

52. Jaoude P, Kufel T, El-Solh AA. Survival Benefit of CPAP favors hypercapnic patients with the overlap syndrome. Lung 2014;192(2):251–8.

53. Kuklisova Z, Tkacova R, Joppa P, et al. Severity of nocturnal hypoxia and daytime hypercapnia predicts CPAP failure in patients with COPD and obstructive sleep apnea overlap syndrome. Sleep Med 2017;30:139–45.

54. Coleman JM 3rd, Wolfe LF, Kalhan R. Noninvasive ventilation in chronic obstructive pulmonary disease. Ann Am Thorac Soc 2019;16(9):1091–8.

55. Raveling T, Bladder G, Vonk JM, et al. Improvement in hypercapnia does not predict survival in COPD patients on chronic noninvasive ventilation. Int J Chron Obstruct Pulmon Dis 2018;13:3625–34.

56. McNicholas WT. COPD-OSA overlap syndrome: evolving evidence regarding epidemiology, clinical consequences, and management. Chest 2017; 152(6):1318–26.

57. Lambert AA, Putcha N, Drummond MB, et al. Obesity is associated with increased morbidity in moderate to severe COPD. Chest 2017;151(1): 68–77.

58. Soler X, Gaio E, Powell FL, et al. High prevalence of obstructive sleep apnea in patients with moderate to severe chronic obstructive pulmonary disease. Ann Am Thorac Soc 2015;12(8):1219–25.

59. Donovan LM, Feemster LC, Udris EM, et al. Poor outcomes among patients with chronic obstructive pulmonary disease with higher risk for undiagnosed obstructive sleep apnea in the LOTT cohort. J Clin Sleep Med 2019;15(1):71–7.

60. Aarrestad S, Tollefsen E, Kleiven AL, et al. Validity of transcutaneous PCO2 in monitoring chronic hypoventilation treated with non-invasive ventilation. Respir Med 2016;112:112–8.

61. Lermuzeaux M, Meric H, Sauneuf B, et al. Superiority of transcutaneous CO2 over end-tidal CO2 measurement for monitoring respiratory failure in nonintubated patients: a pilot study. J Crit Care 2016;31(1):150–6.

62. Murphy PB, Brignall K, Moxham J, et al. High pressure versus high intensity noninvasive ventilation in stable hypercapnic chronic obstructive pulmonary disease: a randomized crossover trial. Int J Chron Obstruct Pulmon Dis 2012;7:811–8.

63. Ekkernkamp E, Storre JH, Windisch W, et al. Impact of intelligent volume-assured pressure support on sleep quality in stable hypercapnic chronic obstructive pulmonary disease patients: a randomized, crossover study. Respiration 2014;88(4): 270–6.

64. Oscroft NS, Chadwick R, Davies MG, et al. Volume assured versus pressure preset noninvasive ventilation for compensated ventilatory failure in COPD. Respir Med 2014;108(10): 1508–15.

65. Orr JE, Coleman J, Criner GJ, et al. Automatic EPAP intelligent volume-assured pressure support is effective in patients with chronic respiratory failure: a randomized trial. Respirology 2019;24(12): 1204–11.

66. McArdle N, Rea C, King S, et al. Treating chronic hypoventilation with automatic adjustable versus fixed epap intelligent volume-assured positive airway pressure support (iVAPS): a randomized controlled trial. Sleep 2017;40(10). https://doi.org/10.1093/ sleep/zsx136.

67. Andrade RGS, Viana FM, Nascimento JA, et al. Nasal vs Oronasal CPAP for OSA treatment: a meta-analysis. Chest 2018;153(3):665–74.

68. Selim BJ, Wolfe L, Coleman JM, et al. Initiation of noninvasive ventilation for sleep related hypoventilation disorders: advanced modes and devices. Chest 2018;153(1):251–65.

69. Hazenberg A, Kerstjens HA, Prins SC, et al. Initiation of home mechanical ventilation at home: a randomised controlled trial of efficacy, feasibility and costs. Respir Med 2014;108(9):1387–95.

70. Duiverman ML, Vonk JM, Bladder G, et al. Home initiation of chronic non-invasive ventilation in COPD patients with chronic hypercapnic respiratory failure: a randomised controlled trial. Thorax 2019; 75(3):244–52.

71. Schwarz EI, Bloch KE. Frontiers in clinical practice of long-term care of chronic ventilatory failure. Respiration 2019;98(1):1–15.

72. Vitacca M, Bianchi L, Guerra A, et al. Tele-assistance in chronic respiratory failure patients: a randomised clinical trial. Eur Respir J 2009;33(2):411–8.

73. Chatwin M, Hawkins G, Panicchia L, et al. Randomised crossover trial of telemonitoring in chronic respiratory patients (TeleCRAFT trial). Thorax 2016; 71(4):305–11.

Management of Rare Causes of Pediatric Chronic Respiratory Failure

Jenny Shi, MD[a,b], Nawal Al-Shamli, MD[a,b], Jackie Chiang, MA, MD[a,b], Reshma Amin, MD, Msc[a,b,*]

KEYWORDS

- Pediatrics • Noninvasive ventilation • Chronic respiratory failure • Spinal muscular atrophy (SMA)
- Congenital central hypoventilation syndrome (CCHS) • Cerebral palsy (CP) • Scoliosis
- Chiari malformations

KEY POINTS

- The need for long-term noninvasive positive pressure ventilation (NiPPV) in children with chronic respiratory failure is rapidly growing.
- NiPPV therapy can play an important role in the management of children with chronic respiratory failure.
- The rapidly growing number of children requiring long-term NiPPV therapy highlights the need for health care providers to become proficient in the management of patients requiring NiPPV, including the indications, types, and pediatric-specific considerations of therapy.
- Future research is needed to devise standardized protocols for the initiation and maintenance of therapy as well as to systematically evaluate its immediate and long-term effects.

INTRODUCTION

In recent decades, the population of children requiring long-term mechanical ventilation (LTMV) because of chronic respiratory failure has expanded exponentially.[1] Prevalence has grown by approximately 5-fold to 10-fold over the last couple of decades, with more children graduating to adult care with LTMV.[1,2] These findings are echoed by other studies worldwide.[3–5] Factors that have contributed to the increase in the demand for LTMV are multifactorial and include advancements in ventilator technology and life-prolonging medical care, as well as the benefits of receiving family-centered care at home.[2] LTMV can be administered invasively or noninvasively via a mask interface.

Respiratory failure is defined as the inability to maintain adequate oxygenation and/or ventilation.[6] Onset can be acute, chronic, or acute on chronic.[6] In patients with more insidious disease, nocturnal hypoventilation may be the first indicator of chronic respiratory failure.[7] Although other investigators find this too limited, the American Academy of Sleep Medicine defines nocturnal hypoventilation in pediatric patients as arterial, transcutaneous, or end-tidal carbon dioxide greater than 50 mm Hg for greater than 25% of the total sleep time.[8] Daytime hypoventilation is defined as arterial P_{CO_2} greater than 45 mm Hg.[8] At present, the gold standard for diagnosis of pediatric sleep disordered breathing (SDB), including nocturnal hypoventilation, in need of noninvasive positive pressure ventilation (NiPPV) is a laboratory-based, technologist-attended

[a] The Division of Respiratory Medicine, Department of Pediatrics, The Hospital for Sick Children, 4539 Hill Wing, 555 University Avenue, Toronto, Ontario M5G 1X8, Canada; [b] The University of Toronto, Toronto, Ontario, Canada
* Corresponding author. Division of Respiratory Medicine, The Hospital for Sick Children, 4539 Hill Wing, 555 University Avenue, Toronto, Ontario M5G 1X8, Canada.
E-mail address: reshma.amin@sickkids.ca

Sleep Med Clin 15 (2020) 511–526
https://doi.org/10.1016/j.jsmc.2020.07.002
1556-407X/20/© 2020 Elsevier Inc. All rights reserved.

polysomnogram (PSG) with identification of SDB before patients become symptomatic.[8]

Primary indications for NiPPV in children include respiratory failure secondary to (1) upper airway obstruction, (2) neuromuscular and musculoskeletal disease, (3) lower respiratory tract disease, and/or (4) control of breathing abnormalities.[9] This article reviews NiPPV for the pediatric population and presents current evidence on the long-term management of select rare causes of pediatric chronic respiratory failure.

NONINVASIVE POSITIVE PRESSURE VENTILATION IN PEDIATRICS

NiPPV therapy refers to the application of positive airway pressure (PAP) using a mask interface without the use of an endotracheal tube or surgical airway.[10] The PAP therapy counteracts the upper airway collapse, enhances minute ventilation, improves oxygenation, and unloads the inspiratory muscles.[10] In pediatrics, the 2 most common types of PAP therapy are continuous PAP (CPAP) and bilevel PAP. CPAP delivers a constant distending pressure throughout the respiratory cycle but does not assist in active inspiration.[9] Therefore, it is not sufficient treatment of chronic respiratory failure. As such, this article focuses on the use of bilevel PAP therapy as NiPPV with backup rate.

Bilevel Positive Airway Pressure Therapy

Bilevel PAP delivers ventilatory support by cycling through a preset inspiratory PAP (IPAP) and expiratory PAP (EPAP).[9] The higher IPAP works to decrease work of breathing, respiratory rate, and hypercapnia, whereas the lower EPAP helps to pneumatically stent the upper airway open, counteract intrinsic positive end-expiratory pressure, and improve oxygenation.[9] A backup rate is always set in pediatrics to ensure a minimum guaranteed breath rate. Bilevel PAP is most effective when its biphasic pressure support is delivered in synchrony with the patient's spontaneous respiratory efforts (if present), which can sometimes be challenging in children because of issues with mask leak and triggering.[10] In the most common setting of a flow-triggered mode with a preset backup rate, the IPAP is delivered when the patient's respiratory effort generates a flow greater than a preset threshold, and the machine is cycled to deliver EPAP when the flow decreases to less than a preset fraction of the peak inspiratory flow.[10] Commonly used devices in North America use preset software to establish flow and trigger cycling. This software has not been validated for use in children. As such, devices in children should only be used if the trigger and cycle can be determined by the physician at the bedside.

Most machines provide a variety of different ventilation modes and, despite similar nomenclature, these modes can vary from one manufacturer to another. Therefore, it is imperative for clinicians to be familiar with the details of the specific modes for each of the different machines being prescribed to patients. (For a detailed review on this important topic, see Michelle Cao and Gaurav Singh's article, "Noninvasive Ventilator Devices and Modes," in this issue.)

Interfaces

Choosing the optimal interface can help ensure the success of NiPPV therapy. The choice should take into account the patient's age, facial anatomy, comfort, and preference.[9] In addition, the ideal interface should aim to minimize unintentional leak and dead space ventilation, be well adhered to the patient's face (with caution to not contribute to midfacial hypoplasia), and have low resistance to airflow.[9] However, there are fewer mask options for children compared with adults. The most common categories of interfaces used in pediatrics are the nasal mask, nasal pillows, oronasal mask, and total face mask.[2] Each interface comes with its own advantages and disadvantages and can be tailored to each patient's individual needs (**Table 1**).

In addition to these conventional, ready-made interfaces, technological advances have made it possible to develop three-dimensional modeled custom masks for children who experience discomfort, nasal obstruction, or side effects from poorly fitting commercially available masks.[11] These custom masks would especially benefit younger children and infants, for whom there are particularly limited options.[12] An improved fit could thereby potentially promote efficacy and adherence by reducing leaks and unintended adverse effects of NiPPV therapy.[13] Although there are some data suggesting that customized masks may reduce nasal skin irritation and apnea-hypopnea index, more research is required to compare the performance between different types of pediatric interfaces.[13,14]

Contraindications

Before initiating NiPPV, patients should be carefully assessed clinically to determine their candidacy to receive therapy. Other than in the acute setting, it is not recommended that children use NiPPV for more than 16 h/d because of the

Table 1
Advantages and disadvantages of different noninvasive ventilation interfaces

Interface Type	Description	Advantages	Disadvantages
Nasal mask	Covers nose from bridge to below nostrils	• Minimizes claustrophobia • Minimizes anatomic dead space • No risk of aspiration	• Increased unintentional leak • Risk of nasal congestion and dryness • Risk of skin irritation • Risk of midface hypoplasia
Oronasal mask	Covers mouth and nose	• Reduces unintentional leak	• Increased claustrophobia • Risk of upper airway obstruction2° mask pressure on the mandible • Risk of nasal congestion and dryness • Risk of skin irritation • Risk of midface hypoplasia
Nasal pillows	Inserts directly into nares	• Minimizes claustrophobia • Minimizes anatomic dead space • No risk of aspiration • No risk of midface hypoplasia • No risk of skin irritation	• Increased unintentional leak • Risk of nasal congestion and dryness • Only available for older children ($\geq$5 y of age)
Total face mask	Covers eyes, nose, and mouth	• Reduces unintentional leak • No midface hypoplasia • Less skin irritation	• Increased claustrophobia • Risk of aspiration • Irritation to eyes and ears
Mouthpiece	Lips form a seal around it	• No claustrophobia • No risk of aspiration • No midface hypoplasia • No skin irritation • Not continuously connected to a device (can be used intermittently)	• Cannot be used while asleep • Requires active patient cooperation

Data from Refs.[9,12,105]

increasing risk of interface-related complications, such as skin breakdown and midface hypoplasia. Alternatives such as oral/mouthpiece ventilation could be considered at that time. In addition, prolonged use of NiPPV, including usage while awake, is also likely to interfere with the patient's communication, development, and overall health-related quality of life.[12] Ideally, NiPPV usage is less than or equal to 12 h/d. Other contraindications to NiPPV include uncontrolled gastroesophageal reflux (which is a common problem with young infants or those with neuromuscular weakness); oral secretions, because of the risk of direct aspiration; uncontrolled bulbar dysfunction or failure to protect the airway; recent upper airway or craniofacial surgery; inability to tolerate NiPPV or interface; inability to fit an interface for the child; insufficient caregiver support; and/or patient preference. In the end, decisions for NiPPV versus long-term invasive mechanical ventilation include challenge discussions about long-term risk and benefits. A close patient, family, and doctor relationship helps to mitigate these challenging situations.

Patient Safety and Caregiver Considerations

Noninvasive positive pressure therapy requires special care and attention in young, weak, and/or developmentally delayed patients who may not be able call for help or replace their masks if accidentally displaced.[9] This requirement is of the highest concern when using oronasal and total face masks in children that are dependent on ventilation, such as those with congenital central hypoventilation syndrome (CCHS). Nocturnal shift nursing and callout mechanisms should be arranged for these patients who are unable to independently remove their masks.[9] Use of an oximeter to provide continuous oxygen saturation monitoring is also recommended in pediatrics as well as the use of NiPPV machine alarms.[15]

Caregiver support and engagement is paramount in pediatrics because children rely heavily on family caregivers for their care. This requirement is also a recognized factor that positively influences the adherence to PAP therapy in pediatrics.[16,17] Young children and children with medical complexity are often completely dependent on their caregivers to apply and remove the face mask, operate the NiPPV machine, and troubleshoot any emerging problems.[18] In the case of medically complex and fragile children, it is recommended that at least 2 primary caregivers are trained, with at least 1 trained caregiver providing eyes-on care for the duration of their NiPPV therapy.[15] Clinicians and therapists need to document that the use of NiPPV by the identified primary caregivers has been effective, with demonstration and repetition of the skill.

This significant care requirement is not only physically and mentally demanding but can also affect a caregiver's ability to work and earn income.[15] Compounded with the expenses of equipment, extra supplies, transportation, home adaptations, home nursing, respite, and more, the financial impact of long-term NiPPV can be considerable.[19] Clinicians should clearly counsel patients and families on the reality of care at home with a child using NiPPV. An honest and open discussion with the families about disease trajectory and the impact of treatment on caregivers, other family members, and the patient is therefore essential before the initiation of therapy. In addition, caregivers should be provided with information on available community resources and opportunities for financial support given the significant physical, emotional, and financial ramifications of NiPPV therapy on the entire family.

Complications

NiPPV therapy use should be carefully monitored and regularly reassessed for potential complications (**Table 2**).

Midface hypoplasia is one of the recognized long-term complications of NiPPV therapy specific to children. It occurs secondary to constant pressure exerted by the face mask on a growing craniofacial skeleton. The risk of developing midface hypoplasia is higher when NiPPV therapy is used for longer daily durations (>10 h/d) and in younger children.[14] It is thought that reducing mask pressure and decreasing daily duration of NiPPV therapy use as well as alternating face mask devices could minimize the risk of developing midface hypoplasia. However, there are limited commercial mask interfaces that can fit small infants and children, particularly those with craniofacial anomalies. In addition, facial size and structure change rapidly in growing children,

making frequent reevaluation of the mask interface crucial.[20] Children at risk for developing midface hypoplasia should have regular maxillomandibular growth evaluation by a craniofacial specialist.[21]

In addition, although all NiPPV interfaces are made with an intentional leak that prevents rebreathing of carbon dioxide, the risk does increase with larger masks.[9] As a result, it is important to use the smallest and best-fitting mask; caregivers should be counseled to always check for the intentional leak after applying oronasal and total face masks.[9]

Adherence

Patient adherence to NiPPV therapy should be regularly reassessed because longer use has been shown to be associated with improvements in daytime sleepiness, quality of life, and neurocognitive function.[22–24] In adults, the threshold for clinical benefit has traditionally been 4 h/night.[23] However, this singular definition cannot be applied to children because sleep patterns evolve with age and the threshold for hours of use or percentage of total sleep time is not known.[9] As a result, there is currently no consensus definition for NiPPV adherence in children. Therefore, clinicians should aim for NiPPV therapy usage by their patients for 100% of the total sleep time. Adherence should be assessed with a combination of patient and/or parental report along with objective data that can be downloaded from the machine.[10] Despite the known benefits of NiPPV therapy, adherence continues to be a major challenge. Average duration of use varies greatly between studies and ranges from approximately 3 to 8 h/night.[25–28] Ramirez and colleagues[28] found that adherence was not related to the patient's age, underlying disease, type of interface, nocturnal gas exchange, or duration of treatment. Instead, factors that are associated with nonadherence include low maternal education, low social support, low caregiver knowledge, being an adolescent, African American ethnicity, unpleasant initial experience, technical difficulties, side effects, and lack of subjective symptom improvement.[17,29] In contrast, factors that were associated positively with adherence include previous positive experiences, subjective symptom improvement, early adaptation to therapy, health education, and family and health care team support.[17] Although there is limited pediatric evidence on effective interventions that promote NiPPV adherence, there have been studies showing that behavior analysis and therapy can be helpful.[30] Other strategies that may improve adherence include peer support groups, education programs,

Table 2
Management of complications of noninvasive ventilation

Complication	Management
Skin irritation	• Ensure mask fit is not too tight • Alternate interfaces • Use skin-protecting barriers (dressings, pads)
Nasal congestion, dryness, nosebleeds	• Humidify circuit • Trial nasal corticosteroid sprays
Eye irritation, dryness	• Ensure proper mask fit • Lubricating eye drops
Gastric distension, emesis, aspiration	• Optimize gastroesophageal reflux management • Avoid concomitant feeds • If fed by gastrostomy tube, vent and/or run slow, continuous feeds • Avoid noninvasive ventilation if uncontrolled emesis
Midface hypoplasia	• Decrease pressures • Decrease daily duration of noninvasive ventilation • Alternate interfaces • Regular assessment by craniofacial specialist
Pneumothorax	• Hospitalization • Decision to continue therapy and/or decrease pressures made on case-by-case basis
Reduced cardiac output	• Caution in patients who are preload dependent
Rebreathing carbon dioxide	• Use smallest mask possible • Ensure proper mask fit • Check intentional leak of oronasal and total face masks before use

Data from Refs.[9,21,22]

initiation of therapy in an inpatient unit, as well as home visit follow-ups.[9,28]

Initiation of Noninvasive Positive Pressure Ventilation Therapy and Follow-up

Mask desensitization is often an essential first step when initiating NiPPV in a child with tactile sensitivity, behavioral disorder, and/or impaired cognition. It may also be required in otherwise healthy children. The approach to mask desensitization should be individualized to the child's maturity level and any relevant comorbidities, such as anxiety or behavior disorders.[31] Principles of

behavioral psychology may help guide training strategies; these include positive reinforcement, graduated exposure, distraction, and escape prevention.[31] Parental buy-in of these strategies is a crucial factor in determining short-term and long-term success of NiPPV therapy.[31]

One approach is to introduce masks in the clinic with nonthreatening play therapy. Patients can begin by practicing with the mask on low pressures while awake. Once they are able to tolerate this at home or have been successfully acclimated to therapy during a brief hospital admission, they can then be brought to the sleep laboratory for a NiPPV initiation study. It is paramount for the clinical team to work closely with patients and their families to ensure ongoing graduated tolerance to therapeutic pressures.

For follow-up, children prescribed NiPPV are reviewed every 3 months in clinic to check for effectiveness and adherence to therapy, including mask fit, general equipment function, and data download. (For an in-depth review of download interpretation and management, see Philip Choi and colleagues' article, "Noninvasive Ventilation Downloads and Monitoring," in this issue.) Frequency of follow-up PSGs may vary based on the underlying medical condition, but most patients prescribed NiPPV undergo annual sleep studies. As per the American Thoracic Society guidelines, children with CCHS undergo sleep studies every 6 months until the age of 3 years.[32] Factors that may increase the frequency of testing include clinical deterioration, rapid growth in height and/or weight, intolerance of therapy, or any change in clinical status that may influence the need for NiPPV therapy (eg, recent upper airway surgery).[9] Predictors that are associated with a change in NiPPV settings during a titration PSG include a shorter window of time since initiation of therapy as well as an underlying primary central nervous system or musculoskeletal disorder.[33]

INDICATIONS FOR NONINVASIVE POSITIVE PRESSURE VENTILATION IN CHILDREN

Indications for home NiPPV therapy in children can be categorized in accordance with the underlying disease pathophysiology: (1) upper airway obstruction, (2) musculoskeletal and/or neuromuscular disease, (3) lower respiratory tract diseases, and/or (4) control of breathing abnormalities (**Table 3**).

Upper Airway Obstruction

Obstructive sleep apnea (OSA) is characterized by repeated episodes of partial (hypopnea) or complete (apnea) upper airway obstruction associated with oxygen desaturation and/or arousals.[34] The prevalence of OSA in healthy children is estimated at 1% to 5%. However, it may exceed 50% in children with certain medical conditions (eg, trisomy 21, neuromuscular diseases, and Chiari malformations).[35] The main factors that predispose children to upper airway collapse can be divided broadly into anatomic and functional factors.[36] Anatomic factors include adenoidal and/or tonsillar hypertrophy, craniofacial abnormalities (eg, Pierre Robin sequence and trisomy 21), and obesity.[36] Functional factors include neurologically based alterations in the upper airway muscle tone.[36] In

healthy children, adenotonsillar hypertrophy is the commonest cause of OSA, and adenotonsillectomy is the mainstay therapy, with curative rates more than 70%.[26] However, success rates decrease significantly in children with underlying comorbidities.[36] Although most children who fail to respond to adenotonsillectomy or are who are not candidates for this surgery can be managed with CPAP, a subset of children require bilevel PAP because of intolerance of the high CPAP pressures needed to control the OSA and/or the presence of ongoing hypoventilation despite maximal CPAP therapy.[35,37]

Neuromuscular Diseases and Chest Wall Anomalies

Neuromuscular diseases (NMDs) are common, with an overall estimated prevalence of 1 in 3000 members of the general population.[38] Children with neuromuscular diseases are at increased risk for developing respiratory complications.[39] Respiratory muscles involved in the onset of respiratory insufficiency can be grouped into inspiratory, expiratory, and oropharyngeal muscles.[40–43] Inspiratory muscle weakness results in lung hypoinflation and atelectasis, leading to ventilation/perfusion mismatch, hypoxemia, and reduced lung compliance.[40–43] Compensatory tachypnea, with small tidal volumes, exacerbates the atelectasis and predisposes to respiratory fatigue.[40–43] Expiratory muscle weakness results in an ineffective cough and retention of secretions, which predispose children to recurrent pneumonia and further atelectasis.[40–43] Bulbar muscle weakness can lead to swallowing difficulties and inadequate clearance of secretions, resulting in recurrent aspiration pneumonia.[40–43] Weakness of facial, pharyngeal, and laryngeal muscles places these children at higher risk for upper airway obstruction, especially in the supine position, which further exacerbates the ventilatory demands.[40–43] Eventually, respiratory fatigue and ventilation insufficiency result in hypoventilation, initially during rapid eye movement sleep but with subsequent progression to diurnal hypoventilation.[40–43]

In patients with chest wall deformity, the ribs and respiratory muscles are at a mechanical disadvantage because of distortion of the chest wall.[44] This disadvantage limits the normal movement of the ribs because some respiratory muscles are overstretched and others are not activated, which subsequently reduces total lung capacity and chest wall compliance. Thus, the respiratory muscles are unable to perform the necessary work to overcome the respiratory load placed on them by the reduced compliance of the

Table 3			
Indications for home noninvasive therapy in children			
Upper Airway Obstruction	**Neuromuscular Disease and Chest Wall Anomalies**	**Lower Respiratory Tract Diseases**	**Control of Breathing Abnormalities**
Upper airway anomalies: • Laryngotracheal stenosis • Vocal cord paralysis • Laryngomalacia • Other upper airway malformation • Neck mass or tumor Craniofacial abnormalities: • Craniosynostosis • Pierre Robin sequence • Trisomy 21 • Goldenhar • Treacher Collins syndrome • Achondroplasia • Beckwith-Wiedemann syndrome Obesity	Neuromuscular disease Cerebral Palsy Myopathies: • Duchenne muscular Dystrophy • Becker's • Congenital myopathy Neuromuscular junction: • Myasthenia gravis Motor neuron diseases • Spinal muscular atrophy Peripheral nerve: • Charcot Marie tooth • Friederich's ataxia Inflammatory myopathies: • Mitochondrial myopathy (MITO) • Carnitine deficiency (CD) • Lactate dehydrogenase deficiency (LDHA) Myelopathies: • Spinal cord injury (above C3) • Spinal cord tumor • Acute flaccid paralysis • Demyelinating disease • GBS • Multiple sclerosis Chest wall disorders • Kyphosis • Scoliosis • Thoracic dystrophies	Chronic cardiopulmonary diseases • Cystic fibrosis • Bronchiectasis • Chronic Lung disease of prematurity • Interstitial lung disease • Pulmonary hypoplasia • Congenital heart disease	Central hypoventilation/central apneas Congenital: • Congenital central hypoventilation syndrome • Rapid-onset obesity with hypothalamic dysregulation (ROHHAD) • Chiari I and Chiari II • Mobius syndrome • Joubert syndrome • Achondroplasia • Prader-Willi syndrome • Inborn errors of metabolism (pyruvate dehydrogenase complex deficiency, Leigh disease carnitine deficiency) Acquired: • Central nervous system infection • Central nervous system tumor • Central nervous system/spinal cord trauma • Central nervous system stroke/hemorrhage • Central nervous system surgery • Medications

Abbreviations: CD, carnitine deficiency; GBS, Guillain-Barré syndrome; LDHA, lactate dehydrogenase A; ROHHAD, rapid-onset obesity with hypothalamic dysregulation.

Adapted from Amin R, Al-Saleh S, Narang I. Domiciliary noninvasive positive airway pressure therapy in children. Pediatr Pulmonol. 2016;51(4):335–348; with permission.

respiratory system. Therefore, the work of breathing increases, leading to muscle fatigue and alveolar hypoventilation.

In general, the respiratory management of children with NMD and chest wall deformity includes invasive and noninvasive ventilation, airway clearance techniques, oral secretions management, nutrition optimization, as well as prompt treatment of lower respiratory infections and prevention of infections by vaccination.[40]

Lower Respiratory Tract Diseases

Infants and children with severe sequelae of chronic lung disease of prematurity, also known as bronchopulmonary dysplasia (BPD), may require chronic NiPPV therapy.[45] BPD develops in about 1.5% of all newborn births and, of infants with severe BPD, 41% require positive pressure ventilation at 36 weeks postmenstrual age.[45,46] Respiratory failure results from combination of multiple mechanisms, including pulmonary hypoplasia, lung tissue scarring, and distortion of lung architecture, leading to decreased tidal volume, increased airway resistance, gas trapping, decreased compliance, and increased vascular resistance.[47] In addition, tracheomalacia and bronchomalacia may develop because of ongoing positive pressure therapy, causing severe air trapping and resulting in a reduction in diaphragm contractility.[47] Some infants with BPD require prolonged mechanical ventilation but overall lung function does improve with growth and postnatal lung development.[47] If LTMV is indicated, invasive ventilation via tracheostomy is recommended because infants have longer, irregular sleeping schedules, in excess of 16 h/d, which makes NiPPV unsafe in the home environment.[48]

End-stage lung disease in children is also encountered in the context of advanced cystic fibrosis (CF), non-CF bronchiectasis, interstitial lung diseases, and conditions of the pulmonary vasculature such as idiopathic pulmonary hypertension.[49] In CF and non-CF bronchiectasis, severe airway obstruction and inflammatory bronchiectatic processes result in sputum retention, hyperinflation, ventilation perfusion mismatch, decrease respiratory muscle strength, and mechanical diaphragmatic dysfunction from lung hyperinflation and malnutrition, leading to respiratory failure.[49] Chronic hypoxemia causes hypoxic vasoconstriction and subsequently pulmonary hypertension and cor pulmonale ensue.[49] A systematic review evaluating the use of NiPPV in CF concluded that noninvasive ventilation, used in addition to oxygen, may improve gas exchange during sleep to a greater extent than oxygen therapy alone in moderate to severe disease.[50]

NiPPV therapy is used in end-stage lung diseases to avoid the need for intubation, facilitate successful discharge from the intensive care unit (ICU), and bridge toward lung transplant.[50] Initiation of therapy needs to be individualized, with consideration of benefits, risks, and the patient's goals of care on a case-by-case basis. Such considerations may include gastroesophageal reflux and risk of aspiration, or advanced CF and risk of pneumothorax.[51] After NiPPV is initiated, these children require ongoing follow-up to monitor effectiveness of therapy and continually weigh benefits against possible risks.

Control of Breathing

Control of breathing abnormalities can result in central hypoventilation and/or central apnea.[52] The controller theory postulates that, in healthy individuals, there is a reference that determines the ideal set point of the system (eg, partial pressure of carbon dioxide [$Paco_2$]).[52] The central respiratory center then integrates and coordinates the extensive sensory input from the neural and peripheral chemoreceptors, intrapulmonary receptors, and chest wall and muscle mechanoreceptors and provides neural input to the respiratory muscle to modulate ventilation to be maintained at the set point.[53] During sleep transitions, the difference between control of breathing in wakefulness and sleep can cause ventilatory instability as $Paco_2$ gradually increases during sleep to around 3 to 8 mm Hg more than awake levels, leading to a new sleep set point.[52] Central apneas subsequently develop if the $Paco_2$ then decreases to less than the eucapnic sleep level (ie, apneic threshold).[52] Furthermore, individuals with higher sensitivity to fluctuations in the ventilatory system (known as high loop gain based on an engineering analogy to describe a feedback system) may be more prone to ventilator instability, resulting in periodic breathing.[54,55] Injury to the respiratory control center can cause further disturbances to ventilation and can be classified as congenital (eg, CCHS) or acquired (eg, posterior fossa mass or medications).[52] Management should be directed to address the underlying cause, if possible, with ventilation support used to treat central sleep apnea (CSA) or hypoventilation.[52]

RARE PEDIATRIC DISEASES
Spinal Muscular Atrophy

Spinal muscular atrophy (SMA) is a rare autosomal recessive neurodegenerative disorder affecting the anterior horn cells in the spinal cord, leading to progressive muscle weakness and atrophy.[56] Despite its rare occurrence, it is the most common cause of infant mortality in developed countries, although recent emerging treatments and disease screening practices are rapidly changing the face of the disease.[56] SMA is a clinically and genetically heterogeneous disease that can be classified into types 0 to 4 by symptom onset and severity.[15,56]

The natural history of respiratory decline in SMA begins with inspiratory and expiratory muscle weakness, although the diaphragm is spared, with or without dysphagia, which results in weak cough and recurrent respiratory infections.[57] The presence of a bell-shaped thorax frequently contributes to these abnormalities. Without intervention, patients develop SDB, followed by daytime hypercapnea, and eventually death.[57]

Combined with nutritional and airway clearance therapies, NiPPV therapy has been shown to reduce respiratory infections; shorten hospital and ICU stays; and improve life expectancy, quality of life, sleep quality, and lung development.[57] It may even be used early on as a preventive strategy.[58] In the palliative setting, NiPPV can also be used to improve quality of life, reduce work of breathing, and facilitate discharge home.[15] Ultimately, the initiation and maintenance of NiPPV should be a collaborative decision with ongoing discussion between the health care team and the patient's family, with respect to the child's goals of care as the disease progresses.

Early initiation of NiPPV therapy is recommended because it has been shown to promote chest remodeling and normal lung development.[58] The use of high-span NiPPV (ie, increased IPAP levels with a delta pressure of at least 10 cm H_2O) is frequently recommended to prevent chest wall stiffness and limitation.[58] Additional goals of therapy include managing any SDB and to ensure respiratory muscle rest overnight. To this end, clinical practice in our center includes an adequate backup rate so that less than 20% of breaths are spontaneously triggered, as well as a guaranteed inspiratory time with every breath. Special safety considerations in children with SMA include their increased risk of gastroesophageal reflux and aspiration, as well as neuromuscular weakness impairing their ability to independently remove masks in case of emesis, reflux, or secretions.[15] Possible solutions to enhance patient safety while using NiPPV include feeding by gastrostomy or gastrojejunal tubes, the use of nasal masks, and/or overnight shift nursing.

Recent years have seen the introduction of disease-modifying agents, nusinersen and onasemnogene abeparvovec. Nusinersen is an antisense oligonucleotide that promotes production of functional survival motor neuron (SMN) protein, but access restrictions and its extraordinary cost limits its availability for many patients.[56] Landmark phase 3 trial have shown nusinersen to be safe, tolerable, and associated with improvements in motor function and overall survival; however, it did not alter dependence on long-term ventilation.[59,60] Early treatment may maximize the drug's benefits, which has given rise to newborn screening pilot programs.[61] However, nusinersen is not curative and its long-term effects are not yet known.[56]

More recently, onasemnogene abeparvovec, a gene replacement therapy, was approved by the US Food and Drug Administration in May 2019 in children less than 2 years old. It has been shown to improve survival and motor function, but its impacts on long-term ventilatory requirements are uncertain.

Congenital Central Hypoventilation Syndrome

CCHS is a rare genetic disease that affects the control of breathing. It is characterized by hypoventilation during sleep and/or wakefulness, autonomic nervous system dysregulation, as well as an increased risk of developing neural crest tumors and/or Hirschsprung disease.[62] The disease can present in infancy, childhood, or adulthood.[63,64] A pathologic mutation in the PHOXB2 gene is diagnostic of CCHS.[32] There are 2 main types of mutation: (1) polyalanine repeat expansion mutations (PARMs), which account for 90% of reported cases; and (2) nonpolyalanine repeat expansion mutations (NPARMs), which present in 10% of reported cases.[32] It is well established that children with PARMs in the range of 20/27 to 20/33 genotypes and most with NPARM mutations require continuous mechanical ventilatory support, whereas those with fewer repeats (20/24–20/26) typically require only nocturnal support.[32]

Individuals with CCHS have a pattern of breathing characterized by diminished tidal volumes and monotonous respiratory rates while awake and sleep[32] Hypoventilation is most pronounced during non–rapid eye movement sleep, during which breathing is primarily regulated by the chemoreceptors. The ventilatory control abnormality in CCHS seems to be in the integration of chemoreceptor input to central ventilatory controllers, rather than abnormalities in the chemoreceptors themselves.[65] Patients with CCHS also have autonomic nervous system dysregulation, which may present as breath-holding spells, episodes of profound sweating, low basal body temperature, abnormalities in blood pressure and cardiac rhythm, gut dysmotility, poor pupillary light response, and absence of physiologic response to exertion and stress.[66] Patients with CCHS may not show fever, tachypnea, or increased work of breathing with acute respiratory infections. CCHS should be suspected in patients with unexplained alveolar hypoventilation or delayed recovery of spontaneous breathing following exposure to sedative agents, anesthesia, or severe respiratory infection.[32]

All patients with CCHS require lifelong ventilation, at least during sleep.[32] The recommended management for infants and young children with CCHS is ventilation via tracheostomy in the first several years of life to optimize neurocognitive outcome.[32] Ventilatory settings are adjusted to achieve end-tidal carbon dioxide between 35 and 40 mm Hg and oxygen saturation greater than or equal to 95%.[32]

Transition to NiPPV is considered around school age in patients with CCHS who are stable and require ventilation during sleep only.[32,67] Tracheostomy decannulation can be considered in patients with CCHS who are able to manage secretions, have intact cough reflex, need suction of the trachea less than or equal to once a day, tolerate tracheostomy capping during the day with adequate gas exchange, have normal upper airways on bronchoscopy assessment, and for motivated children and families.[68] NiPPV can be provided via bilevel PAP in the conventional spontaneous/timed mode or pressure control mode depending on device. In addition, volume-assured pressure support (VAPS) can also be used. In a small pediatric cohort, VAPS has been shown to achieve better control of carbon dioxide levels throughout the night because it autotitrates the pressures to achieve a constant, preset alveolar ventilation.[69] When using VAPS mode in the setting of CCHS, they should be adjusted so that the starting pressures are adequate and the time to achieving adequate ventilation is minimized.

Diaphragm pacing is an option for ambulatory children who are on ventilation via tracheostomy during both wakefulness and sleep; it offers the ability to be liberated from the ventilator during the daytime.[32] In addition, diaphragm pacing may aid tracheostomy decannulation in stable individuals who are ventilator dependent during sleep.[32,65,70]

In addition to respiratory complications, patients with CCHS are at increased risk for neurocognitive delay, cardiac rhythm disorders, and sudden death.[32] As such, annual PSG, 72-hour Holter recording, echocardiogram, and neurocognitive assessment are recommended to all patients with CCHS.[32] Certain CCHS genotypes are also associated with the risk of developing Hirschsprung disease and neural crest tumors.[32] NiPPV use resulting in aerophagia with colonic distention can be problematic for those individuals with Hirschsprung disease. For patients with PHOX2B NPARMs and longer PARMs (20/28–20/33), close surveillance of neural crest tumors is recommended.[32] In addition, counseling patients and families on the serious adverse events associated with the use of sedating medications and alcohol, including coma and death, is paramount.[71]

Cerebral Palsy

Cerebral palsy (CP) encompasses a heterogeneous group of nonprogressive, central motor disorders that are caused by abnormalities during development of the fetal or infantile brain.[72] CP is the leading cause of childhood disability in the United States, with a median estimated prevalence of 2.4 per 1000 live births.[72] Prevalence increases with decreasing gestational age, and the severity of functional limitation can vary based on the underlying cause and disease subtype.[72] Respiratory disease is the leading cause of morbidity and mortality in children with CP.[73] Cause is multifactorial, including scoliosis, chest wall deformities, impaired airway clearance, oropharyngeal motor dysfunction, recurrent aspiration, and respiratory tract infections.[73] This article focuses on the role of NiPPV therapy in managing hypoventilation secondary to upper airway obstruction and scoliosis.[73]

Children with CP are at increased risk of both nocturnal and diurnal upper airway obstruction, which may exist independently or concurrently.[74] Obstruction can be multifactorial, with factors including maxillary hypoplasia, enlarged inferior nasal turbinates, adenotonsillar hypertrophy, hypotonia of palate and constrictor muscles, glossoptosis, retrognathia, oropharyngeal hypotonia and pseudobulbar palsy, redundant aryepiglottic folds, upper airway inflammation from gastroesophageal reflux, and laryngeal dystonia.[74] In addition, children with CP may have pseudobulbar palsy, which can cause an uncoordinated pharyngeal dilator reflex, which normally stimulates pharyngeal muscle contraction to maintain airway patency just before diaphragmatic contraction.[75] In addition to careful history and physical examination, clinical assessment may include lateral neck radiograph, upper airway endoscopy, PSG, and blood gas analysis.[76] The physical examination may be confusing because the use of baclofen pumps may reduce the amount of spasticity peripherally but, because the pumps do not treat cranial muscles, severe spasticity may be prominent in these areas, causing airway obstruction. Oral baclofen can be considered in these patients to prevent upper airway obstruction.

Although there is a paucity of literature studying the use of NiPPV in treating SDB in children with CP, the limited literature available does support a treatment benefit with respect to improved sleep quality, daytime functioning, and quality of life, as well as reduced respiratory morbidity and mortality.[77] A retrospective study comparing patients with CP who received adenotonsillectomy or CPAP against an untreated group found improved caregiver concerns, sleep disturbance, daytime functioning, and quality of life.[78] CPAP may therefore be considered in children with upper airway obstruction and OSA alone, and bilevel PAP may be necessary if there is comorbid hypoventilation from restrictive lung disease or altered control of breathing.[76] It is especially important for these patients to have optimal gastroesophageal reflux management before initiating NiPPV.[74] Ultimately, the decision to pursue NiPPV therapy for children with CP needs to be individualized based on potential benefits and risks, patient preferences, as well as burden of care in the context of the patient's care goals. Future goals and directions for NiPPV for SDB in children with developmental delay could include home-based high-flow therapy, which may be better tolerated by patients and more easily administered by caregivers.

Scoliosis

In growing children, scoliosis can result in thoracic cage deformity and thus interfere with lung development.[73] Restrictive lung disease consequently develops with decreased total lung capacity, decreased chest wall and lung compliance, increased airway resistance, respiratory muscle weakness, and diaphragmatic dysfunction.[73] The decrease in lung volume is primarily determined by angle of scoliosis (>70°), number of vertebrae involved (7 or more), location of the curve (cephalad), and loss of normal thoracic kyphosis.[79] The hypoinflation and atelectasis eventually lead to irreversible atrophy of the lungs and further reduction of the lung volume.[79] The inability to generate sustained increased work of breathing may then result in eventual respiratory failure. Persistent hypoventilation and hypoxemia could also lead to pulmonary hypertension and cor pulmonale.[73] In general, a Cobb angle greater than 90° predisposes patients to cardiorespiratory failure.[79]

Scoliosis is generally managed conservatively, with postural therapy and braces, and/or surgically with spinal fusion.[73] However, bracing may cause further restriction and may not be tolerated well in those patients who already have significant lung restriction. Surgery correction can help prevent progression of scoliosis, preserve pulmonary function, prevent progression to pulmonary hypertension, and improve quality of life and cosmetic appearance.[15] These benefits need to be weighed in the context of the child's growth potential and against the moderately high surgical complication rate in children with additional comorbidities such as CP or other neuromuscular diseases.[73] Initiation of NiPPV therapy before surgery and continuation following extubation should be considered to help patients wean off invasive ventilation and shorten hospital stay.[15] These children should undergo a PSG before their procedure and NiPPV initiation, then have ongoing follow-up to guide possible weaning of therapy.[80]

Research is lacking on the benefit of NiPPV therapy for children with scoliosis, but there is good evidence based on adult studies that NiPPV can significantly improve survival because it reduces hypercapnia and improves oxygenation and vital capacity.[81,82] Thus, long-term NiPPV therapy should be considered for any child with chronic respiratory failure secondary to scoliosis and resultant restrictive lung disease.[15]

Chiari Malformations

Chiari malformations (CMs) are a group of disorders characterized by caudal displacement of the posterior part of cerebellum either alone or together with lower medulla, through the foramen magnum into the spinal canal.[83] Chiari malformations are commonly classified into 3 main groups, of which Chiari malformation type I (CM-I) is the most common.[83–85]

CM-I is increasingly diagnosed early in symptomatic and asymptomatic children because of readily available MRI.[86] Symptomatic CM-I presents mainly with neurologic or SDB symptoms caused by compression of brain stem and lower cranial nerves as well as the disruption of cerebrospinal fluid flow.[86] Children with CM-I are at an increased risk for developing neurocognitive deficits.[86] In addition, catastrophic events such as cardiorespiratory arrest and death during sleep have been reported.[86,87] Thus, early diagnosis and management of CM-I is essential. The prevalence of SDB in pediatric patients with CM-I is high, ranging between 24% and 70% (5-fold to 10-fold higher than the general pediatric population).[88–91] SDB in CM-I commonly manifests as OSA, CSA, or mixed apneas with or without hypoventilation, with most showing a predominantly obstructive apnea.[89,91,92] Therefore, CM-I should be considered not only in cases of CSA but also in cases of unexplained OSA or OSA that is resistant to conventional treatment, including the presence of persistent headache after therapy.

CM-II is commonly diagnosed prenatally or at birth because of the presence of myelomeningocele, frequently accompanied by hydrocephalus.[93] Patients with CM-II typically experience long-term comorbidities, including brain stem dysfunction (eg, swallowing difficulties and vocal cord paresis), respiratory complications, bowel and bladder dysfunction, musculoskeletal problems (eg, scoliosis and hip dislocation), neurodevelopmental delay, tethered cords, and seizures.[94] The prevalence of SDB in children with CM-II exceeds 50%.[93–95] Among 109 children with myelomeningocele from a single center, 83 underwent PSG. SDB was documented in 62%

(mild sleep apnea in 42% and moderate to severe sleep apnea in 20%).[95] CSA, OSA, and hypoventilation were all documented in patients with CM-II.[93,94] SDB is also associated with an increased risk of sudden death in children with CM-II.[96,97] Therefore, routine evaluation of SDB in this population is suggested.[94] In addition, the authors recommend head computed tomography and an in-laboratory sleep study for patients with spina bifida because of the risk of CSA with CMs.

The 2 main pathophysiologic mechanisms in CMs leading to OSA and CSA are poor upper airway muscle tone and abnormal control of breathing, respectively.[98–101] OSA results from the mechanical compression and/or stretch of the respiratory nuclei in the medulla and lower cranial nerves controlling pharyngeal and dilator laryngeal muscles leading to poor upper airway muscle tone and upper airway collapse during sleep.[98–101] CSA is caused by various mechanisms resulting in dysfunction of the respiratory centers. These mechanisms include depression of the reticular activating system, compromised blood supply caused by direct compression of brain stem and its vasculature, damaged central chemoreceptors with decrease responsiveness to carbon dioxide, impaired afferent input from the carotid bodies to the medulla caused by compression or stretch of glossopharyngeal nerve, and compression of phrenic motor neurons in the anterior horn of the cervical spinal cord because of a syrinx.[98–101]

At present, there are no published guidelines on when patients with CM-I should undergo PSG.[91] In a prospective study by Losurdo and colleagues,[89] 53 consecutive children and adolescents with CM-I, only 7 patients reported SDB symptoms, whereas 13 patients were confirmed to have SDB on PSG. None of patients with CSA reported SDB symptoms.[89] Such symptoms are therefore not an adequate screen for SDB in this population, especially in children with CSA, who would be potentially missed if symptoms alone were an indication for PSG.[102]

Surgical interventions, including adenotonsillectomy and posterior fossa decompression, are first-line treatment of SDB in children with CMs.[103] NiPPV may be initiated as a bridge to surgical intervention. Surgical outcomes can be variable, and some patients experience only partial resolution of their SDB, whereas others experience a worsening of SDB requiring noninvasive respiratory support.[104] Therefore, long-term follow-up PSG is indicated to reevaluate the SDB after surgical interventions.[103] Long-term NiPPV may be required in those children with persistent SDB despite surgical intervention and/or in children in whom surgical intervention is not indicated or feasible.[91] Regardless of how or why the CMs came to attention, PSG should be performed before Chiari repair given the high risk of SDB in these patients.

SUMMARY

NiPPV therapy can play an important role in the management of children with chronic respiratory failure. The rapidly growing number of children requiring long-term NiPPV therapy highlights the need for health care providers to become proficient in the management of patients requiring NiPPV, including the indications, types, and pediatric-specific considerations of therapy. Future research is needed to devise standardized protocols for the initiation and maintenance of therapy as well as to systematically evaluate its immediate and long-term effects.

DISCLOSURE

The authors have no relationships with any commercial company that has a direct financial interest in the subject matter or materials discussed in this article or with a company making a competing product.

REFERENCES

1. McDougall CM, Adderley RJ, Wensley DF, et al. Long-term ventilation in children: longitudinal trends and outcomes. Arch Dis Child 2013;98(9): 660–5.
2. Amin R, Sayal P, Syed F, et al. Pediatric long-term home mechanical ventilation: twenty years of follow-up from one Canadian center. Pediatr Pulmonol 2014;49(8):816–24.
3. Chau SK, Yung AWY, Lee SL. Long-term management for ventilator-assisted children in Hong Kong: 2 decades' experience. Respir Care 2017; 62(1):54–64.
4. Wallis C, Paton JY, Beaton S, et al. Children on long-term ventilatory support: 10 Years of progress. Arch Dis Child 2011;96(11):998–1002.
5. Graham RJ, Fleegler EW, Robinson WM. Chronic ventilator need in the community: a 2005 pediatric census of Massachusetts. Pediatrics 2007;119(6). https://doi.org/10.1542/peds.2006-2471.
6. Roussos C, Koutsoukou A. Respiratory failure. Eur Respir J 2003;22(Supplement 47):3s–14s.
7. Ambrosino N, Casaburi R, Chetta A, et al. 8th International conference on management and rehabilitation of chronic respiratory failure: the long summaries - Part 3. Multidiscip Respir Med 2015; 10. https://doi.org/10.1186/s40248-015-0028-x.

8. Berry RB, Budhiraja R, Gottlieb DJ, et al. Rules for scoring respiratory events in sleep: update of the 2007 AASM manual for the scoring of sleep and associated events. J Clin Sleep Med 2012;8(5):597–619.

9. Amin R, Al-Saleh S, Narang I. Domiciliary noninvasive positive airway pressure therapy in children. Pediatr Pulmonol 2016;51(4):335–48.

10. Perrem L, Mehta K, Syed F, et al. How to use noninvasive positive airway pressure device data reports to guide clinical care. Pediatr Pulmonol 2020;55(1):58–67.

11. Carroll A, Amirav I, Marchand R, et al. Three-dimensional modeled custom-made noninvasive positive pressure ventilation masks in an infant. Am J Respir Crit Care Med 2014;190(8):950.

12. Castro-Codesal ML, Olmstead DL, MacLean JE. Mask interfaces for home non-invasive ventilation in infants and children. Paediatr Respir Rev 2019;32:66–72.

13. Cheng Y-L, Hsu D-Y, Lee H-C, et al. Clinical verification of patients with obstructive sleep apnea provided with a customized cushion for continuous positive airway pressure. J Prosthet Dent 2015;113. https://doi.org/10.1016/j.prosdent.2014.01.030.

14. Fauroux B, Lavis JF, Nicot F, et al. Facial side effects during noninvasive positive pressure ventilation in children. Intensive Care Med 2005;31(7):965–9.

15. Amin R, MacLusky I, Zielinski D, et al. Pediatric home mechanical ventilation: a Canadian Thoracic Society clinical practice guideline executive summary. Can J Respir Crit Care Sleep Med 2017;1(1):7–36.

16. Parmar A, Messiha S, Baker A, et al. Caregiver support and positive airway pressure therapy adherence among adolescents with obstructive sleep apnea. Paediatr Child Health 2019;pxz107. https://doi.org/10.1093/pch/pxz107.

17. Ennis J, Rohde K, Chaput JP, et al. Facilitators and barriers to noninvasive ventilation adherence in youth with nocturnal hypoventilation secondary to obesity or neuromuscular disease. J Clin Sleep Med 2015;11(12):1409–16.

18. Cohen E, Kuo DZ, Agrawal R, et al. Children with medical complexity: an emerging population for clinical and research initiatives. Pediatrics 2011;127(3):529–38.

19. Edwards JD, Panitch HB, Constantinescu A, et al. Survey of financial burden of families in the U.S. with children using home mechanical ventilation. Pediatr Pulmonol 2018;53(1):108–16.

20. Kirk VG, O'Donnell AR. Continuous positive airway pressure for children: a discussion on how to maximize compliance. Sleep Med Rev 2006;10(2):119–27.

21. Li KK, Riley RW, Guilleminault C. An unreported risk in the use of home nasal continuous positive airway pressure and home nasal ventilation in children. Chest 2000;117(3):916–8.

22. Sawyer AM, Gooneratne NS, Marcus CL, et al. A systematic review of CPAP adherence across age groups: clinical and empiric insights for developing CPAP adherence interventions. Sleep Med Rev 2011;15(6):343–56.

23. Weaver TE, Maislin G, Dinges DF, et al. Relationship between hours of CPAP use and achieving normal levels of sleepiness and daily functioning. Sleep 2007;30(6):711–9.

24. Antic NA, Catcheside P, Buchan C, et al. The effect of CPAP in normalizing daytime sleepiness, quality of life, and neurocognitive function in patients with moderate to severe OSA. Sleep 2011;34(1):111–9.

25. Uong EC, Epperson M, Bathon SA, et al. Adherence to nasal positive airway pressure therapy among school-aged children and adolescents with obstructive sleep apnea syndrome. Pediatrics 2007;120(5). https://doi.org/10.1542/peds.2006-2731.

26. Marcus CL, Beck SE, Traylor J, et al. Randomized, double-blind clinical trial of two different modes of positive airway pressure therapy on adherence and efficacy in children. J Clin Sleep Med 2012;8(1):37–42.

27. Marcus CL, Rosen G, Ward SLD, et al. Adherence to and effectiveness of positive airway pressure therapy in children with obstructive sleep apnea. Pediatrics 2006;117(3):e442–51.

28. Ramirez A, Khirani S, Aloui S, et al. Continuous positive airway pressure and noninvasive ventilation adherence in children. Sleep Med 2013;14(12):1290–4.

29. King MS, Xanthopoulos MS, Marcus CL. Improving positive airway pressure adherence in children. Sleep Med Clin 2014;9(2):219–34.

30. Koontz KL, Slifer KJ, Cataldo MD, et al. Improving pediatric compliance with positive airway pressure therapy: the impact of behavioral intervention. Sleep 2003;26(8):1010–5.

31. Slifer KJ, Kruglak D, Benore E, et al. Behavioral training for increasing Preschool children's adherence with positive airway pressure: a preliminary study. Behav Sleep Med 2007;5(2):147–75.

32. Weese-Mayer DE, Berry-Kravis EM, Ceccherini I, et al. An official ATS clinical policy statement: congenital central hypoventilation syndrome. Am J Respir Crit Care Med 2010;181(6):626–44.

33. Al-Saleh S, Sayal P, Stephens D, et al. Factors associated with changes in invasive and noninvasive positive airway pressure therapy settings during pediatric polysomnograms. J Clin Sleep Med 2017;13(2):183–8.

34. Sateia MJ. International classification of sleep disorders-third edition: highlights and modifications. Chest 2014;146(5):1387–94.

35. Marcus CL, Chapman D, Ward SD, et al. Clinical practice guideline: diagnosis and management of childhood obstructive sleep apnea syndrome. Pediatrics 2002;109(4):704–12.

36. Amin R, Holler T, Narang I, et al. Adenotonsillectomy for obstructive sleep apnea in children with complex chronic conditions. Otolaryngol Neck Surg 2018;158(4):760–6.

37. Padman R, Hyde C, Foster P, et al. The pediatric use of bilevel positive airway pressure therapy for obstructive sleep apnea syndrome: a retrospective review with analysis of respiratory parameters. Clin Pediatr (Phila) 2002;41(3):163–9.

38. Emery AE. Population frequencies of inherited neuromuscular diseases–a world survey. Neuromuscul Disord 1991;1(1):19–29.

39. Perrin C, Unterborn JN, Ambrosio CD', et al. Pulmonary complications of chronic neuromuscular diseases and their management. Muscle Nerve 2004;29(1):5–27.

40. Hull J, Aniapravan R, Chan E, et al. British Thoracic Society guideline for respiratory management of children with neuromuscular weakness. Thorax 2012;67(Suppl 1):i1–40.

41. Farrero E, Antón A, Egea CJ, et al. Guidelines for the management of respiratory complications in patients with neuromuscular disease. Arch Bronconeumol 2013;49(7):306–13.

42. Allen J. Pulmonary complications of neuromuscular disease: a respiratory mechanics perspective. Paediatr Respir Rev 2010;11(1):18–23.

43. Mehta S. Neuromuscular disease causing acute respiratory failure. Respir Care 2006;51(9):1016–23. Available at: http://www.ncbi.nlm.nih.gov/pubmed/16934165.

44. Bergofsky EH. Respiratory failure in disorders of the thoracic cage. Am Rev Respir Dis 1979;119(4):643–69.

45. Deakins KM. Bronchopulmonary dysplasia. Respir Care 2009;54(9):1252–62. Available at: http://www.ncbi.nlm.nih.gov/pubmed/19712501.

46. Malkar MB, Gardner WP, Mandy GT, et al. Respiratory severity score on day of life 30 is predictive of mortality and the length of mechanical ventilation in premature infants with protracted ventilation: respiratory Severity Scores in Prolonged Ventilated Premature Infants. Pediatr Pulmonol 2015;50(4):363–9.

47. Madurga A, Mižíková I, Ruiz-Camp J, et al. Recent advances in late lung development and the pathogenesis of bronchopulmonary dysplasia. Am J Physiol Lung Cell Mol Physiol 2013;305(12):L893–905.

48. Parrilla C, Scarano E, Guidi ML, et al. Current trends in paediatric tracheostomies. Int J Pediatr Otorhinolaryngol 2007;71(10):1563–7.

49. Ringholz F, Devins M, McNally P. Managing end stage lung disease in children. Paediatr Respir Rev 2014;15(1):75–80 [quiz: 80-81].

50. Moran F, Bradley JM, Piper AJ. Non-invasive ventilation for cystic fibrosis. Cochrane Database Syst Rev 2017;(2):CD002769.

51. Flume PA. Pneumothorax in cystic fibrosis. Chest 2003;123(1):217–21.

52. McLaren AT, Bin-Hasan S, Narang I. Diagnosis, management and pathophysiology of central sleep apnea in children. Paediatr Respir Rev 2019;30:49–57.

53. Caruana-Montaldo B, Gleeson K, Zwillich CW. The control of breathing in clinical practice. Chest 2000;117(1):205–25.

54. Khoo MCK. Determinants of ventilatory instability and variability. Respir Physiol 2000;122(2–3):167–82.

55. Dempsey JA, Smith CA. Pathophysiology of human ventilatory control. Eur Respir J 2014;44(2):495–512.

56. Vukovic S, McAdam L, Zlotnik-Shaul R, et al. Putting our best foot forward: clinical, treatment-based and ethical considerations of nusinersen therapy in Canada for spinal muscular atrophy. J Paediatr Child Health 2019;55(1):18–24.

57. Schroth MK. Special considerations in the respiratory management of spinal muscular atrophy. Pediatrics 2009;123.

58. Bach JR, Bianchi C. Prevention of pectus excavatum for children with spinal muscular atrophy type 1. Am J Phys Med Rehabil 2003;82(10):815–9.

59. Mercuri E, Darras BT, Chiriboga CA, et al. Nusinersen versus sham control in later-onset spinal muscular atrophy. N Engl J Med 2018;378(7):625–35.

60. Finkel RS, Mercuri E, Darras BT, et al. Nusinersen versus sham control in infantile-onset spinal muscular atrophy. N Engl J Med 2017;377(18):1723–32.

61. Kariyawasam DST, Russell JS, Wiley V, et al. The implementation of newborn screening for spinal muscular atrophy: the Australian experience. Genet Med 2019. https://doi.org/10.1038/s41436-019-0673-0.

62. Amin R, Riekstins A, Al-Saleh S, et al. Presentation and treatment of monozygotic twins with congenital central hypoventilation syndrome. Can Respir J 2011;18(2):87–9.

63. Matera I. PHOX2B mutations and polyalanine expansions correlate with the severity of the respiratory phenotype and associated symptoms in both congenital and late onset Central Hypoventilation syndrome. J Med Genet 2004;41(5):373–80.

64. Weese-Mayer DE, Berry-Kravis EM, Zhou L. Adult identified with congenital central hypoventilation syndrome–mutation in PHOX2b gene and late-onset CHS. Am J Respir Crit Care Med 2005; 171(1):88.

65. Kasi A, Perez I, Kun S, et al. Congenital central hypoventilation syndrome: diagnostic and management challenges. Pediatr Heal Med Ther 2016;7: 99–107.

66. Weese-Mayer DE, Silvestri JM, Huffman AD, et al. Case/control family study of autonomic nervous system dysfunction in idiopathic congenital central hypoventilation syndrome. Am J Med Genet 2001; 100(3):237–45.

67. Moraes TJ, MacLusky I, Zielinski D, et al. Section 11: central hypoventilation, congenital and acquired. Can J Respir Crit Care Sleep Med 2018; 2(sup1):78–82.

68. Heffner JE. The technique of weaning from tracheostomy. Criteria for weaning; practical measures to prevent failure. J Crit Illn 1995;10(10):729–33.

69. Khayat A, Medin D, Syed F, et al. Intelligent volume-assured pressured support (iVAPS) for the treatment of congenital central hypoventilation syndrome. Sleep Breath 2017;21(2):513–9.

70. Diep B, Wang A, Kun S, et al. Diaphragm pacing without tracheostomy in congenital central hypoventilation syndrome patients. Respiration 2015; 89(6):534–8.

71. Chen ML, Turkel SB, Jacobson JR, et al. Alcohol use in congenital central hypoventilation syndrome. Pediatr Pulmonol 2006;41(3):283–5.

72. Oskoui M, Coutinho F, Dykeman J, et al. An update on the prevalence of cerebral palsy: a systematic review and meta-analysis. Dev Med Child Neurol 2013;55(6):509–19.

73. Boel L, Pernet K, Toussaint M, et al. Respiratory morbidity in children with cerebral palsy: an overview. Dev Med Child Neurol 2019;61(6):646–53.

74. Wilkinson DJ, Baikie G, Berkowitz RG, et al. Awake upper airway obstruction in children with spastic quadriplegic cerebral palsy. J Paediatr Child Health 2006;42(1–2):44–8.

75. Seddon PC, Khan Y. Respiratory problems in children with neurological impairment. Arch Dis Child 2003;88(1):75–8.

76. Kontorinis G, Thevasagayam MS, Bateman ND. Airway obstruction in children with cerebral palsy: need for tracheostomy? Int J Pediatr Otorhinolaryngol 2013;77(10):1647–50.

77. Grychtol R, Chan EY. Use of non-invasive ventilation in cerebral palsy. Arch Dis Child 2018; 103(12):1170–7.

78. Hsiao KH, Nixon GM. The effect of treatment of obstructive sleep apnea on quality of life in children with cerebral palsy. Res Dev Disabil 2008;29(2): 133–40.

79. Kearon C, Viviani GR, Kirkley A, et al. Factors determining pulmonary function in adolescent idiopathic thoracic scoliosis. Am Rev Respir Dis 1993; 148(2):288–94.

80. LeBlanc M, Mérette C, Savard J, et al. Incidence and risk factors of insomnia in a population-based sample. Sleep 2009;32(8):1027–37.

81. Buyse B, Meersseman W, Demedts M. Treatment of chronic respiratory failure in kyphoscoliosis: oxygen or ventilation? Eur Respir J 2003;22(3):525–8.

82. Simonds AK, Elliott MW. Outcome of domiciliary nasal intermittent positive pressure ventilation in restrictive and obstructive disorders. Thorax 1995;50(6):604–9.

83. Sarnat HB. Disorders of segmentation of the neural tube: chiari malformations. Handb Clin Neurol 2008;87:89–103.

84. Sarnat HB. Cerebellar networks and neuropathology of cerebellar developmental disorders. Handb Clin Neurol 2018;154:109–28.

85. Choi SS, Tran LP, Zalzal GH. Airway abnormalities in patients with Arnold-Chiari malformation. Otolaryngol Neck Surg 1999;121(6):720–4.

86. Rogers JM, Savage G, Stoodley MA. A systematic review of cognition in chiari i malformation. Neuropsychol Rev 2018;28(2):176–87.

87. Martinot A, Hue V, Leclerc F, et al. Sudden death revealing Chiari type 1 malformation in two children. Intensive Care Med 1993;19(2):73–4.

88. Dauvilliers Y, Stal V, Abril B, et al. Chiari malformation and sleep related breathing disorders. J Neurol Neurosurg Psychiatry 2007;78(12): 1344–8.

89. Losurdo A, Dittoni S, Testani E, et al. Sleep disordered breathing in children and adolescents with Chiari malformation type I. J Clin Sleep Med 2013;9(4):371–7.

90. Botelho RV, Bittencourt LRA, Rotta JM, et al. A prospective controlled study of sleep respiratory events in patients with craniovertebral junction malformation. J Neurosurg 2003;99(6):1004–9.

91. Khatwa U, Ramgopal S, Mylavarapu A, et al. MRI findings and sleep apnea in children with Chiari I malformation. Pediatr Neurol 2013;48(4): 299–307.

92. Dhamija R, Wetjen NM, Slocumb NL, et al. The role of nocturnal polysomnography in assessing children with Chiari type I malformation. Clin Neurol Neurosurg 2013;115(9):1837–41.

93. Alsaadi MM, Iqbal SM, Elgamal EA, et al. Sleep-disordered breathing in children with Chiari malformation type II and myelomeningocele: apnea in children with spinal bifida. Pediatr Int 2012;54(5): 623–6.

94. Patel DM, Rocque BG, Hopson B, et al. Sleep-disordered breathing in patients with myelomeningocele. J Neurosurg Pediatr 2015;16(1):30–5.

95. Waters KA, Forbes P, Morielli A, et al. Sleep-disordered breathing in children with myelomeningocele. J Pediatr 1998;132(4):672–81.

96. Jernigan SC, Berry JG, Graham DA, et al. Risk factors of sudden death in young adult patients with myelomeningocele. J Neurosurg Pediatr 2012; 9(2):149–55.

97. Kirk VG, Morielli A, Brouillette RT. Sleep-disordered breathing in patients with myelomeningocele: the missed diagnosis. Dev Med Child Neurol 2007; 41(1):40–3.

98. Rabec C, Laurent G, Baudouin N, et al. Central sleep apnoea in Arnold-Chiari malformation: evidence of pathophysiological heterogeneity. Eur Respir J 1998;12(6):1482–5.

99. De Backer WA. Central sleep apnoea, pathogenesis and treatment: an overview and perspective. Eur Respir J 1995;8(8):1372–83.

100. Hanly PJ. Mechanisms and management of central sleep apnea. Lung 1992;170(1):1–17.

101. Bokinsky GE, Hudson LD, Weil JV. Impaired peripheral chemosensitivity and acute respiratory failure in arnold-chiari malformation and syringomyelia. N Engl J Med 1973;288(18):947–8.

102. Amin R, Sayal P, Sayal A, et al. The association between sleep-disordered breathing and magnetic resonance imaging findings in a pediatric cohort with chiari 1 malformation. Can Respir J 2015; 22(1):31–6.

103. Zolty P, Sanders MH, Pollack IF. Chiari malformation and sleep-disordered breathing: a review of diagnostic and management issues. Sleep 2000; 23(5):637–43. Available at: http://www.ncbi.nlm.nih.gov/pubmed/10947031.

104. Leu RM. Sleep-related breathing disorders and the chiari 1 malformation. Chest 2015;148(5):1346–52.

105. Amaddeo A, Frapin A, Fauroux B. Long-term noninvasive ventilation in children. Lancet Respir Med 2016;4(12):999–1008.

Noninvasive Ventilation in Amyotrophic Lateral Sclerosis

Jessica A. Cooksey, MD[a], Amen Sergew, MD[b],*

KEYWORDS

- Amyotrophic lateral sclerosis • Noninvasive ventilation • Bulbar ALS
- Noninvasive positive pressure ventilation

KEY POINTS

- Amyotrophic lateral sclerosis (ALS) is a devastating neurodegenerative disease involving upper and lower motor neurons.
- Progressive weakness involving the respiratory muscles leads to respiratory failure and death.
- Home noninvasive ventilation (NIV) improves survival and quality of life, especially in those with intact bulbar function.
- Following NIV initiation, it is important to monitor symptomatic response and surrogates for gas exchange, such as nocturnal oximetry and remote monitoring of home NIV. Additionally, when available, transcutaneous CO2 monitoring and sleep studies can be considered in patients with persistent issues.

INTRODUCTION

Amyotrophic lateral sclerosis (ALS) is a devastating neurodegenerative disease that affects upper and lower motor neurons, leading to progressive weakness and, ultimately, paralysis of skeletal muscles. Onset of weakness in ALS can occur first in the limbs, bulbar muscles (muscles that coordinate speech, mastication, and swallowing) or, much less commonly, in the respiratory muscles. Irrespective of the initial distribution of affected muscles, weakness progresses to involve the diaphragms, leading first to disrupted sleep, then respiratory insufficiency, and ultimately respiratory failure and death. Respiratory failure is the leading cause of death in ALS, accounting for more than 80% of mortality seen in the disease.[1] There is currently no cure for ALS, and in the absence of treatment, the median time from symptom onset to death is 3 years.[2] Although the ultimate outcome of ALS is similar regardless of which muscles are affected first, the pattern of onset is an important prognostic indicator. Patients with bulbar weakness at the time of symptom onset have been reported to have shorter median survival times.[2,3] Other predictors of poorer prognosis include older age at onset and more rapid rate of decline in pulmonary function.[2,3]

Currently, there are a few interventions that have the potential to improve outcomes in ALS. Riluzole, which inhibits glutaminergic neurotransmission, has been shown to prolong survival by about 3 months.[4,5] Edaravone, a free radical scavenger, confers modest improvements in functional outcomes in selected patients but has not been shown to affect mortality.[6–8] Home noninvasive ventilation (NIV), which is interchangeably called noninvasive positive pressure ventilation, has been shown to improve survival and quality of life, although a survival benefit has been inconsistently reported in patients with significant bulbar dysfunction.[9]

[a] Northwestern University, 1475 East Belvidere Road, Suite 185, Grayslake, IL 60030, USA; [b] Division of Pulmonary, Critical Care and Sleep Medicine, Section of Critical Care Medicine, Department of Medicine, National Jewish Health, 1400 Jackson Street, B140, Denver, CO 80207, USA
* Corresponding author.
E-mail address: sergewa@njhealth.org

Sleep Med Clin 15 (2020) 527–538
https://doi.org/10.1016/j.jsmc.2020.08.004
1556-407X/20/Published by Elsevier Inc.

IMPACT OF NONINVASIVE VENTILATION ON AMYOTROPHIC LATERAL SCLEROSIS
Benefits of Noninvasive Ventilation on Survival and Quality of Life

Several observational studies have demonstrated that NIV confers mortality and quality of life benefits in ALS.[10–17] In the only randomized, controlled trial of NIV in ALS published to date, this finding was confirmed. Bourke and colleagues[9] randomized patients with ALS to NIV or standard care when they developed orthopnea with maximum inspiratory pressure less than 60 cm H_2O, symptomatic hypercapnia (defined as an Epworth Sleepiness Scale score of 10 or higher), or morning headache accompanied by hypercapnia on an arterial blood gas. Among all patients, median survival was 48 days longer among those treated with NIV than in those who received standard care. This benefit was driven by patients with relatively intact bulbar function. No mortality benefit was seen in patients with severe bulbar dysfunction. Among those with preserved bulbar function, treatment with NIV led to a 205-day improvement in median survival. Quality of life, sleep-related quality of life, and the duration of time during which quality of life remained at least 75% of baseline were significantly higher in the group treated with NIV. This suggests that patients with preserved bulbar function lived longer and did so with reasonably preserved quality of life. These quality of life differences were greater in patients with preserved bulbar function, although patients with severe bulbar dysfunction did show a benefit on measures of dyspnea and sleep-related quality of life.

Patterns of use of positive airway pressure (PAP) were different among patients with preserved bulbar function versus those with severe bulbar dysfunction. Mean NIV use among patients with preserved bulbar function was 9.3 hours per day, whereas among those with severe bulbar dysfunction, mean use was 3.8 hours per day. Overall, participants randomized to NIV received bilevel PAP with a mean inspiratory PAP (IPAP) of 15 cm H_2O pressure and mean expiratory PAP (EPAP) of 4 cm H_2O pressure. Patients with preserved bulbar function tolerated pressures that were 23% higher than those tolerated by patients with severe bulbar dysfunction. This study could not answer definitively whether a survival benefit was not seen among patients with severe bulbar dysfunction because they were less tolerant of PAP or because PAP does not confer a survival advantage in this subgroup of patients. It was noted, however, that hours of PAP use did not correlate with improved survival among patients with severe bulbar dysfunction, suggesting that for patients with severe bulbar dysfunction, improving NIV adherence may not improve survival. Other observational series have reported a survival benefit of NIV in patients with bulbar dysfunction, although it has been reported to be more modest in patients without bulbar dysfunction.[16,17] A single retrospective cohort study reported better survival in patients with bulbar-onset disease than those with limb-onset disease.[18]

Other Benefits of Noninvasive Ventilation: Sleep Quality, Oxygenation, Ventilation, Lung Function, and Energy Expenditure

NIV has also been shown to have other important impacts in ALS. It improves not just subjective measures of sleep-related quality of life, but also objective polysomnographic measures of sleep quality.[19,20] It has been shown to increase the time spent in rapid eye movement sleep and slow wave sleep, and to reduce the microarousal index.[19,20] Nocturnal oxygenation and transcutaneous carbon dioxide are also improved with NIV.[19–21] As with mortality and quality of life measures, objective improvements in sleep quality, nocturnal oxygenation, and ventilation have been disproportionately described in patients without significant bulbar dysfunction. In addition to improving subjective measures of dyspnea, NIV has been shown in two studies to slow the rate of decline in vital capacity.[10,15] In a study that used indirect calorimetry to measure energy expenditure, NIV was shown to reduce resting energy expenditure.[22] This suggests that NIV has the potential to slow the weight loss that typifies ALS and portends a poor prognosis.[23]

INDICATIONS FOR NONINVASIVE VENTILATION IN AMYOTROPHIC LATERAL SCLEROSIS
Society Guidelines

Drawing on much of the evidence detailed previously, the current American Academy of Neurology guidelines on the care of the patient with ALS recommend considering the initiation of NIV in patients with respiratory insufficiency to prolong survival, slow the rate of forced vital capacity (FVC) decline, and enhance quality of life.[24]

The issue of when in the course of disease to initiate NIV is an evolving one. In the early studies of NIV in ALS, NIV was typically started in symptomatic patients with advanced neuromuscular weakness. For example, in Bourke and colleagues,[9] patients had to have orthopnea with an maximum inspiratory pressure less than 60 cm H_2O or symptomatic daytime hypercapnia. Current Medicare guidelines on the timing of initiation of NIV in neuromuscular disease largely reflect this inclination, although there is mounting evidence that waiting for symptomatic respiratory insufficiency and development of the frank gas exchange abnormalities that characterize advanced neuromuscular disease is not optimal, and patients may benefit from earlier initiation of NIV. In contrast to current practice in the United States, the European Federation of Neuroscience guidelines recommend considering initiation of NIV earlier in disease, when the FVC falls less than 80% predicted.[25]

Centers for Medicare and Medicaid Services Guidelines

The current Centers for Medicare and Medicaid Services (CMS) clinical indications for the use of respiratory-assist device therapy (RAD) in neuromuscular disease arise from a consensus conference report published in 1999 by the National Association for Medical Direction of Respiratory Care.[26] These guidelines were drafted in response to rising rates of use and consequent rising costs associated with provision of NIV for a variety of disorders, in the absence of clear guidelines to direct appropriate use. These consensus guidelines recommend that "appropriate symptoms attributable to nocturnal hypoventilation should first be identified" in patients with neuromuscular disease.[26] In terms of specific clinical criteria, the current CMS RAD guidelines largely reflect the National Association for Medical Direction of Respiratory Care consensus conference report, and recommend the initiation of NIV if any of the following criteria are met:

- FVC <50% predicted
- Maximum inspiratory pressure <60 cm H_2O pressure or sniff nasal pressure <40 cm H_2O pressure
- Arterial blood gas (performed while awake) with $Paco_2$ ≥45 mm Hg
- Nocturnal oxyhemoglobin saturation ≤88% for ≥5 minutes (with a minimum recording time of 2 hours on the patient's prescribed fraction of inspired oxygen)

The CMS RAD criteria further require that the clinician document the following:

- The presence of neuromuscular disease
- Chronic obstructive pulmonary disease does not contribute significantly to the patient's pulmonary limitation

For neuromuscular disease, the decision to use a machine that is only able to deliver a spontaneous mode of ventilation or a machine able to deliver a back-up respiratory rate is left to the judgment of the prescribing clinician in the current CMS RAD guidelines. It should be noted that different criteria apply for other sleep-related hypoventilatory disorders, such as obesity hypoventilation syndrome (discussed in Roop Kaw and Marta Kaminska's article, "Obesity Hypoventilation: Traditional Versus Nontraditional Populations," in this issue) and hypercapnic chronic obstructive pulmonary disease (discussed in Jeremy E. Orr and colleagues' article, "Management of Chronic Respiratory Failure in Chronic Obstructive Pulmonary Disease: High-Intensity and Low-Intensity Ventilation," in this issue). The CMS RAD guidelines apply to devices that are able to deliver NIV with or without a back-up respiratory rate, but which do not have internal batteries or the ability for the patient to readily switch between different modes of ventilation, such as nighttime bilevel PAP via a mask and daytime mouthpiece ventilation. Devices with an internal battery and with the ability to provide different modes of ventilation for daytime and nighttime are classified as home mechanical ventilators and are regulated slightly differently by CMS.[27]

Although the one available randomized controlled trial of NIV in ALS and most observational data suggest that NIV is not as well tolerated and the benefits more modest in bulbar ALS than in nonbulbar ALS, the CMS RAD guidelines do not make a distinction between bulbar and nonbulbar disease. Nor should the clinician necessarily make a distinction in the decision to offer NIV to a patient, given that there is still demonstrated benefit, albeit more modest, in those patients with significant bulbar dysfunction. Adjustments to the NIV prescription, however, may be advisable in patients with significant bulbar dysfunction, given that in most published series, patients with bulbar dysfunction have been noted to tolerate lower pressures than patients without bulbar dysfunction.

EARLY SCREENING AND INITIATION OF NONINVASIVE VENTILATION

Initial reports of NIV in ALS examined primarily patients with advanced disease and gas exchange abnormalities. Subsequent studies have demonstrated that outcomes may be improved with provision of NIV earlier in the disease. Limited data suggest that NIV adherence remains reasonable with early initiation of NIV.

Impact of Early Initiation of Noninvasive Ventilation on Survival

Several studies have reported an added survival benefit when NIV is initiated before FVC falls less than 50% predicted.[17,28–30] In a retrospective cohort study of 474 patients, Khamankar and colleagues[17] reported an overall survival benefit of NIV in bulbar and nonbulbar ALS, although the impact was smaller in patients with bulbar dysfunction. In that cohort, improved survival correlated with earlier initiation of NIV (FVC $\geq$80% predicted), and with increased hours of nightly use of NIV and concomitant use of a cough-assist device for airway clearance. Median survival among patients who started NIV when FVC was less than 50% predicted was 20.3 months, whereas among patients who started NIV when FVC was greater than or equal to 80% predicted, median survival was 25.36 months. Another retrospective cohort study examined early (FVC <80% predicted) versus very early (FVC $\geq$80% predicted) initiation of NIV, and reported a 4-month survival benefit with initiation of NIV with FVC greater than or equal to 80% predicted.[29]

Impact of Early Initiation of Noninvasive Ventilation on Forced Vital Capacity

In a pilot, randomized, sham-controlled clinical trial, Jacobs and colleagues[31] randomized patients with FVC greater than 50% predicted to either bilevel PAP set at IPAP of 8 cm H_2O pressure and EPAP of 4 cm H_2O pressure (without titration) or sham. In the sham group, participants received continuous PAP 4 cm H_2O pressure via a nasal mask with an enlarged exhalation port that effectively reduced the measured delivered pressure to less than 1 cm H_2O. Participants in the sham group were converted to active NIV when they developed symptoms of respiratory insufficiency or their FVC fell less than 50% predicted. At the time of study enrollment, median FVC was 76.5% predicted in the active NIV group and 79.5% predicted in the sham group. This pilot study was powered primarily to look at NIV adherence, not survival or respiratory function, but did find that the rate of decline in FVC was slower in the group treated with early NIV.[31]

Impact of Early Initiation of Noninvasive Ventilation on Adherence

A retrospective cohort study reported no difference in NIV adherence rates with initiation of NIV when FVC was less than 80% versus when FVC greater than 80% predicted.[32]

MODES OF NONINVASIVE VENTILATION IN AMYOTROPHIC LATERAL SCLEROSIS
Fixed Bilevel Positive Airway Pressure

Home NIV modes and devices are discussed in depth in Gaurav Singh and Michelle Cao's article,

"Noninvasive Ventilator Devices and Modes," in this issue. Home NIV is typically delivered via a single limb mask interface, with a vented mask that allows for CO_2 escape connected to a machine that is able to provide separately adjustable IPAP and EPAP settings. The most straightforward of these is fixed bilevel PAP, in which the EPAP level is set to maintain upper airway patency (eg, in the case of concomitant ALS and obstructive sleep apnea) and the IPAP is set to provide pressure support to maintain an adequate tidal volume (V_T). Fixed bilevel PAP is available in spontaneous (S) mode (no backup respiratory rate), spontaneous/timed (ST) mode (backup respiratory rate available, activated only if patient's respiratory rate falls lower than set backup rate), and timed (T) mode (breaths delivered at a set rate, independent of patient triggering). The timed mode (T) is infrequently used, because it is not designed for patient-device synchrony.[33] For patients with ALS, a backup respiratory rate is recommended.[34]

Volume-Assured Pressure Support

Volume-assured pressure support (VAPS) is a mode of bilevel PAP in which the IPAP and therefore the pressure support is adjusted automatically to achieve a target level of ventilation. The clinician sets a target V_T (average VAPS, Respironics, Murrysville, PA), or a target alveolar ventilation (V_A) (intelligent VAPS, ResMed, San Diego, CA) based on the patient's ideal body weight. The device algorithms calculate an average V_T or V_A over several breaths, and adjust the pressure support accordingly within a range determined by the clinician, to achieve the target V_T or V_A. The theoretic advantage of these modalities in the setting of progressive neuromuscular weakness is that the device automatically increases the pressure support over time as patients inevitably weaken and require more support to maintain adequate V_T. This has the potential to be particularly advantageous for patients who are not able to travel to clinic for frequent reassessment of the adequacy of their settings, either for reasons of distance or physical disability.

Some devices that are capable of providing VAPS modes of ventilation must be set with a fixed EPAP. In the absence of upper airway obstruction, patients with ALS generally benefit from minimal EPAP (eg, EPAP 4 cm H_2O pressure), to help minimize work of breathing.[33] Patients with issues with upper airway patency may benefit from increased EPAP, and EPAP requirements may vary throughout the night or from night to night. In this case, there are some machines that can provide automatically adjusting EPAP levels, which detect airflow limitation and adjust EPAP accordingly with a goal of maintaining upper airway patency.

Evidence for Particular Modes of Noninvasive Ventilation

In a randomized crossover trial of VAPS (iVAPS, ResMed) versus standard pressure support for patients with hypoventilation, slightly lower pressure support (8.3 cm H_2O pressure vs 10.0 cm H_2O pressure) was required with VAPS to achieve similar nocturnal oxygenation and transcutaneous CO_2 (TCO_2), with no differences in sleep quality and slightly better adherence to VAPS (5 hours 40 minutes vs 4 hours 20 minutes).[35] In a retrospective review of VAPS versus pressure support, fewer patients achieved their target V_T with pressure support, and the rapid shallow breathing index (respiratory rate/V_T) was higher with pressure support, suggesting increased work of breathing.[36]

Patient-Device Synchrony

In addition to selecting the mode of ventilation, clinicians have the option to adjust features of the pressure waveform, such as inspiratory time (T_i), rise time, trigger sensitivity, and cycle sensitivity to optimize synchrony between the patient and the machine.[33] This is particularly important in ALS, because progressive diaphragmatic weakness can make it difficult for patients to trigger and cycle, and longer T_i can help optimize gas exchange. Selection of these settings should be performed by an experienced clinician and/or respiratory therapist, and should be guided by patient comfort. In general, patients with ALS benefit from a high trigger sensitivity, low cycle sensitivity, slow rise time, and long T_i.[33] Appropriate mask fitting for comfort and to minimize unintentional mask leak is also essential.

Noninvasive Ventilation: Summary and Suggested Initial Settings

Irrespective of the mode of NIV selected, particular attention should be paid to the following:

- Ensuring an adequate V_T, with a target of 8 mL/kg ideal body weight
- Provision of a backup respiratory rate and high trigger sensitivity to ensure adequate minute ventilation and maximize patient-device synchrony
- Conversion to a device with an internal battery and the ability to provide mouthpiece ventilation at the point at which the patient requires respiratory support during wakefulness
- Appropriate follow-up and monitoring to assess adherence and adequacy of gas exchange

In an excellent review on the initiation of NIV for sleep-related hypoventilation disorders, Selim and colleagues[33] provide suggested initial settings, summarized in **Table 1**. Additionally, Gaurav Singh and Michelle Cao's article, "Noninvasive Ventilator Devices and Modes"; and Philip Choi and colleagues' article, "Noninvasive Ventilation Downloads and Monitoring," in this issue discuss noninvasive ventilator devices and modes, and long-term follow-up of NIV (downloads and troubleshooting).

For Respironics respiratory-assist devices (eg, DreamStation) and home ventilator (Trilogy), VAPS is considered add-on software. The mode of NIV must first be selected[33]:

- Spontaneous (S)
- Spontaneous timed (ST): mandatory T_i delivered only with timed breaths and not with spontaneous breaths
- Timed (T): mandatory T_i delivered with all breaths and is not used because it is not designed for patient-device synchrony
- Pressure control (PC): mandatory T_i delivered with spontaneous and timed breaths

Patients with ALS should typically receive PC AVAPS or PC ST, because it ensures that they receive consistent, adequate T_i with all breaths.

For the ResMed respiratory assist device (AirCurve 10 ST, AirCurve 10 ST-A) and home ventilator (Astral), the devices are set in iVAPS without first setting an additional mode. In this mode, T_i is delivered with spontaneous and timed breaths.

Noninvasive Ventilation During Wakefulness/Daytime Ventilation

When patients with ALS develop dyspnea during wakefulness, it is appropriate to transition to a ventilator with an internal battery. These devices are portable, allowing patients to safely and comfortably travel outside the home with ventilatory support. Daytime support is provided via a mask using a bilevel PAP or VAPS mode. It can also be delivered using mouthpiece ventilation in a volume- or pressure-controlled mode.[33] Devices with internal batteries are generally capable of providing multiple programs (eg, nighttime bilevel PAP via a mask and daytime volume-controlled ventilation via a mouthpiece).

NONINVASIVE VENTILATION FAILURE: CAUSES AND SUGGESTED SOLUTIONS

Adherence to NIV has been shown to correlate with improved mortality in ALS.[10,12] Several authors have reported that severe bulbar dysfunction

Table 1
Suggested NIV settings and titration for patients with ALS

Impact on respiratory mechanics	↓ Muscle capacity ↑ Chest wall resistance
Target tidal volume (mL)	Target tidal volume 8 mL/kg ideal body weight
IPAP (cm H_2O)	Intermediate IPAP (or best tolerated) Adjust IPAP to a PS for tidal volume goal in BPAP-ST Allow IPAP min at a higher baseline Set IPAP max higher than the 90%/95% delivered value (for AVAPS or iVAPS, to allow for automatic increase in IPAP with further weakening)
EPAP (cm H_2O)	Low EPAP to reduce work of breathing and improve triggering

Respiratory rate (bpm)	Adjust to goal minute ventilation based on ABG, $TcCO_2$, or both
	   Respironics: use fixed RR, not autoset, to avoid mimicking a high RR, low V_T pattern (thereby increasing work of breathing)
	   ResMed: use "intelligent" backup rate, backup shifts between two-thirds of the set rate during spontaneous breaths, and the set rate during periods of apnea

Trigger sensitivity	High trigger sensitivity to support a weak respiratory muscle effort
	   Respironics: flow trigger at 1–3 L/min; do not use autotrak function because it is not validated in neuromuscular weakness
	   ResMed: trigger high or very high

Rise time	Default or slow rise time
	   Respironics: 3 (300 ms)–6 (600 ms)
	   ResMed: 500–900 ms
	Patients with significant bulbar dysfunction are likely to need a slower rise time; those with minimal bulbar symptoms benefit from faster rise time

Ti (ms)	Long Ti or long Ti minimum to maximize tidal volume and gas exchange (↑I:E) Ti/Ttot 50% Respironics: Ti applies to mandatory (timed) breaths only in fixed or adjusting bilevel PAP mode; in pressure control mode, Ti applies to mandatory (timed) and spontaneous breaths ResMed: Ti applies to mandatory (timed) and spontaneous breaths

Cycle sensitivity	Default or low cycle sensitivity (late cycle) to provide a longer inhalation time (maximize tidal volume and gas exchange by high I:E)
	   Respironics: manual at 10%–15% of peak flow; do not use autotrak function because it is not validated in neuromuscular weakness
	   ResMed: cycle low or very low

Titration	Adjust PS (BPAP-ST), expiratory tidal volume (AVAPS), or Va (iVAPS) based on ABG (pH, $PaCO_2$), $TcCO_2$, overnight oximetry, serum bicarbonate, work of breathing, patient comfort, or a combination Patients with significant bulbar dysfunction may be less tolerant of higher pressures (and therefore less tolerant of higher V_T or Va if VAPS mode is selected)

Abbreviations: ABG, arterial blood gas; ALS, Amyotrophic lateral sclerosis; AVAPS, Average Volume Assured Pressure Support; Va, alveolar ventilation; BPAP-ST (bilevel positive airway pressure - spontaneous/timed mode); BPAP, bilevel PAP; IPAP, inspiratory positive airway pressure; iVAPS, intelligent volume-assured pressure support; I:E inspiratory:expiratory; Ti: inspiratory time; NIV, non-invasive ventilation; PS, pressure support; PaCO2, partial pressure of carbon dioxide in arterial blood; RR, respiratory rate; TcCO2, transcutaneous carbon dioxide; VT, tidal volume.

Adapted from Selim BJ, Wolfe L, Coleman JM, 3rd, Dewan NA. Initiation of Noninvasive Ventilation for Sleep Related Hypoventilation Disorders: Advanced Modes and Devices. Chest. 2018;153(1):251-65; with permission.

is a risk factor for NIV failure.[10,11,16,37–39] Predictors of NIV failure in bulbar patients include the severity of bulbar function and the degree of nocturnal hypoxemia.[16] Failure was noted in one study of mostly patients with bulbar ALS to be linked to upper airways obstruction, which was a marker of poor prognosis.[40] Additionally, bulbar patients can have more difficulty with leak from nasal masks because of incomplete mouth closure, especially during sleep.

Factors that can lead to NIV intolerance include sialorrhea with associated drooling, choking, and aspiration and viscous bronchial secretions, which can lead to recurrent infections.[16,38,41] Frontotemporal dementia has been shown to decrease survival in patients with ALS and also leads to NIV noncompliance in patients with ALS with bulbar and limb-onset.[42]

Spasticity is a common feature of ALS.[43] Although large muscle spasms are a more frequently described characteristic of ALS, laryngospasm has also been described.[44–46] Daytime episodes of laryngospasm are distressing for patients and caregivers, and nighttime episodes can contribute to poor tolerance of NIV, particularly in patients with significant bulbar dysfunction. Several authors have described the use of low-dose benzodiazepines as needed for laryngospasm.[44,46]

Suggested Solutions: Communication

Factors that can impact NIV success include improved communication regarding the goals of NIV. At the time of NIV initiation, patients' and their caregivers' understanding of the benefits of NIV in ALS can lead to improved adherence.[41]

Suggested Solutions: Inpatient Initiation of Noninvasive Ventilation

In-patient initiation of NIV, either overnight in-laboratory titration or with multiple days in the hospital with close involvement of respiratory therapists, has been shown to improve tolerance. In one study, this entailed a prolonged hospitalization with a mean of 12 days to reach normalization of nocturnal oximetry and arterial blood gas.[47] Unfortunately, this is not feasible in some health care systems because of reimbursement issues. In that case, home setup or a PAP nap titration (which entails a PAP titration during a brief daytime clinic visit or daytime visit to the sleep laboratory) are the alternatives. When initiating NIV in the outpatient setting, factors linked with the improvement of NIV tolerance include discussion of potential obstacles at the time of initiation and providing in-home support for patients.[41]

Suggested Solutions: Improved Airway Clearance and Bulbar Symptoms

For severe bulbar patients, consider delaying NIV initiation until airway clearance and sialorrhea have been addressed. Mechanical insufflation/exsufflation initiation can improve airway clearance. In patients with refractory sialorrhea, severe laryngospasm, and recurrent infections, invasive ventilation is considered. Baclofen or dextromethorphan/quinidine (Nuedexta) do not improve the respiratory components of the Revised ALS Functional Rating Scale but do improve the bulbar component significantly[48] and may be useful adjunct therapies at the time of initiation of NIV. Consider low pressures, such as an IPAP 6 to 8 cm H_2O and an EPAP of 3 to 5 cm H_2O in bulbar patients at the time of NIV initiation.[9,44] Following NIV initiation, bulbar patients need close follow-up with careful attention to mask fit and airway clearance.

LONG-TERM MONITORING OF NONINVASIVE VENTILATION IN AMYOTROPHIC LATERAL SCLEROSIS

Once NIV has been initiated in a patient with ALS, follow-up can include an evaluation of symptomatic response and assessment of objective improvement in gas exchange. A detailed discussion of long-term monitoring of home NIV appears in Philip Choi and colleagues' article, "Noninvasive Ventilation Downloads and Monitoring," in this issue. Briefly, this is accomplished with nocturnal oximetry, remote monitoring of home NIV, TCO_2 monitoring, and sleep studies. Our recommendations in regards to long-term monitoring of NIV are summarized in **Fig. 1**.

Nocturnal Oximetry

Nocturnal oximetry is a widely available modality that is useful for long-term monitoring of NIV. Ventilatory asynchrony can occur during sleep and can result in nocturnal hypoxemia despite minimal symptoms.[49] Optimization of nocturnal oxygenation with NIV has also been shown to correlate with improved mortality.[50] Nocturnal oximetry can evaluate for not only the presence and extent of desaturation, but also the patterns of desaturation, which may also hint at the cause of ventilatory asynchrony.[51] For example, intermittent desaturations (ie, an elevated oxygen desaturation index) can suggest upper airway obstruction and are generally caused by oropharyngeal collapse similar to obstructive sleep apnea. These can often be resolved with increased EPAP.[52] In a retrospective observational study, Gonzalez-

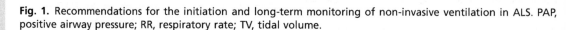

Initiate NIV:
- Location:
  - Overnight titration in sleep lab
  - In-patient titration over multiple days
  - PAP nap
  - In-home titration
- Weekly review of downloads for the first month
- Screening serum bicarbonate
- Nocturnal oximetry after one month

Long-term monitoring:
- Every 3 mo or with worsened symptoms or adherence:
  - Review downloads: TV, RR, leak, average hours of nightly use, % patient triggered breaths
  - Check serum bicarbonate
  - Nocturnal Oximetry
- Consider transcutaneous CO2 monitoring If available

Persistent NIV Failure Despite Adjustments:
- Consider a home sleep study (polygraphy) or polysomnography

Fig. 1. Recommendations for the initiation and long-term monitoring of non-invasive ventilation in ALS. PAP, positive airway pressure; RR, respiratory rate; TV, tidal volume.

Bermejo and colleagues[50] reported on the use of nocturnal oximetry to ascertain the effectiveness of home NIV. In this study, nocturnal oximetry with home sleep study, spirometry, and arterial blood gas were evaluated in the first month then every 3 months for the first year following initiation of NIV. Group 1 had "corrected ventilation" defined as tolerating NIV, nocturnal oximetry less than 90% for less than 5% of the time, and improved symptoms and blood gases in the first month. Group 2 did not meet these criteria in the first month. Following this, adjustments were made to optimize NIV use at month 1 and then every 3 months thereafter. The only significant difference between the two groups was the nocturnal oximetry results in the first month. The 12-month survival was 75% in the group 1 patients, whereas for group 2 patients, it was 43%. This difference was noted despite similar improvements in daytime symptoms and daytime blood gas results.[50] Group 2 patients who underwent adjustment of their NIV settings at months 1 and 3, resulting in appropriate ventilation in month 6, had no significant mortality difference at 12 months when compared with group 1. If adequate ventilation was not achieved by month 6 in group 2, mortality was higher than in group 1. Taken together, these findings highlight the importance of frequent assessment of nocturnal oxygenation with nocturnal oximetry, especially in the first 6 months following initiation of NIV.

Remote Monitoring

Remote monitoring of NIV devices has also advanced the care of patients on home NIV. Remote access provides data downloads of NIV machines without an in-person visit, via an internal or external modem associated with the patient's machine and a cloud-based data storage system maintained by the device manufacturers. Various factors are important to monitor ventilation adequacy, such as the exhaled V_T, respiratory rate, leak, and the percent of patient triggering breaths.[51,52] The downloaded data also document adherence and patterns of use. Additionally, evaluation of the flow and pressure curve tracings can help identify some causes of asynchrony and where adjustments should be made to the settings or device.[53] Adjustments are made remotely and on RAD machines. For regulatory reasons, adjustments cannot be made remotely on home ventilators, such as the ResMed Astral or Respironics Trilogy. For those devices, remote downloads are obtained, but adjustments must be made in person.

A research group in Portugal demonstrated the benefits of remote monitoring. The control group was 20 patients with ALS that had a clinic visit 2 to 3 weeks after initiation of NIV then every 3 months thereafter. Another 20 patients were assigned to the treatment group and had a modem that allowed for data transmission weekly or whenever patients reported difficulties. Based on these data, NIV parameters could be adjusted remotely. Both groups were followed from the time of NIV initiation to 3 years or death. The remote monitoring group had fewer office visits and emergency room or in-hospital admissions. In this group, there was also a trend toward a survival benefit ($P = .13$).[47]

Transcutaneous CO₂ Monitoring

TCO_2 monitoring has been shown to correlate well with blood gas analysis.[54] Although it does not provide a detailed evaluation of a patient's acid base balance, it can help delineate between hypoxia caused by ventilation/perfusion mismatch and that caused by hypoventilation. This is useful especially in younger patients with intact cardiovascular systems where desaturation is less likely during hypoventilation. TCO_2 monitoring can also help identify NIV-induced hyperventilation, which can lead to central apneas and glottic closures.[51] Despite these benefits, TCO_2 is less used than nocturnal oximetry because of cost and limited availability.

Polysomnography

There are significant variations among centers on the use of polysomnography (PSG) for NIV initiation and titration in ALS and no guidelines exist that address this subject. PSGs have been shown to help in the initiation and titration of NIV, leading to improvement of oxygen saturation, hypercapnia, and apnea-hypopnea-index. This results in improved daytime sleepiness, depression, and quality of life.[19,20,55,56]

Patients with ALS can have fragmented sleep because of arousals related to limited ability to change positions and pain. One group of researchers conducted a split-night PSG on all of their patients with ALS and found that almost half had incomplete testing mainly because of poor sleep efficiency and absence of rapid eye movement sleep.[57] In preparing for a PSG in patients with ALS, taking measures to address ALS-specific concerns may improve the success rate and usefulness in PSGs.

Measures to create comfort for this patient population may include a Hoyer lift, a call bell that is easily accessible, other aids to address pain and positioning during sleep, and allowing bed partners or caretakers to also spend the night. Sialorrhea can also impact sleep and a suction machine for these patients is helpful. An experienced and attentive staff can increase the success of a PSG. An in-depth discussion of how to tailor a sleep laboratory for various neuromuscular diseases is provided in Justin A. Fiala and John M. Coleman III's article, "Tailoring the Sleep Laboratory for Chronic Respiratory Failure," in this issue.

One single-centered study evaluated the use of PSG on treatment-naive patients of which 88% had neuromuscular weakness.[58] All of the patients initially had a daytime titration with a PAP nap in a modified sleep laboratory using a protocol that took a minimum of 4 hours. This was followed by 2 to 3 weeks of acclimatization with patients using NIV in their homes. After this period, patients returned for a full night PSG titration or a sham titration (where no adjustments were made to settings). The patients who underwent PSG titration had a lower incidence of ventilator asynchrony. Adherence improved in patients with poor adherence before PSG (defined as use <4 hours per day during the acclimatization period). There was a mean increase in NIV use by 95 min/d in the group who had a PSG and a decrease in use of 23 minutes in the sham group ($P = .01$).[58]

Respiratory Polygraphy (Home Sleep Testing)

Respiratory polygraphy (home sleep testing) may present a more cost-effective and less time consuming alternative to PSG. Polygraphy excludes the use of electroencephalogram, electrooculogram, and chin electromyogram, which are used in PSGs for sleep-wake differentiation and the analysis of sleep architecture. One study evaluated patients with ALS with polygraphy and found that it was useful in patients with FVC greater than 75% because it helped to detect nocturnal hypoventilation, resulting in earlier initiation of NIV.[59] Polygraphy, similar to PSG (but not nocturnal oximetry), provides the ability to identify issues with upper airway patency. If impaired upper airway patency is identified, adjustments are made to improve compliance and ventilation.[60]

Overall, PSG or polygraphy can be considered in patients who have persistent symptoms and other causes of NIV failure. Given the significant cost, limitation of resources, and the burden on patients and their families associated with these tests, identifying the appropriate patients for PSG and polygraphy is important.

SUMMARY

ALS is a progressive neurodegenerative disease that affects upper and lower motor neurons and has limited treatment options. Ultimately, the involvement of the diaphragm leads to respiratory failure and NIV is the main intervention used for the management of this. NIV can improve survival, quality of life, and dyspnea symptoms. Bulbar patients have more difficulty with NIV tolerance and therefore with adherence. Even with better adherence, the benefits of NIV are less robust in bulbar patients as compared with those with limb-onset ALS. Fixed or adjusting bilevel PAP is used for NIV. Once initiated, close monitoring with nocturnal oximetry, remote downloads from the home NIV machine, measurement of serum bicarbonate, and TCO_2 monitoring should be conducted, especially in bulbar patients. Adjusting the various settings on the machine (eg, IPAP, EPAP, T_i, rise time, trigger sensitivity, and cycle sensitivity) can help improve synchrony, adherence, and efficacy with regard to symptoms and gas exchange. PSG and respiratory polygraphy have the potential to identify asynchrony and, in the case of PSG, to make real-time adjustment to settings to improve synchrony, thereby improving NIV success. These are rarely done because of cost and inconvenience for patients and their caregivers. During later disease, transitioning to a home ventilator with an internal battery is imperative for safety and portability.

DISCLOSURE

The authors have no disclosures or conflicts of interest.

REFERENCES

1. Gordon PH, Corcia P, Lacomblez L, et al. Defining survival as an outcome measure in amyotrophic lateral sclerosis. Arch Neurol 2009;66(6):758–61.
2. Haverkamp LJ, Appel V, Appel SH. Natural history of amyotrophic lateral sclerosis in a database population. Validation of a scoring system and a model for survival prediction. Brain 1995;118(Pt 3):707–19.
3. Ringel SP, Murphy JR, Alderson MK, et al. The natural history of amyotrophic lateral sclerosis. Neurology 1993;43(7):1316–22.
4. Bensimon G, Lacomblez L, Meininger V. A controlled trial of riluzole in amyotrophic lateral sclerosis. ALS/Riluzole Study Group. N Engl J Med 1994;330(9):585–91.
5. Lacomblez L, Bensimon G, Leigh PN, et al. Dose-ranging study of riluzole in amyotrophic lateral sclerosis. Amyotrophic Lateral Sclerosis/Riluzole Study Group II. Lancet 1996;347(9013):1425–31.
6. Abe K, Itoyama Y, Sobue G, et al. Confirmatory double-blind, parallel-group, placebo-controlled study of efficacy and safety of edaravone (MCI-186) in amyotrophic lateral sclerosis patients. Amyotroph Lateral Scler Frontotemporal Degener 2014;15(7–8):610–7.
7. Yoshino H, Kimura A. Investigation of the therapeutic effects of edaravone, a free radical scavenger, on amyotrophic lateral sclerosis (phase II study). Amyotroph Lateral Scler 2006;7(4):241–5.
8. Writing G, Edaravone ALSSG. Safety and efficacy of edaravone in well defined patients with amyotrophic lateral sclerosis: a randomised, double-blind, placebo-controlled trial. Lancet Neurol 2017;16(7):505–12.
9. Bourke SC, Tomlinson M, Williams TL, et al. Effects of non-invasive ventilation on survival and quality of life in patients with amyotrophic lateral sclerosis: a randomised controlled trial. Lancet Neurol 2006;5(2):140–7.
10. Bourke SC, Bullock RE, Williams TL, et al. Noninvasive ventilation in ALS: indications and effect on quality of life. Neurology 2003;61(2):171–7.
11. Aboussouan LS, Khan SU, Meeker DP, et al. Effect of noninvasive positive-pressure ventilation on survival in amyotrophic lateral sclerosis. Ann Intern Med 1997;127(6):450–3.
12. Kleopa KA, Sherman M, Neal B, et al. Bipap improves survival and rate of pulmonary function decline in patients with ALS. J Neurol Sci 1999;164(1):82–8.
13. Pinto AC, Evangelista T, Carvalho M, et al. Respiratory assistance with a non-invasive ventilator (Bipap) in MND/ALS patients: survival rates in a controlled trial. J Neurol Sci 1995;129(Suppl):19–26.
14. Hirose T, Kimura F, Tani H, et al. Clinical characteristics of long-term survival with noninvasive ventilation and factors affecting the transition to invasive ventilation in amyotrophic lateral sclerosis. Muscle Nerve 2018;58(6):770–6.
15. Leonardis L, Dolenc Groselj L, Vidmar G. Factors related to respiration influencing survival and respiratory function in patients with amyotrophic lateral sclerosis: a retrospective study. Eur J Neurol 2012;19(12):1518–24.
16. Sancho J, Martinez D, Bures E, et al. Bulbar impairment score and survival of stable amyotrophic lateral sclerosis patients after noninvasive ventilation initiation. ERJ Open Res 2018;4(2). https://doi.org/10.1183/23120541.00159-2017.
17. Khamankar N, Coan G, Weaver B, et al. Associative increases in amyotrophic lateral sclerosis survival duration with non-invasive ventilation initiation and usage protocols. Front Neurol 2018;9:578.
18. Berlowitz DJ, Howard ME, Fiore JF Jr, et al. Identifying who will benefit from non-invasive ventilation in amyotrophic lateral sclerosis/motor neurone disease in a clinical cohort. J Neurol Neurosurg Psychiatry 2016;87(3):280–6.
19. Boentert M, Brenscheidt I, Glatz C, et al. Effects of non-invasive ventilation on objective sleep and nocturnal respiration in patients with amyotrophic lateral sclerosis. J Neurol 2015;262(9):2073–82.
20. Vrijsen B, Buyse B, Belge C, et al. Noninvasive ventilation improves sleep in amyotrophic lateral sclerosis: a prospective polysomnographic study. J Clin Sleep Med 2015;11(5):559–66.
21. Katzberg HD, Selegiman A, Guion L, et al. Effects of noninvasive ventilation on sleep outcomes in amyotrophic lateral sclerosis. J Clin Sleep Med 2013;9(4):345–51.
22. Georges M, Morelot-Panzini C, Similowski T, et al. Noninvasive ventilation reduces energy expenditure in amyotrophic lateral sclerosis. BMC Pulm Med 2014;14:17.
23. Shimizu T, Nagaoka U, Nakayama Y, et al. Reduction rate of body mass index predicts prognosis for

survival in amyotrophic lateral sclerosis: a multi-center study in Japan. Amyotroph Lateral Scler 2012;13(4):363–6.

24. Miller RG, Jackson CE, Kasarskis EJ, et al. Quality Standards Subcommittee of the American Academy of N Neurology. Practice parameter update: the care of the patient with amyotrophic lateral sclerosis: drug, nutritional, and respiratory therapies (an evidence-based review): report of the Quality Standards Subcommittee of the American Academy of Neurology. Neurology 2009;73(15):1218–26.

25. EFNS Task Force on Diagnosis and Management of Amyotrophic Lateral Sclerosis:, Andersen PM, Abrahams S, Borasio GD, et al. EFNS guidelines on the clinical management of amyotrophic lateral sclerosis (MALS): revised report of an EFNS task force. Eur J Neurol 2012;19(3):360–75.

26. Clinical indications for noninvasive positive pressure ventilation in chronic respiratory failure due to restrictive lung disease, COPD, and nocturnal hypoventilation: a consensus conference report. Chest 1999;116(2):521–34.

27. Sahni A, Wolfe L. Sleep strategies: noninvasive ventilation: redefining insurance guidelines. 2019. American College of Chest Physicians web site. Available at: https://wwwmdedgecom/chestphysician/article/206771/sleep-medicine/noninvasive-ventilation-redefining-insurance-guidelines. Accessed March 6, 2020.

28. Lechtzin N, Scott Y, Busse AM, et al. Early use of non-invasive ventilation prolongs survival in subjects with ALS. Amyotroph Lateral Scler 2007;8(3):185–8.

29. Vitacca M, Montini A, Lunetta C, et al. Impact of an early respiratory care programme with non-invasive ventilation adaptation in patients with amyotrophic lateral sclerosis. Eur J Neurol 2018;25(3):556-e33.

30. Carratu P, Spicuzza L, Cassano A, et al. Early treatment with noninvasive positive pressure ventilation prolongs survival in amyotrophic lateral sclerosis patients with nocturnal respiratory insufficiency. Orphanet J Rare Dis 2009;4:10.

31. Jacobs TL, Brown DL, Baek J, et al. Trial of early noninvasive ventilation for ALS: a pilot placebo-controlled study. Neurology 2016;87(18):1878–83.

32. Vitacca M, Banfi P, Montini A, et al. Does timing of initiation influence acceptance and adherence to NIV in patients with ALS? Pulmonology 2020;26(1):45–8.

33. Selim BJ, Wolfe L, Coleman JM 3rd, et al. Initiation of noninvasive ventilation for sleep related hypoventilation disorders: advanced modes and devices. Chest 2018;153(1):251–65.

34. McKim DA, Road J, Avendano M, et al, Canadian Thoracic Society Home Mechanical Ventilation Committee. Home mechanical ventilation: a Canadian Thoracic Society clinical practice guideline. Can Respir J 2011;18(4):197–215.

35. Kelly JL, Jaye J, Pickersgill RE, et al. Randomized trial of 'intelligent' autotitrating ventilation versus standard pressure support non-invasive ventilation: impact on adherence and physiological outcomes. Respirology 2014;19(4):596–603.

36. Nicholson TT, Smith SB, Siddique T, et al. Respiratory pattern and tidal volumes differ for pressure support and volume-assured pressure support in amyotrophic lateral sclerosis. Ann Am Thorac Soc 2017;14(7):1139–46.

37. Servera E, Sancho J, Banuls P, et al. Bulbar impairment score predicts noninvasive volume-cycled ventilation failure during an acute lower respiratory tract infection in ALS. J Neurol Sci 2015;358(1–2):87–91.

38. Vandenberghe N, Vallet AE, Petitjean T, et al. Absence of airway secretion accumulation predicts tolerance of noninvasive ventilation in subjects with amyotrophic lateral sclerosis. Respir Care 2013;58(9):1424–32.

39. Gruis KL, Brown DL, Schoennemann A, et al. Predictors of noninvasive ventilation tolerance in patients with amyotrophic lateral sclerosis. Muscle Nerve 2005;32(6):808–11.

40. Georges M, Attali V, Golmard JL, et al. Reduced survival in patients with ALS with upper airway obstructive events on non-invasive ventilation. J Neurol Neurosurg Psychiatry 2016;87(10):1045–50.

41. Baxter SK, Baird WO, Thompson S, et al. The initiation of non-invasive ventilation for patients with motor neuron disease: patient and carer perceptions of obstacles and outcomes. Amyotroph Lateral Scler Frontotemporal Degener 2013;14(?):105–10.

42. Olney RK, Murphy J, Forshew D, et al. The effects of executive and behavioral dysfunction on the course of ALS. Neurology 2005;65(11):1774–7.

43. Hobson EV, McDermott CJ. Supportive and symptomatic management of amyotrophic lateral sclerosis. Nat Rev Neurol 2016;12(9):526–38.

44. Jackson CE, McVey AL, Rudnicki S, et al. Symptom management and end-of-life care in amyotrophic lateral sclerosis. Neurol Clin 2015;33(4):889–908.

45. Braun AT, Caballero-Eraso C, Lechtzin N. Amyotrophic lateral sclerosis and the respiratory system. Clin Chest Med 2018;39(2):391–400. https://doi.org/10.1016/j.ccm.2018.01.003.

46. van der Graaff MM, Grolman W, Westermann EJ, et al. Vocal cord dysfunction in amyotrophic lateral sclerosis: four cases and a review of the literature. Arch Neurol 2009;66(11):1329–33.

47. Volanti P, Cibella F, Sarva M, et al. Predictors of noninvasive ventilation tolerance in amyotrophic lateral sclerosis. J Neurol Sci 2011;303(1–2):114–8.

48. Smith R, Pioro E, Myers K, et al. Enhanced bulbar function in amyotrophic lateral sclerosis: the

Nuedexta treatment trial. Neurotherapeutics 2017; 14(3):762–72.

49. Fanfulla F, Taurino AE, Lupo ND, et al. Effect of sleep on patient/ventilator asynchrony in patients undergoing chronic non-invasive mechanical ventilation. Respir Med 2007;101(8):1702–7.

50. Gonzalez-Bermejo J, Morelot-Panzini C, Arnol N, et al. Prognostic value of efficiently correcting nocturnal desaturations after one month of non-invasive ventilation in amyotrophic lateral sclerosis: a retrospective monocentre observational cohort study. Amyotroph Lateral Scler Frontotemporal Degener 2013;14(5–6):373–9.

51. Janssens JP, Borel JC, Pepin JL, et al. Nocturnal monitoring of home non-invasive ventilation: the contribution of simple tools such as pulse oximetry, capnography, built-in ventilator software and autonomic markers of sleep fragmentation. Thorax 2011;66(5):438–45.

52. Rabec C, Georges M, Kabeya NK, et al. Evaluating noninvasive ventilation using a monitoring system coupled to a ventilator: a bench-to-bedside study. Eur Respir J 2009;34(4):902–13.

53. Rabec C, Rodenstein D, Leger P, et al. Ventilator modes and settings during non-invasive ventilation: effects on respiratory events and implications for their identification. Thorax 2011;66(2):170–8.

54. Rafiq MK, Bradburn M, Proctor AR, et al. Using transcutaneous carbon dioxide monitor (TOSCA 500) to detect respiratory failure in patients with amyotrophic lateral sclerosis: a validation study. Amyotroph Lateral Scler 2012;13(6):528–32.

55. Butz M, Wollinsky KH, Wiedemuth-Catrinescu U, et al. Longitudinal effects of noninvasive positive-pressure ventilation in patients with amyotrophic lateral sclerosis. Am J Phys Med Rehabil 2003; 82(8):597–604.

56. Mustfa N, Walsh E, Bryant V, et al. The effect of noninvasive ventilation on ALS patients and their caregivers. Neurology 2006;66(8):1211–7.

57. Loewen AH, Korngut L, Rimmer K, et al. Limitations of split-night polysomnography for the diagnosis of nocturnal hypoventilation and titration of non-invasive positive pressure ventilation in amyotrophic lateral sclerosis. Amyotroph Lateral Scler Frontotemporal Degener 2014;15(7–8):494–8.

58. Hannan LM, Rautela L, Berlowitz DJ, et al. Randomised controlled trial of polysomnographic titration of noninvasive ventilation. Eur Respir J 2019;53(5). https://doi.org/10.1183/13993003.02118-2018.

59. Prell T, Ringer TM, Wullenkord K, et al. Assessment of pulmonary function in amyotrophic lateral sclerosis: when can polygraphy help evaluate the need for non-invasive ventilation? J Neurol Neurosurg Psychiatry 2016;87(9):1022–6.

60. Gonzalez-Bermejo J, Perrin C, Janssens JP, et al. Proposal for a systematic analysis of polygraphy or polysomnography for identifying and scoring abnormal events occurring during non-invasive ventilation. Thorax 2012;67(6):546–52.

Phrenic Nerve Involvement in Neuralgic Amyotrophy (Parsonage-Turner Syndrome)

Ellen Farr, MD[a], Dom D'Andrea, BS[b], Colin K. Franz, MD, PhD[c],*

KEYWORDS

- Parsonage-Turner syndrome • Neuralgic amyotrophy • Brachial neuritis • Brachial plexus
- Phrenic nerve • Diaphragm muscle • Neuromuscular respiratory weakness • Phrenic neuropathy

KEY POINTS

- Neuralgic amyotrophy is usually characterized by its abrupt, painful onset associated with a variety of nerve injury patterns that typically affect a brachial distribution and may include the phrenic nerve.
- Phrenic nerve involvement is frequently overlooked even after the diagnosis is made because the severity of symptoms can vary and are nonspecific. All patients should be screened.
- Nocturnal noninvasive ventilation options should be considered to manage phrenic neuropathy from neuralgic amyotrophy.
- Functional recovery from phrenic neuropathy is slow and may take up to 2 to 3 years to plateau.
- Regular monitoring of diaphragm function during this period with tests such as spirometry and diaphragm ultrasound should be offered.

INTRODUCTION

Parsonage-Turner syndrome is also known as neuralgic amyotrophy (NA), acute idiopathic brachial plexus neuritis, or scapular belt syndrome. It is a painful, multifocal, peripheral nerve disorder causing both paresis and sensory loss. It was originally referred to as Parsonage-Turner syndrome as it was named for the resident and neurologist who characterized the condition in a case series of 136 patients in 1948[1] but had been previously described in the literature dating back to 1897.[2–4]

The initial presentation involves sudden onset of severe pain in the neck, shoulder, and/or arm, which can persist anywhere from a few hours to 1 month. In a cohort of 99 patients with NA, the pain was reported as a constant "sharp," "stabbing," "throbbing," or "aching."[5] Within 2 to 4 weeks the patient experiences profound weakness in the affected limb, and sensory abnormalities occur up to 80% of the time.[5,6] After 1 month, atrophy can be seen in the affected muscles,[7] and recovery of strength and muscle bulk can take up to 3 years.[5]

The reported incidence of NA varies. The annual incidence has been estimated as 1 to 3 cases per 100,000.[8–10] This is almost certainly an underestimation due to poor general awareness of NA by physicians, and difficulties in differentiating between similarly presenting diagnoses such as adhesive capsulitis, cervical spondylopathy, rotator cuff tears, and nerve compression.[11] A prospective study in the Netherlands from 2015 showed an incidence closer to 1 in 1000.[12] NA tends to

a Shirley Ryan AbilityLab, McGaw Medical Center, Northwestern University, 355 East Erie Street, 26N (Biologics), Chicago, IL 60611, USA; b Shirley Ryan AbilityLab, 355 East Erie Street, 26N (Biologics), Chicago, IL 60611, USA; c Shirley Ryan AbilityLab, Feinberg School of Medicine, Northwestern University, 355 East Erie Street, 26N (Biologics), Chicago, IL 60611, USA
* Corresponding author.
E-mail address: cfranz@sralab.org

Sleep Med Clin 15 (2020) 539–543
https://doi.org/10.1016/j.jsmc.2020.08.002
1556-407X/20/© 2020 Elsevier Inc. All rights reserved.

predominantly affect men and occurs most often in the third and seventh decades of life. No association has been noted thus far between a patient's handedness and the affected side.[5] There are 2 forms of NA: idiopathic and hereditary. Idiopathic NA has been associated with a variety of preceding exposures such as surgery, trauma, viral infection, vaccination, and heavy exercise.[1,5,13–17] Hereditary NA is an autosomal dominant disorder that is associated with a mutation in the SEPT9 gene and predisposes to recurrent attacks of peripheral nerve damage.[18] Recurrence and recovery rates differ between the 2 groups. The hereditary form is more severe with a 75% recurrence rate and reduced recovery. One study noted 67% of patients with hereditary NA rated their recovery as less than 50% after 3 years.[19,20]

The typical pattern of presentation in NA is patchy and at times asymmetric.[5] In their seminal paper, Parsonage and Turner claimed that the long thoracic nerve was most affected[1]; however, others noted that patients with a single peripheral nerve involvement had radial, thoracic, or suprascapular neuropathies equally, whereas those with multiple nerves involved were found to have axillary and suprascapular most commonly.[5] The frequency of upper limb involvement is how the condition became known as scapular belt syndrome or brachial plexus neuritis; however, pathology outside of the brachial plexus is not uncommon with lumbar plexus, phrenic nerve, and autonomic nerve involvement in up to 10% of patients.[19] The varied presentation of the condition and involvement of multiple individual nerves suggests that NA may actually be a disease of multiple mononeuropathies.

The diagnosis can be made clinically, but additional studies are useful to support the diagnosis and rule out mimics such as cervical radiculopathy or Pancoast tumor. Improvements in MRI have made it possible to identify neuritis at the level of the nerve root, plexus, and/or proximal nerve branches. The reliability of MRI or neuromuscular ultrasound to identify neuritis from NA in smaller nerve branches is unclear. The gold standard of anatomic localization still hinges on electromyography (EMG) and nerve conduction studies, but even this is limited, as needle EMG cannot always distinguish a multiple mononeuropathy pattern from a more proximal lesion (ie, plexopathy). Peripheral nerve ultrasound and improvements in MRI technology will likely contribute to an increasing role for imaging modalities in the future.

PHRENIC NERVE INVOLVEMENT

Despite being known more as a disease of the brachial plexus, the phrenic nerve can be affected in 6% to 14% of patients with NA.[5,19,21] A recent study reported that idiopathic disease has a lower incidence of phrenic involvement, around 7%, whereas patients with the hereditary form have phrenic neuropathies 14% of the time, but figures may underestimate phrenic involvement, as not all patients included were screened for diaphragm dysfunction, and dysfunction can be found in some individuals who are asymptomatic or with nonspecific symptoms.[19] Unilateral and bilateral phrenic nerves can be affected, and the injured nerve does not have to be ipsilateral to the affected limb.[5] Patients with phrenic nerve involvement usually present with orthopnea, exertional dyspnea, and dyspnea when immersed in water, similar to patients with respiratory compromise from other neuromuscular causes.[22–24] The presenting symptoms occur with equal frequency in patients with unilateral versus bilateral disease, except for orthopnea, which occurs more commonly in bilaterally impaired diaphragms.[21] Patients with unilateral diaphragm paralysis are more likely to present with orthopnea when other comorbid conditions are present such as obesity, lung disease, or heart disease.[22]

With regard to pulmonary function testing, as expected, patients with bilateral phrenic involvement are more impaired. The greatest differences are demonstrated between supine and sitting vital capacities (VC) with a greater than 30% decrease when supine in those with bilaterally damaged nerves. In unilaterally affected patients, this difference between supine and seated VC was between 10% and 30%.[21,22]

Recovery of the phrenic nerve depends on the type of damage incurred and the location of the lesion. Nerve involvement in NA can be demyelinating and/or axonal in character (**Fig. 1**). Although not specifically described in NA, Seddon's original classification of peripheral nerve lesions distinguished between "neuropraxia" (demyelinating) and the more severe "axonotmesis" (axonal) pathology.[25] Neuropraxia is characterized by focal conduction block associated with demyelination, yet more rapid recovery possible within several weeks because the distal axon does not undergo Wallerian degeneration. In contrast, axonotmesis lesions are characterized by axon damage within the nerve and distal Wallerian degeneration, which often results in incomplete and delayed (months to years) functional recovery, because axon regeneration is a slow inefficient process that occurs at a rate of 1 to 2 mm/d.[26] Previous studies on NA rarely distinguish between axonotmesis and neuropraxia, but in general report phrenic functional recovery happens within 1 to 3 years of their initial episode.[27] Improvement in symptoms does not

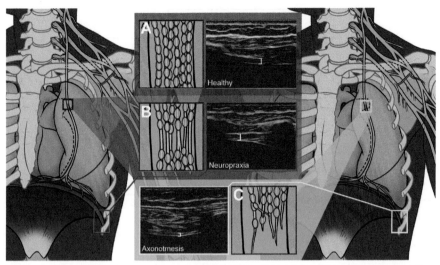

Fig. 1. Graphical representation of the 2 types of phrenic nerve injury in NA and their corresponding diaphragm findings on ultrasound. B-mode ultrasound images were obtained of the diaphragm at the ninth intercostal space between the mid- and anterior axillary lines at end expiration (functional residual capacity). Diaphragm thickness on each example noted in white brackets. (A) Example of a healthy phrenic nerve demonstrating normal diaphragm thickness. (B) Example of a phrenic nerve with neuropraxia or demyelinating injury demonstrating diaphragm with retained muscle bulk. The orange box shows corresponding sonographic view of the left hemidiaphragm. (C) Example of a phrenic nerve with axonotmesis or axonal injury demonstrating diaphragm atrophy. The yellow box shows corresponding sonographic view of the left hemidiaphragm.

necessarily represent improvement in diaphragm radiographic appearance. For example, the follow-up of several patients with diaphragmatic paresis noted that these patients had functionally improved 2.5 to 4 years after onset of the condition but were still noted to have elevated or immobile hemidiaphragms.[5]

The most accepted technique to characterize nerve injury type (axonal vs demyelination) is by needle EMG. However, needle EMG of the diaphragm has nontrivial risks such as pneumothorax[28] so there can be reluctance to order it. A noninvasive test that is entering more widespread use in the diagnosis of phrenic nerve dysfunction is diaphragmatic ultrasound.[29] Ultrasound is an easily accessible bedside test that can evaluate the diaphragm in real time. It also has the potential to identify a complete axonal (axonotmesis) lesion based on the presence of severe, early onset diaphragm muscle atrophy,[29] but further work will be required to establish the validity of this approach (see **Fig. 1**).

TREATMENT

Respiratory muscle weakness is common in patients with neuromuscular disease, which has been well studied in specific disorders such as Duchenne muscular dystrophy and amyotrophic lateral sclerosis, as recently reviewed.[30] Less is known about NA specifically, but as other neuromuscular disorders, it is categorized as a restrictive thoracic disorder for Medicare reimbursement for noninvasive ventilation (NIV). Screening for sleep and respiratory disturbances should be performed in all patients with NA (**Fig. 2**). When appropriate, objective measurements such as spirometry, point of care diaphragm ultrasound, or overnight pulse oximetry can be very helpful. Briefly, the minimum requirement for coverage includes symptoms that suggest hypoventilation plus any of the following: awake arterial blood gas CO2 levels greater than 45 mm Hg, oxygen saturation of less than 88% for at least 5 min of nocturnal recording, maximum inspiratory pressure less than 60 cm H2O, or forced vital capacity less than 50% predicted performed in the upright or supine position.[31]

Sleep disturbances are common in the phrenic variant of NA. When supine, the abdominal contents exert more pressure on the weakened diaphragm making inspiration more difficult, especially during rapid eye movement sleep when the diaphragm is the only active inspiratory muscle. For unclear reasons, the functional prognosis of patients with phrenic nerve involvement seems to be less favorable than other brachial plexus nerve symptoms.[27] If no improvement is seen following 2 to 3 years of supportive treatments with NIV, surgical plication of the diaphragm can be considered for phrenic lesions to partially

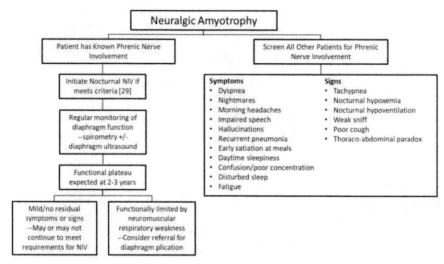

Fig. 2. Management approach to phrenic neuropathy in NA.

restore lost function in unilateral disease.[32] Before undergoing plication, all patients with NA should review recurrence and recovery rates (outlined earlier) with the referring neuromuscular specialist.

There is insufficient data to recommend a specific pharmacologic approach to the acute phase of NA, but it is common practice to consider a course of high-dose corticosteroids if the diagnosis is made within the first month after symptom onset.[9] This approach has validity based on the current understanding on NA pathophysiology. Attempts to conduct clinical trials in acute NA have been stymied for logistical reasons; for example, one trial was stopped after 3 years in 2007 because very few patients were diagnosed and referred within the required first month.[33] The severity of pain, particularly at the onset of NA, seems to respond best to nonsteroidal antiinflammatory drugs combined with long-acting opioids.[19] If pain persists over the longer term, treatments should be targeted to the pain generator (ie, musculoskeletal vs neuropathic), and referral to an interdisciplinary pain management center should be considered.[34]

SUMMARY AND FUTURE DIRECTIONS

Improvements for diagnosis and management of NA are ongoing. Acute treatments have yet to be well studied, as overall awareness of the disease is low and thus diagnosis is often delayed. Presently, there is only one US clinical trial for NA, and it involves rehabilitative management after peripheral dysfunction.[10] Better recognition of diaphragmatic dysfunction in this patient population is also important, as evaluation is only performed when specific symptomatology is noted, which

may delay diagnosis and treatment. Because of the relatively high involvement of the phrenic nerve with NA, the authors recommend screening all patients with NA for signs and symptoms of neuromuscular respiratory dysfunction (see **Fig. 2**). These patients respond well to conservative treatment with NIV. Unlike many other neuromuscular conditions that are steadily progressive, NA is usually a monophasic illness followed by a protracted recovery (over 2–3 years). Thus, regular monitoring with spirometry and diaphragmatic ultrasounds are some of the best options to monitor for improvements and determine the appropriateness for diaphragm plication surgery in unilateral involvement.

DISCLOSURE

The authors have no disclosures.

REFERENCES

1. Parsonage MJ, Turner JW. Neuralgic amyotrophy; the shoulder-girdle syndrome. Lancet 1948;1:973–8.
2. Allen IM. The neurological complication of serum treatment. Lancet 1931;2:1128–31.
3. Dyke SC. Peripheral nerve lesions, after ant-tetnic serum. Lancet 1918;1:570.
4. Feinberg J. Fall von Erb-Klumpke scher Lahmung nach influenza. Centralbl 1897;16:588–637.
5. Tsairis P, Dyck PJ, Mulder DW. Natural history of brachial plexus neuropathy. Report on 99 patients. Arch Neurol 1972;27:109–17.
6. Hussey AJ, O'Brien CP, Regan PJ. Parsonage-Turner syndrome - case report and literature review. Hand (N Y) 2007;2(4):218–21.

7. Feinberg JH, Radecki J. Parsonage-turner syndrome. HSS J 2010;6(2):199–205.

8. Beghi E, Kurland LT, Mulder DW, et al. Brachial plexus neuropathy in the population of Rochester, Minnesota. Ann Neurol 1985;18:320–3.

9. Van Eijk JJ, Groothuis JT, Van Alfen N. Neuralgic amyotrophy: an update on diagnosis, pathophysiology, and treatment. Muscle Nerve 2016;53(3):337–50.

10. MacDonald BK, Cocerell OC, Sander JW, et al. The incidence and lifetime prevalence of neurologic disorders in a prospective community-based study in the UK. Brain 2000;123:665–76.

11. Monteiro Dos Santos RB, Dos Santos SM, Carneiro Leal FJ, et al. Parsonage-Turner syndrome. Rev Bras Ortop 2015;50(3):336–41.

12. van Alfen N, van Eijk JJ, Ennik T, et al. Incidence of neuralgic amyotrophy (Parsonage Turner syndrome) in a primary care setting–a prospective cohort study. PLoS One 2015;10(5):e0128361.

13. Dillin L, Hoaglund FT, Scheck M. Brachial neuritis. J Bone Joint Surg 1985;67A:878–80.

14. Magee KR, DeJong RN. Paralytic brachial neuritis. JAMA 1960;174:1258–62.

15. McCarty EC, Tsairis P, Warren RF. Brachial neuritis. Clin Orthop 1999;368:37–43.

16. Weikers NJ, Mattson RH. Acute parlytic brachial neuritis. A clinical and electrodiagnostic study. Neurology 1969;18:1153–8.

17. Odell JA, Kennelly K, Stauffer J. Phrenic nerve palsy and Parsonage-Turner syndrome. Ann Thorac Surg 2011;92(1):349–51.

10. Kuhlenbaumer G, Hannibal MC, Nolic E, et al. Mutations in SEPT9 cause hereditary neuralgic amyotrophy. Nat Genet 2005;37:1044–6.

19. van Alfen N, van Engelen BG. The clinical spectrum of neuralgic amyotrophy in 246 cases. Brain 2006;129(Pt 2):438–50.

20. Seror P. Neuralgic amyotrophy. An update. Joint Bone Spine 2017;84:153–8.

21. van Alfen N, Doorduin J, Marieke H, et al. Phrenic neuropathy and diaphragm dysfunction in neuralgic amyotrophy. Neurology 2018;91(9):e843–9.

22. McCool FD, Tzelepis GE. Dysfunction of the diaphragm. N Engl J Med 2012;366:932–42.

23. Skatrud J, Iber C, McHugh W, et al. Determinants of hypoventilation during wakefulness and sleep in diaphragmatic paralysis. Am Rev Respir Dis 1980;121:587–93.

24. Stradling JR, Warley AR. Bilateral diaphragm paralysis and sleep apnoea without diurnal respiratory failure. Thorax 1988;43:75–7.

25. Seddon HJ. A classification of nerve injuries. Br Med J 1942;2(4260):237–9.

26. Seddon HJ, Medawar PB, Smith H. Rate of regeneration of peripheral nerves in man. J Physiol 1943;102(2):191–215.

27. Hughes PD, Polkey MI, Moxham J, et al. Long-term recovery of diaphragm strength in neuralgic amyotrophy. Eur Respir J 1999;13:379–84.

28. Honet JC. Pneumothorax and EMG. Arch Phys Med Rehabil 1988;69:149.

29. Boon AJ, Sekiguchi H, Harper CJ, et al. Sensitivity and specificity of diagnostic ultrasound in the diagnosis of phrenic neuropathy. Neurology 2014;83(14):1264–70.

30. Sahni AS, Wolfe L. Respiratory care in neuromuscular diseases. Respir Care 2018;63(5):601–8.

31. Medicare C. Respiratory assist device: Medical review documentation checklist. Available at: https://www.cgsmedicare.com/jc/mr/pdf/mr_checklist_rad_e0471.pdf. Accessed January 31, 2020.

32. Freeman RK, Van Woerkom J, Vyverberg A, et al. Long-term follow-up of the functional and physiologic results of diaphragm plication in adults with unilateral diaphragm paralysis. Ann Thorac Surg 2009;88(4):1112–7.

33. Clinical Trials.gov. Neuralgic amyotrophy: Central Reorganization and rehabilitation after peripheral dysfunction. Available at: https://clinicaltrials.gov/ct2/show/NCT03441347?cond=Neuralgic+Amyotrophy&draw=2&rank=1. Accessed January 9, 2020.

34. Scholten PM, Harden RN. Assessing and treating patients with neuropathic pain. PM R 2015;(11 Suppl):S257–69.

Noninvasive Ventilator Devices and Modes

Gaurav Singh, MD, MPH[a,b], Michelle Cao, DO[c,d],*

KEYWORDS

- Noninvasive positive pressure ventilation (NIPPV) • Home mechanical ventilation • Pressure control
- Volume-assured pressure support (VAPS) • Chronic respiratory failure • Hypoventilation
- Neuromuscular disease

KEY POINTS

- Noninvasive ventilation is increasingly being used to treat patients with chronic respiratory failure, including neuromuscular diseases, restrictive thoracic disorders, obstructive lung diseases, and other hypoventilation conditions.
- A thorough understanding of advanced respiratory devices and, in particular, modes of ventilation and other relevant settings aids in managing such patients.
- Pressure-limited modes of ventilation such as spontaneous/timed and pressure control are more commonly used with noninvasive ventilation because of enhanced patient comfort and leak compensation.
- Volume-assured pressure support is a supplementary volume-targeted and pressure-limited function available on certain devices that maintains a target ventilation by continuously adjusting inspiratory pressure.
- Evidence supporting superiority of particular ventilation modes for different diseases is limited, but spontaneous/timed is commonly used in practice and in studies showing efficacy for relevant clinical outcomes.

INTRODUCTION

Although domiciliary mechanical ventilation has been implemented in the care of patients with chronic respiratory failure (CRF) for nearly a century, initially with negative pressure ventilators and subsequently with positive pressure applied invasively via tracheostomy, use of noninvasive positive pressure ventilation (NIPPV) is a modern paradigm.[1] Following the introduction of nasal continuous positive airway pressure (CPAP) for obstructive sleep apnea (OSA),[2] the first descriptions of home NIPPV for CRF ensued in the 1980s.[3-8] Since then, there has been an exponential increase in the number and sophistication of ventilator devices for home use. This increase has matched the growing indications for NIPPV, including neuromuscular diseases (NMDs), restrictive thoracic disorders, obstructive lung diseases, and other hypoventilation conditions. The prevalence of home mechanical ventilation has steadily increased worldwide in the past few decades.[8-13] The basis for this evolution includes not only improvements in gas exchange, hospitalizations, mortality, symptoms, quality of life, and health care costs but also patient preference and comfort. The growing need for NIPPV

[a] Pulmonary, Critical Care, and Sleep Medicine Section, Department of Medicine, Veterans Affairs Palo Alto Health Care System, 3801 Miranda Avenue, Mail Code 111P, Palo Alto, CA 94304, USA; [b] Division of Pulmonary, Allergy, and Critical Care Medicine, Department of Medicine, Stanford University, 300 Pasteur Drive, Palo Alto, CA 94304, USA; [c] Division of Neuromuscular Medicine, Department of Neurology, Stanford University, 213 Quarry Road, Mail Code 5979, Palo Alto, CA 94304, USA; [d] Division of Sleep Medicine, Department of Psychiatry, Stanford University, 213 Quarry Road, Mail Code 5979, Palo Alto, CA 94304, USA
* Corresponding author. Stanford University, 213 Quarry Road, Mail Code 5979, Palo Alto, CA 94304.
E-mail address: michellecao@stanford.edu

Sleep Med Clin 15 (2020) 545–555
https://doi.org/10.1016/j.jsmc.2020.08.005

necessitates a more comprehensive understanding of these devices, including selection of modes of ventilation and additional settings required to effectively and safely care for patients with CRF in the outpatient setting.

This article provides an overview of home NIPPV devices and modes. Given the rapidly increasing number of manufacturers and devices capable of NIPPV, it is beyond the scope of this focused review to cover specific details of each manufacturer or device. The goal is to provide a foundation for NIPPV modes, from which practitioners can extrapolate applications to various devices. For illustrative purposes, the focus is on 2 common manufacturers in the United States, Philips Respironics and ResMed, along with their most current devices indicated for NIPPV. These manufacturers are specifically discussed because they use volume-assured pressure support (VAPS) technology in some of their devices. Readers are encouraged to contact these and other manufacturers along with durable medical equipment providers to learn more about the specifics of different available NIPPV devices.

DISTINGUISHING PORTABLE VENTILATORS FROM RESPIRATORY ASSIST DEVICES

It is important to differentiate portable ventilators from respiratory assist devices (RADs), because this has implications for patient care, as well as for insurance approval, reimbursement, and health care costs. Although the size and weight of portable ventilators have traditionally exceeded those of RADs, they have progressively become more compact. Likewise, RADs have evolved expanded functionality. Consequently, the differences among these devices are increasingly becoming blurred.

According to the Centers for Medicare and Medicaid Services (CMS), RADs are bilevel positive airway pressure (PAP) devices that are used for restrictive thoracic disorders, NMD, chronic obstructive pulmonary disease (COPD), other hypoventilation conditions, and central sleep apnea. Ventilators are indicated for restrictive thoracic disorders, NMD, and CRF consequent to severe hypercapnic COPD.[14] Thus, there is an overlap in the medical conditions for which RADs and ventilators can be used, although there is a wide spectrum of disease for the indicated disorders. In general, portable ventilators can be considered rather than RADs based on increasing severity of disease, including progressive nature of the ailment, for which more prolonged use and closer monitoring may be required. Specific indications for which ventilators may be more appropriate than RADs include need for daytime use in addition to nocturnal or intermittent use, requirement for an internal battery in case of power outages, alarms for closer monitoring (ie, respiratory rate, minute ventilation, apneas, pressures, leak, and disconnect), and need for higher pressures than RADs are capable of supplying. In addition, ventilators may be indicated for patients with overlap syndrome with alveolar hypoventilation and OSA, where a volume-targeted mode of ventilation combined with auto-titrating expiratory PAP (EPAP) feature to maintain dynamic upper airway patency.

Prior criteria stipulated that RADs were indicated in situations in which intermittent and short durations of respiratory support were deemed feasible, with disruption or failure of therapy not being immediately life threatening. In contrast, ventilators were indicated for scenarios in which more continuous or prolonged use was deemed necessary, with interruption or failure of therapy placing the patient at risk of serious harm or death.[15] Revised CMS criteria for ventilators do not include such language. Instead, the decision to use a ventilator is based on the specific circumstances and details of the individual patient's medical condition. The clinician must ensure there is sufficient information in the medical record to justify use of a portable ventilator.[14] Documentation should incorporate essential objective and historical elements, including some, but not necessarily all, of the following: spirometry, blood gases showing hypercapnia, exacerbations, admissions, desaturation and dyspnea with activity/ambulation, prior/current treatments, and tried/failed treatments including RADs devices (or an explanation indicating that a RAD device would be inappropriate if not tried previously).

NONINVASIVE VENTILATION VERSUS INVASIVE VENTILATION

Modes of ventilation are similar with regard to invasive ventilation and NIPPV, so the same general principles used with invasive ventilation in the intensive care unit setting can be applied in the outpatient setting with NIPPV. However, some key differences need to be kept in mind when considering noninvasive ventilation instead of invasive mechanical ventilation. NIPPV typically uses a single-limb or passive respiratory circuit. The single-limb tubing connects the ventilator to a mouthpiece or a mask interface that is donned by the patient. Mask options include nasal pillows, nasal, oronasal or full face, total face, and helmet mask. Because NIPPV is designed as an open system, there is an intentional leak that occurs through an exhalation port located in the mask interface or respiratory circuit tubing (ie, venting), which minimizes rebreathing of carbon dioxide (CO_2). There is also potential for unintentional leak with use of a mask, either around the mask or caused by mouth opening when using a nasal interface. Intentional leak with an open circuit makes measurements of end-tidal CO_2 unreliable, although transcutaneous CO_2 ($TcCO_2$) can be used with improved accuracy.[16] Pressure modes are better at accommodating leak (ie, leak compensation) compared with volume modes of ventilation.[17]

Although a passive circuit may be used with invasive ventilation, another option includes double-limb or active circuit, consisting of inspiratory and expiratory limbs, with the latter being used for elimination of CO_2. This closed system allows better control of leak; more precise monitoring of ventilatory parameters, including tidal volumes and end-tidal CO_2; higher and more precise delivery of the fraction of inspired oxygen; and increased ventilatory capacity. An active dual-limb circuit with volume cycled ventilation and a positive end expiratory pressure (PEEP) of 0 occasionally may be used noninvasively in patients with respiratory muscle weakness, such as NMD.[18]

AVAILABLE DEVICES FOR NONINVASIVE POSITIVE PRESSURE VENTILATION IN THE OUTPATIENT SETTING

This article focuses on the most current models from 2 major manufacturers of RADs and home ventilators suitable for domiciliary NIPPV, Philips Respironics and ResMed. **Table 1** lists such RADs and portable ventilators for ambulatory uses, along with available modes of ventilation. Ventilator modes and specific differences between Philips Respironics and ResMed are discussed later.

IMPORTANT/GENERAL SETTINGS/CONCEPTS

Before a detailed discussion of ventilation modes, a basic understanding of relevant ventilation parameters is informative. Three phase variables in mechanical ventilation control the inspiratory components of a mechanical breath: trigger, target, and cycle. The trigger variable determines the initiation of a mechanical breath, which is prompted either by the patient (referred to as a spontaneous breath and may be triggered by flow, volume, or pressure) or ventilator (termed a mandatory breath, which is triggered by time). In assisted ventilation, the device augments spontaneous patient-triggered breathing. In assist/control (AC)

ventilation, mandatory breaths are either time triggered, or patient triggered. The target or limit variable is typically either volume (ie, tidal volume) or pressure (ie, inspiratory pressure). With a volume target, the inspiratory pressure is determined by the mechanics of the lung and chest wall. With a pressure target, the tidal volume is determined by the compliance of the respiratory system and patient assistance. The cycle or termination variable causes cessation of the inspiratory phase and is determined most commonly by flow or time, but volume and pressure are also possible. Older modes of ventilation remain on these devices, although they are no longer used, such as controlled ventilation, where mandatory breaths are time triggered.

Alternating with the inhalation phase of mechanical ventilation is an exhalation phase that is governed by an expiratory phase variable referred to as EPAP, PEEP, or CPAP, depending on the particular RAD or ventilator and mode of ventilation used. This variable is a constant pressure applied throughout the exhalation phase that maintains upper airway patency (eg, for OSA or NMD) and improves oxygenation by recruiting and preventing collapse of alveoli, with both mechanisms also permitting adequate ventilation and elimination of CO_2. It also decreases respiratory work to trigger inspiration in patients with intrinsic PEEP (eg, COPD). After inhalation is triggered, the amount of time it takes to transition from EPAP or PEEP to the target inspiratory PAP (IPAP) is called the rise time (the pressurization time). The inspiratory time (Ti) is the total amount of time spent in the inhalation phase of respiration, until cycling to the exhalation phase. The clinician typically sets the duration of both rise time and Ti based on disease state (eg, shorter for COPD and longer for NMD) and patient comfort, and rise time can only be a certain fraction of Ti. In addition, the difference between IPAP and EPAP is the pressure support (PS) or driving pressure, which is the main factor assisting in ventilation and elimination of CO_2. Caution should be applied to distinguish IPAP and PS, because either may be set as the higher pressure in relation to EPAP, depending on the specific RAD or ventilator.

MODES OF NONINVASIVE VENTILATION

This article discusses in detail only the commonly used pressure-targeted modes, because they are used with more regularity compared with volume-targeted modes with NIPPV because of enhanced patient comfort, patient-ventilator synchrony, and leak compensation with the former.[17] These modes are all fundamentally bilevel forms of

Table 1
Common respiratory assist devices, portable ventilators, and modes of ventilation

Device	Pressure Modes	Volume Modes	Hybrid/Additive Modes
		Mode of Ventilation	
RADs			
Philips Respironics Dream Station BiPAP ST	CPAP, S, ST	NA	NA
Philips Respironics Dream Station BiPAP-AVAPS	CPAP, S, ST, PC	NA	NA
ResMed AirCurve 10 ST	CPAP, S, ST, T	NA	NA
ResMed AirCurve 10 ST-A	CPAP, S, ST, T	NA	iVAPS
ResMed Stellar 100/150	CPAP, S, ST, T, PAC	NA	iVAPS
Portable Ventilators			
Philips Respironics Trilogy 100	CPAP, S, ST, T, PC, PC-SIMV, PC-MPV	AC, SIMV, VC, AC-MPV	AVAPS, AVAPS-AE
Philips Respironics Trilogy Evo	CPAP, PSV, ST, SIMV-PC, AC-PC, MPV-PC	AC-VC, SIMV-VC, MPV-VC	AVAPS, AVAPS-AE
ResMed Astral 100/150	CPAP, ST, PAC, PAVC, P-SIMV, PS, MPV:PAVC, MPV:PS/SVt	AVC, V-SIMV, MPV:AVC	iVAPS Auto-EPAP

Abbreviations: AC, assist control; AVAPS, average VAPS; AVC, volume control assist control; BiPAP, bilevel positive airway pressure; iVAPS, intelligent VAPS; MPV, mouthpiece ventilation; NA, not available; P, pressure; PAC, pressure control assist control; PAVC, pressure-assist volume control; PC, pressure control; PS, pressure support; PSV, pressure support ventilation; S, spontaneous; SIMV, synchronized intermittent mandatory ventilation; ST, spontaneous/timed; SVt, safety tidal volume; T, timed; V, volume; VC, volume control.

ventilation (**Table 2**). Other modes are mentioned briefly for completeness, including volume modes, which are more commonly used with invasive ventilation.

Spontaneous Mode

Spontaneous (S) mode is the simplest mode on bilevel PAP. Inspiratory effort by the patient initiates a ventilator-assisted breath that increases the pressure from EPAP to IPAP at a rate determined by the rise time, with flow cycling back to EPAP. There is no backup respiratory rate in the event that the patient's spontaneous respiration decreases. IPAP and EPAP are fixed pressures and therefore tidal volume is variable breath by breath. Although considered a noninvasive ventilatory mode, without the backup respiratory rate, it is not recommended for patients with chronic respiratory insufficiency or failure, or for patients in whom control of ventilation is recommended. S mode is similar to S/timed (T) mode without the backup rate or a fixed Ti, although some

manufacturers may still use a Ti minimum and Ti maximum with S mode (discussed later).

Spontaneous/Timed Mode

Similar to S mode, inspiratory effort by the patient initiates a ventilator-assisted breath that increases the pressure from EPAP to IPAP at a rate determined by the rise time, with flow cycling back to EPAP. In contrast with S mode, ST mode ensures delivery of mandatory, timed breaths by the device if the patient's spontaneous respiratory rate decreases below a set backup rate. In this case, the rise time determines the rate at which the pressure increases from EPAP to IPAP, but the Ti controls the duration of time spent at IPAP, before cycling back to EPAP. There are some relevant functional differences in Ti for different manufacturers in the ST mode (discussed later). The purpose of the ST mode is to ensure a minimum number of breaths per minute (ie, minute ventilation) if a patient is unable to do so spontaneously.

Table 2
Settings for common pressure modes of ventilation used with noninvasive positive pressure ventilation devices

	Philips Respironics	ResMed
S	EPAP, IPAP, rise time	EPAP, IPAP, rise time, Ti min, Ti max
ST	EPAP, IPAP, rise time, Ti, BUR	EPAP, IPAP, rise time, Ti min, Ti max, BUR
PC	EPAP, IPAP, rise time, Ti, BUR	EPAP, IPAP, rise time, Ti, BUR
VAPS	Vt, EPAP, IPAP min, IPAP max, rise time, Ti, BUR, AVAPS rate	Va, EPAP, PS min, PS max, rise time, Ti min, Ti max, BUR
VAPS-AE	Vt, EPAP min, EPAP max, IPAP min, IPAP max, rise time, Ti, BUR, AVAPS rate	Va, EPAP min, EPAP max, PS min, PS max, rise time, Ti min, Ti max, BUR

Abbreviations: AVAPS, average volume-assured pressure support; BUR, backup rate; max, maximum; min, minimum; Ti, inspiratory time; Va, alveolar ventilation; Vt, tidal volume.

Pressure Control Mode

When used with NIPPV devices, pressure control (PC) mode is similar to ST mode, with the exception being that the set Ti is applied to every delivered breath, whether triggered spontaneously by the patient or mandatory and timed by the device. Consequently, the length of inhalation phase is consistent, and the cycle variable is time rather than flow. The advantage of PC compared with ST mode is ensuring a guaranteed Ti with every breath and thus relatively constant tidal volume from breath to breath, which may better support patients who do not have adequate respiratory muscle strength to generate sufficient Ti and hence tidal volume on their own (ie, NMD). Disadvantages of a fixed Ti with every breath include air trapping in those prone to it (ie, COPD), and patient-ventilator dyssynchrony if Ti is set shorter or longer than the patient's desired Ti.

Volume-Assured Pressure Support

Although sometimes classified as a hybrid mode of ventilation because it incorporates features of both volume and pressure ventilation, VAPS is more precisely described as a supplementary volume-targeted and pressure-limited function. This feature is available with some RADs or ventilators only when using a passive circuit and S, ST, T, or PC modes (ie, exclusive to pressure-limited, open ventilation). Rather than using a fixed IPAP with these modes of ventilation, addition of VAPS allows an IPAP or PS range to be programmed, with the goal of achieving a specific tidal volume or alveolar ventilation, depending on the manufacturer. Therefore, typically a flow, pressure, or time trigger increases pressure from a fixed EPAP to an inspiratory pressure between a set IPAP or PS minimum and IPAP or PS maximum, with rise time and Ti elements determined by the underlying pressure-limited mode. The IPAP or PS constantly adjust within the set range to achieve targeted ventilation goals. Similar to ST and PC modes, a backup rate may be used with VAPS. The unique advantage of VAPS is ensuring at least a minimum target ventilation with the minimum necessary inspiratory pressure needed, regardless of lung compliance, airway resistance, or patient dyssynchrony.

Auto-Expiratory Positive Airway Pressure

The feature that autotitrating EPAP (AE) provides in addition to VAPS is an automatically titratable EPAP. An EPAP minimum and EPAP maximum are programmed with proactive pressure adjustments to maintain upper airway patency. This method may be beneficial in hypercapnic patients with CRF with concomitant OSA, such as individuals with overlap syndrome and obesity hypoventilation syndrome (OHS). However, patients with restrictive lung disease or weakness, as with NMD, may not tolerate AE because of sensitivity to pressure variations and potential for glottis closure.[17] AE may avoid the need to obtain laboratory-based polysomnography to titrate EPAP or to gradually titrate it in the outpatient setting. Another advantage is ensuring adequate but comfortable pressures to maintain upper airway patency in various sleep positions and stages.

Mouthpiece Ventilation

Mouthpiece ventilation (MPV) is a strictly daytime mode of noninvasive ventilation. It is exclusively available on various portable ventilators, and not available on RADs. MPV has been best used in neuromuscular disease, in particular Duchenne muscular dystrophy. Its application has been shown to successfully avoid or delay tracheostomy in patients with progressive respiratory failure by improving respiratory mechanics and hypercapnia.[19,20] In contrast with nocturnal modes of NIPPV, which deliver continuous airflow by mask interface, MPV is an on-demand or intermittent mode of ventilation and allows patient autonomy, whereby the patient initiates a breath supported by the device when the patient feels that additional ventilatory support is needed. MPV uses a plastic mouthpiece rather than a mask interface. Unlike daytime nasal ventilation, the mouthpiece allows the face to be free from a mask interface, and the patient may engage in verbal communication as long as speech is not significantly impaired (ie, severe bulbar weakness). MPV also allows breath staking as a means of lung volume recruitment in neuromuscular disease. MPV can be used with pressure (PC) or volume modes (AC), and can be programmed to timed inspiration, or on-demand ventilation in which the patient initiates the breath as much or as little as needed per patient's preference. In general, the inspiratory pressure is titrated to deliver about 2 to 3 times a normal tidal volume if set in PC mode, or, if in AC mode, the determined volume is programmed. Inspiratory time can be used to ensure a full inhalation cycle before spontaneous exhalation. MPV on Philips Respironics home ventilator is called kiss trigger, in which inspiratory airflow is delivered when the patient's lip touches the mouthpiece. MPV is an on-demand mode and inspiratory effort is not required to deliver a breath. Similarly, MPV on ResMed home ventilator is called touch trigger, where engagement of the mouthpiece by the patient's lip triggers the device to deliver a breath. In both devices, patient effort is not required to initiate a breath, but initiation is triggered by kissing or touching the mouthpiece.

Other Modes

CPAP is a constant pressure applied throughout the respiratory cycle, both during inspiration and expiration. It is rarely used for CRF, because it does not assist in ventilation, and it is more appropriate for OSA (a sleep-related upper airway patency disorder). It is important not to confuse OSA or use the term loosely with conditions causing hypercapnic respiratory insufficiency or failure.

PS or PS ventilation (PSV) may be identical to S mode, but it can also be used with a guaranteed tidal volume.

T mode is a pressure-limited and time-cycled modality that uses a fixed respiratory rate and Ti, with spontaneous breaths not being supported. This mode is uncommonly used in clinical practice, because it is uncomfortable in awake, spontaneously breathing patients.

AC uses a set respiratory rate, Ti, and either a pressure limit (ie, PC-AC) or volume limit, which is termed volume control (VC; used with AC it is VC-AC). As opposed to T mode, additional patient-triggered breaths are permitted and are identical to mandatory breaths (ie, supplying the set volume or pressure).

Synchronized intermittent mandatory ventilation (SIMV) is similar to AC, but mandatory breaths are synchronized with the patient's inspiratory effort, and additional breaths are generally assisted spontaneous breaths that are pressure supported (ie, tidal volume determined by patient effort and lung mechanics). The mandatory breaths with SIMV may be pressure limited (ie, SIMV-PC) or volume limited (ie, SIMV-VC).

IMPORTANT DIFFERENCES BETWEEN PHILIPS RESPIRONICS AND ResMed

It is important to highlight some key differences pertinent to ventilation settings among the manufacturers, current devices, and primary modes discussed earlier.

Rise Time and Inspiratory Time

Philips Respironics uses a single-digit numerical scale for rise time (the lower the setting, the shorter the rise time), whereas ResMed uses absolute values in milliseconds. Philips Respironics uses a fixed, programmed Ti for only mandatory breaths in ST mode and all delivered breaths (ie, mandatory and spontaneous) in PC mode, including with the VAPS feature activated (the new Trilogy Evo by Philips is an exception that can use a minimum and maximum Ti). This manufacturer does not provide Ti for S mode. ResMed uses a Ti range (ie, Ti minimum and Ti maximum) for S and ST modes, including with its VAPS feature. Therefore, inhalation cannot cease before Ti minimum, nor can it persist for longer than Ti maximum. ResMed uses a fixed Ti with T and PC modes.

Trigger and Cycle Sensitivity

Philips Respironics RADs do not have the ability to program trigger or cycle sensitivity, because these functions are automated (ie, Digital Auto-Trak).

The portable ventilators from this manufacturer do have an adjustable flow trigger using absolute values in liters per minute or Auto-Trak (with 2 different sensitivity options). The Philips Respironics ventilators also have a flow cycle sensitivity based on percentage of peak inspiratory flow. ResMed RADs use a qualitative measure for both trigger and cycle sensitivity, ranging from very low to very high (the higher the setting, the more readily triggering and cycling occur). ResMed ventilators have an adjustable flow trigger using absolute values in liters per minute, and there is also a flow cycle sensitivity based on percentage of peak inspiratory flow.

Volume-Assured Pressure Support

Both Philips Respironics and ResMed devices have VAPS functionality on some RADs, along with the option of AE on the ventilators, but there are some notable differences between the manufacturers. Philips Respironics uses average VAPS (AVAPS) to achieve a target tidal volume by adjusting inspiratory pressure between a set IPAP minimum and IPAP maximum. AVAPS is a PS function that can be activated on the primary modes discussed earlier and it is not a standalone mode (with the exception of AVAPS-AE, a stand-alone mode on the Philips Trilogy ventilator). ResMed uses intelligent volume-assured PS (iVAPS) to target alveolar ventilation (ie, excluding anatomic dead space), which is determined by patient height and thus ideal body weight, by adjusting PS between PS minimum and PS maximum. The rapidity by which the IPAP changes on Philips Respironics devices is determined by the AVAPS rate, which has a numerical range (the higher the rate, the greater the change in IPAP) and can be set based on disease state. ResMed devices do not have an equivalent feature. Regarding backup respiratory rate, Philips Respironics is capable of using either a set rate or automatic rate, which is 2 breaths/min less than the average of the patient's most recent spontaneous respiratory rate. ResMed's intelligent backup rate targets the patient's spontaneous respiratory rate and automatically adjusts the backup rate based on whether the patient is breathing less often than two-thirds of the targeted spontaneous respiratory rate or is apneic (in which case it is the set rate) versus effectively triggering (in which case it is two-thirds the set rate). Thus, the backup rate is not activated until the patient's respiratory rate decreases below two-thirds of the targeted threshold, thereby maintaining spontaneous triggering.

SELECTING APPROPRIATE NONINVASIVE POSITIVE PRESSURE VENTILATION MODE BASED ON DISEASE STATE

There is limited evidence available to guide the selection of optimal noninvasive mode for various disease states. Most available data suggest that there are no differences in relevant outcomes, particularly between volume and pressures modes of ventilation,[21] as well as with use of VAPS compared with traditional fixed pressure modes.[22,23] Factors that should be considered include patient comfort, patient-ventilator synchrony, maintenance of CO_2 levels within an appropriate range, and avoidance of harm. The most recent and best available evidence for ventilation modes and relevant clinical outcomes based on randomized controlled trials (RCTs), meta-analyses, and society guidelines are discussed next.

Neuromuscular Diseases and Restrictive Thoracic Disorders

Most of the evidence for NIPPV for NMD is derived from studies investigating its effects on patients with amyotrophic lateral sclerosis (ALS). Even so, data from RCTs are limited, with the most robust study being published nearly 15 years ago. This study by Bourke and colleagues[24] showed a survival benefit and improvement in quality-of-life measures with use of NIPPV in patients with ALS without severe bulbar weakness. The mode of ventilation used in this study was ST. Guidelines for management of Duchenne muscular dystrophy advocate using devices with a backup rate to prevent apneas.[25] As such, the most commonly used mode of ventilation for NMD is ST. However, use of PC or VAPS with either ST or PC modes may alternatively be used, although evidence is limited. Retrospective data have been published that a sufficient Ti time with extended Ti minimum can be beneficial in ALS.[26]

Similar to NMD, rigorous evidence evaluating the efficacy of NIPPV for restrictive thoracic disorders is sparse. A meta-analysis of small clinical trials that included 6 studies with at least some participants having chest wall deformities (ie, kyphoscoliosis, postpoliomyelitis, and thoracoplasty) evaluated the effect of NIPPV on various outcome measures, including gas exchange, lung function, sleep parameters, and tolerance of PAP.[27] Although there was significant heterogeneity, outcomes were not significantly different in studies comparing volume with pressure modes of ventilation. All these studies used the ST mode for NIPPV. As with NMD, PC or VAPS with either

ST or PC modes may be acceptable alternatives, but, again, data are sparse.

Chronic Obstructive Pulmonary Disease

In prior decades, the evidence regarding efficacy of NIPPV for COPD has been conflicting but mostly unsupportive of any benefits.[28,29] However, more recent RCTs using high-intensity PS with the specific goal of reducing the arterial partial pressure of CO_2 (P_aCO_2) in chronically hypercapnic patients with COPD have shown improvement in survival[30] and hospital readmissions.[31] Both of these studies used high PS (ie, approximate EPAP of 4–5 cm H_2O and IPAP of 22–24 cm H_2O) as well as high backup rates (ie, about 14–16 breaths/min) to maintain control of patient ventilation and achieve significant reductions in CO_2 levels. Therefore, the ST mode of ventilation using high-intensity PS showed improvements in clinically meaningful outcomes among patients with COPD with compensated hypercapnic respiratory failure. A small randomized crossover trial comparing high-intensity (high pressure, high backup rate) with high-pressure (high pressure, low backup rate) NIPPV did not show superiority with a high-intensity rather than high-pressure strategy with regard to treatment compliance, gas exchange, or sleep quality.[32] Although sample size was small, it raises the question of whether high-pressure NIPPV may be as effective as high-intensity NIPPV in improving ventilatory and clinical end points. In the United States, initial coverage for hypercapnic COPD starts with a bilevel PAP device in S mode (no backup rate). A backup rate device is approved if the provider can provide supportive evidence that hypoventilation or nocturnal hypoxemia (requires facility-based polysomnogram or home sleep study on bilevel PAP in S mode) persisted despite treatment with bilevel PAP in S mode. This policy precludes implementation of high-intensity NIPPV as the initial treatment approach.

Although use of VAPS may provide minor improvement in CO_2 reduction compared with conventional fixed pressure modes, enhancements in adherence, tolerance, comfort, quality-of-life measures, or sleep quality have been comparable. Because of the lack of certainty about the effects of the newer hybrid modes, heterogeneity across studies for algorithms and brands of devices, and potential for leak causing inaccuracy in measurements of tidal volume and thus resulting in hypoventilation, recent guidelines advocate using a fixed PS as the initial choice of ventilation mode among patients with COPD requiring home NIPPV.[33] COPD is discussed in detail in Jeremy E. Orr and colleagues' article, "Management of Chronic Respiratory Failure in Chronic Obstructive Pulmonary Disease: High-Intensity and Low-Intensity Ventilation," in this issue.

Obesity Hypoventilation Syndrome

Recent guidelines recommend using CPAP rather than NIPPV as the initial PAP modality of choice during sleep in stable outpatients with OHS and concomitant severe OSA (ie, apnea hypopnea index $\geq$30 events/h).[34] These recommendations, which are derived to a great extent from Pickwick Study results,[34] are based on lack of significant, consistent, sustained differences in adherence, sleepiness, health-related quality-of-life measures, exercise capacity, waking gas exchange, cardiovascular events, and mortality between CPAP and NIPPV. However, CPAP may be less effective in patients with less severe OSA, advanced age, worse lung function, and more pronounced ventilatory failure on presentation. Accordingly, patients who are hospitalized with respiratory failure thought to be caused by OHS should be discharged with NIPPV for at least 3 months, followed by further diagnostic testing and sleep laboratory–based PAP titration in the outpatient setting. Optimal NIPPV settings are uncertain and should be the same as those used during hospitalization.[35]

NIPPV can also be considered for CPAP failure (ie, worsening hypercapnia or persistent hypoxemia despite use of CPAP). Studies comparing ST with VAPS, including with AE, do not show significant differences in gas exchange, quality-of-life measures, or sleep quality.[36,37] OHS is discussed in detail in Roop Kaw and Marta Kaminska's article, "Obesity Hypoventilation: Traditional Versus Nontraditional Populations," in this issue.

INITIAL SETTINGS AND TITRATION

Table 3 provides general recommended modes and settings for different disorders. Note that polysomnography is not required for management of these conditions or for prescription of a RAD or ventilator, but it may help with titration of settings. Alternatively, titration can be accomplished in the outpatient setting by analyzing device downloads, $TcCO_2$, blood gases analysis, and serum bicarbonate levels. This S/T may be necessary for patients with limited mobility, such as those with NMD, and there are studies showing the feasibility of this practice in patients with NMD, restrictive thoracic disorder, OHS,[38] as well as COPD.[39]

Table 3
General recommended settings based on disease state

Setting	NMD, Restrictive Thoracic Disorders	Hypercapnic COPD	OHS with CPAP Failure
Mode	ST, PC, ± VAPS	ST	S or ST
EPAP	Low (4–6 cm H_2O)	Low (4–6 cm H_2O)	Medium-high ($\geq$7 cm H_2O, or minimum EPAP needed to maintain upper airway patency)
Auto-EPAP	No	Optional	Optional
IPAP/PS or Vt	IPAP minimum $\geq$5 more than EPAP PS $\geq$ 10 Vt 6–8 mL/kg (ideal body weight)	IPAP $\geq$ 18 cm H_2O or PS $\geq$ 15	IPAP $\geq$ 10 cm H_2O or PS $\geq$ 10
Rise time	Medium or slow	Fast	Medium or slow
Ti	1.0–1.5 s	0.5–1.0 s	1.0–2.0 s
BUR	12–14 breaths/min	12–18 breaths/min	Optional (12–14 breaths/min)
AVAPS rate	Medium or fast	Medium	Medium or fast
Trigger sensitivity	High	Medium	Medium
Cycle sensitivity	Low	High	Medium

SUMMARY

Advanced respiratory devices used for NIPPV to manage ventilation in patients with CRF have exponentially increased in number, use, and sophistication, because they provide significant improvements in quality of life and outcomes in such populations. A fundamental understanding of ventilation modes and additional settings used for NIPPV assists practitioners in adapting to different available devices and providing optimal patient care. Although evidence is limited regarding the optimal approach, an appreciation of the advantages as well as shortcomings of different ventilation modes is valuable in tailoring treatment to individual patients with different disease states and pathophysiology. Future comparative studies may provide further insights on mode selection for different disorders requiring ventilatory support.

DISCLOSURE

The authors have no financial conflicts of interest.

REFERENCES

1. Hind M, Polkey MI, Simonds AK. AJRCCM: 100-year-anniversary. Homeward bound: a centenary of home mechanical ventilation. Am J Respir Crit Care Med 2017;195(9):1140–9.
2. Sullivan CE, Issa FG, Berthon-Jones M, et al. Reversal of obstructive sleep apnoa by continuous positive airway pressure applied through the nares. Lancet 1981;1(8225):862–5.
3. Garay SM, Turino GM, Goldring RM. Sustained reversal of chronic hypercapnia in patients with alveolar hypoventilation syndromes. Long-term maintenance with noninvasive nocturnal mechanical ventilation. Am J Med 1981;70(2):269–74.
4. Bach JR, O'Brien J, Krotenberg R, et al. Management of end stage respiratory failure in Duchenne muscular dystrophy. Muscle Nerve 1987;10(2):177–82.
5. Kerby GR, Mayer LS, Pingleton SK. Nocturnal positive pressure ventilation via nasal mask. Am Rev Respir Dis 1987;135(3):738–40.
6. Bach JR, Alba AS, Bohatiuk G, et al. Mouth intermittent positive pressure ventilation in the management of postpolio respiratory insufficiency. Chest 1987; 91(6):859–64.
7. Bach JR, Alba A, Mosher R, et al. Intermittent positive pressure ventilation via nasal access in the management of respiratory insufficiency. Chest 1987; 92(1):168–70.
8. Bach JR, Alba AS, Shin D. Management alternatives for post-polio respiratory insufficiency. Assisted

ventilation by nasal or oral-nasal interface. Am J Phys Med Rehabil 1989;68(6):264–71.

9. King AC. Long-term home mechanical ventilation in the United States. Respir Care 2012;57(6):921–30.

10. Escarrabill J, Tebé C, Espallargues M, et al. Variability in home mechanical ventilation prescription. Arch Bronconeumol 2015;51(10):490–5.

11. Gouda P, Chua J, Langan D, et al. A decade of domiciliary non-invasive ventilation in the west of Ireland. Ir J Med Sci 2017;186(2):505–10.

12. Melloni B, Mounier L, Laaban JP, et al. Home-based care evolution in chronic respiratory failure between 2001 and 2015 (Antadir Federation Observatory). Respiration 2018;96(5):446–54.

13. Povitz M, Rose L, Shariff SZ, et al. Home mechanical ventilation: a 12-year population-based retrospective cohort study. Respir Care 2018;63(4):380–7.

14. Centers for Medicare & Medicaid Services. Ventilators. Available at: https://www.cms.gov/Research-Statistics-Data-and-Systems/Computer-Data-and-Systems/Electronic-Clinical-Templates/DMEPOS-Templates/DMEPOS-Ventilators. Accessed February 28, 2020.

15. Centers for Medicare and Medicaid Services. Decision memo for noninvasive positive pressures RADs for COPD (CAG-00052N). Available at: https://www.cms.gov/medicare-coverage-database/details/nca-decision-memo.aspx?NCAId=56&ver=&viewAMA=Y&bc=AAAAAAAAIAAA&. Accessed February 28, 2020.

16. Aarrestad S, Tollefsen E, Kleiven AL, et al. Validity of transcutaneous PCO_2 in monitoring chronic hypoventilation treated with non-invasive ventilation. Respir Med 2016;112:112–8.

17. Crimi C, Pierucci P, Carlucci A, et al. Long-term ventilation in neuromuscular patients: review of concerns, beliefs, and ethical dilemmas. Respiration 2019;97(3):185–96.

18. Bach JR. Noninvasive respiratory management of patients with neuromuscular disease. Ann Rehabil Med 2017;41(4):519–38.

19. McKim D, Griller N, LeBlanc K, et al. Twenty-four hour noninvasive ventilation in Duchenne muscular dystrophy: a safe alternative to tracheostomy. Can Respir J 2013;20(1):e5–9.

20. Toussaint M, Steens M, Wasteels G, et al. Diurnal ventilation via mouthpiece: survival in end-stage Duchenne patients. Eur Respir J 2006;28:549–55.

21. Arellano-Maric MP, Gregoretti C, Duiverman M, et al. Long-term volume-targeted pressure-controlled ventilation: sense or nonsense? Eur Respir J 2017; 49(6) [pii:1602193].

22. Piper AJ. Advances in non-invasive positive airway pressure technology. Respirology 2019. https://doi.org/10.1111/resp.13631.

23. McArdle N. Volume-targeted pressure support and automatic EPAP for chronic hypoventilation syndromes: an advance in-home ventilation or just more noise? Respirology 2019;24(10):944–51.

24. Bourke SC, Tomlinson M, Williams TL, et al. Effects of non-invasive ventilation on survival and quality of life in patients with amyotrophic lateral sclerosis: a randomised controlled trial. Lancet Neurol 2006; 5(2):140–7.

25. Birnkrant DJ, Bushby K, Bann CM, et al. Diagnosis and management of Duchenne muscular dystrophy, part 2: respiratory, cardiac, bone health, and orthopaedic management. Lancet Neurol 2018;17(4):347–61.

26. Nicholson TT, Smith SB, Siddique T, et al. Respiratory pattern and tidal volume differ for pressure support and volume assured pressure support in amyotrophic lateral sclerosis. Ann Am Thorac Soc 2017;14(7):1139–46.

27. Annane D, Orlikowski D, Chevret S. Nocturnal mechanical ventilation for chronic hypoventilation in patients with neuromuscular and chest wall disorders. Cochrane Database Syst Rev 2014;(12):CD001941.

28. Struik FM, Lacasse Y, Goldstein R, et al. Nocturnal non-invasive positive pressure ventilation for stable chronic obstructive pulmonary disease. Cochrane Database Syst Rev 2013;(6):CD002878.

29. Duiverman ML. Noninvasive ventilation in stable hypercapnic COPD: what is the evidence? ERJ Open Res 2018;4(2) [pii:00012-2018].

30. Köhnlein T, Windisch W, Köhler D, et al. Non-invasive positive pressure ventilation for the treatment of severe stable chronic obstructive pulmonary disease: a prospective, multicentre, randomised, controlled clinical trial. Lancet Respir Med 2014;2(9):698–705.

31. Murphy PB, Rehal S, Arbane G, et al. Effect of home noninvasive ventilation with oxygen therapy vs oxygen therapy alone on hospital readmission or death after an acute COPD exacerbation: a randomized clinical trial. JAMA 2017;317(21):2177–86.

32. Murphy PB, Brignall K, Moxham J, et al. High pressure versus high intensity noninvasive ventilation in stable hypercapnic chronic obstructive pulmonary disease: a randomized crossover trial. Int J Chron Obstruct Pulmon Dis 2012;7:811–8.

33. Ergan B, Oczkowski S, Rochwerg B, et al. European Respiratory Society guidelines on long-term home non-invasive ventilation for management of COPD. Eur Respir J 2019;54(3) [pii:1901003].

34. Mokhlesi B, Masa JF, Brozek JL, et al. Evaluation and management of obesity hypoventilation syndrome. An official American Thoracic Society clinical practice guideline. Am J Respir Crit Care Med 2019; 200(3):e6–24.

35. Masa JF, Mokhlesi B, Benítez I, et al. Long-term clinical effectiveness of continuous positive airway pressure therapy versus non-invasive ventilation therapy in patients with obesity hypoventilation syndrome: a multicentre, open-label, randomised controlled trial. Lancet 2019;393(10182):1721–32.

36. Royer CP, Schweiger C, Manica D, et al. Efficacy of bilevel ventilatory support in the treatment of stable patients with obesity hypoventilation syndrome: systematic review and meta-analysis. Sleep Med 2019; 53:153–64.

37. Patout M, Gagnadoux F, Rabec C, et al. AVAPS-AE versus ST mode: a randomized controlled trial in patients with obesity hypoventilation syndrome. Respirology 2020. https://doi.org/10.1111/resp.13784.

38. Pallero M, Puy C, Güell R, et al. Ambulatory adaptation to noninvasive ventilation in restrictive pulmonary disease: a randomized trial with cost assessment. Respir Med 2014;108(7):1014–22.

39. Duiverman ML, Vonk JM, Bladder G, et al. Home initiation of chronic non-invasive ventilation in COPD patients with chronic hypercapnic respiratory failure: a randomised controlled trial. Thorax 2019. https://doi.org/10.1136/thoraxjnl-2019-213303.

Tailoring the Sleep Laboratory for Chronic Respiratory Failure

Justin A. Fiala, MD, John M. Coleman III, MD*

KEYWORDS

- Polysomnography • PSG • Sleep laboratory • Hypoventilation • COPD • Neuromuscular disease
- Obesity

KEY POINTS

- The clinical sleep laboratory is a highly regulated space, but standard regulations are often not enough when performing sleep studies on patients with chronic respiratory failure.
- Patients with neuromuscular disease, advanced chronic obstructive pulmonary disease, and/or obesity hypoventilation syndrome represent 3 commonly encountered populations for whom specific polysomnogram protocols may be indicated.
- Documentation of polysomnographic findings in formal reports should emphasize the diagnostic criteria most pertinent to the primary diagnosis underlying each patient's chronic respiratory failure.

INTRODUCTION

For decades, the sleep laboratory was the primary location for diagnosis and treatment of sleep apnea. This era of rapid growth saw the creation of guidelines and regulatory parameters for establishing and running a sleep laboratory. These included stipulations for ensuring patient safety and accessibility as well as certification criteria for the sleep technicians performing the studies.[1] The increased utilization of the polysomnography (PSG) saw sleep laboratory numbers grow exponentially until the early 2000s when the development of home sleep testing (HST) offered a less onerous method of diagnostic testing for OSA. This shift away from the in-lab PSG sent a ripple effect through sleep medicine, with significant implications for the role of the sleep laboratory.[2]

Although HST altered the landscape of diagnostic testing in sleep medicine, the sleep laboratory remains an indispensable tool for sleep practitioners. Specifically, there are patient populations and disease processes for which portable HST remains inadequate. These patients tend to have increased medical complexity and/or complicated sleep issues that require the additional data provided by an in-lab PSG. Perhaps unsurprisingly, this shift toward more complex patients and disease processes has forced sleep laboratories to adapt, both in their physical design and in the technologies and diagnostic protocols used. This review addresses the best practices for optimizing the sleep laboratory to meet the unique needs of patients with chronic respiratory failure—specifically associated with neuromuscular disease (NMD), chronic obstructive pulmonary disease (COPD), obesity hypoventilation syndrome (OHS), and congenital hypoventilation syndromes.

PHYSICAL SLEEP LABORATORY

A sleep laboratory is tightly regulated and must meet standards of patient and provider safety, as well as secure handling of personal and protected health-related information. The 2 main

Division of Pulmonary and Critical Care Medicine, Department of Medicine, Northwestern University Feinberg School of Medicine, 676 North Street Clair Street, Suite 1400, Chicago, IL 60611, USA
* Corresponding author.
E-mail address: colemanjm@northwestern.edu

Sleep Med Clin 15 (2020) 557–568
https://doi.org/10.1016/j.jsmc.2020.08.009
1556-407X/20/© 2020 Elsevier Inc. All rights reserved.

regulatory agencies involved are the American Academy of Sleep Medicine (AASM)[3] and the Joint Commission on Accreditation of Healthcare Organizations.[4]

Importantly, the list provided in **Box 1** is far from exhaustive. Indeed, when tailoring the sleep laboratory for chronic respiratory failure, additional equipment and technical requirements are essential to provide the highest level of care for patients undergoing sleep testing. Paramount among these expanded requirements is ensuring that all patient rooms have doorways wide enough to accommodate a motorized or manual wheelchair, as impaired mobility is common in the patient populations requiring in-lab PSGs.

Furthermore, patients with NMD, congenital abnormalities, or severe obesity may be unable to get in and out of the bed on their own and will require a transfer mechanism, including mechanical patient lifts (eg, Hoyer lift), slide boards, or transfer belts. Once situated in bed, it is necessary to ensure the presence of bedside rails or a hanging bar to assist patients with repositioning during sleep. In addition, traditional call mechanisms (ie, call buttons) may be ineffective if a patient lacks the strength to push the button or if significant dysarthria prevents the patient from using the bedside intercom. In such cases, advanced communication devices may provide a reasonable workaround. Patients with impaired mobility may also be unable to autonomously change position in bed, so the use of an air mattress or pressure relief system is recommended. Sleep laboratories serving patients with NMD and congenital syndromes associated with sleep-disordered

breathing should also ensure that PSG monitoring equipment be available in a full range of sizes, as significant muscle wasting and other disease-specific changes in body habitus may require use of smaller than expected equipment. Lastly, as many patients with impaired mobility depend on a round-the-clock caregiver, when feasible, providing them with a comfortable place to sleep is recommended.

For patients with severe, morbid obesity, a bariatric mattress may be required, and the bedframe for the bariatric mattress should include the additional functionalities of raising and lowering the bed for easy accessibility and adjustment. Lastly, sleep laboratories serving obese patients must also ensure the availability of oversized monitoring equipment, including abdominal and thoracic effort belts, blood pressure cuffs, and mask interfaces.

Patients with COPD typically have fewer physical constraints but due to the presence of underlying lung disease may require access to supplemental oxygen therapy, either with wall oxygen or access to tanks.

MODIFIED POLYSOMNOGRAPHY PROTOCOLS FOR NONOBSTRUCTIVE SLEEP APNEA HYPOVENTILATION AND SLEEP-DISORDERED BREATHING

An attended, in-lab, full (level 1) PSG remains the diagnostic standard for patients with significant cardiopulmonary or neurologic comorbidities and/or reasonably high suspicion for chronic hypoventilation.[5] Accordingly, a patient's clinical scenario (particularly their past medical/surgical history and results of any previous cardiopulmonary testing) is crucial for determining whether an in-lab study is warranted. Home sleep testing is effective in many people when screening for traditional OSA but is less accurate with medically complex patients.

Boxes 2 and **3** were compiled using current US insurance guidelines for approved in-lab PSG indications. The authors recommend that sleep practitioners integrate the following criteria into their routine patient assessments in order to determine the appropriateness of an in-lab PSG:

Patients who have (or are suspected to have) any of the indications or comorbidities listed in **Boxes 2** and **3**, respectively, should be referred for a full PSG, as the limited data provided by HST would be insufficient for detecting unstable breathing patterns or hypoventilation.[5]

In cases of uncertainty, the European Respiratory Society recommends that spirometric and/or venous bicarbonate screening be performed, as

---

Box 1
Sleep laboratory bedroom necessities for accreditation

Physical characteristics of a sleep laboratory bedroom must include each of the following for accreditation:

- Single occupancy
- Private, comfortable, and quiet
- Hard, floor-to-ceiling walls
- Privacy door with access to common area
- Designated space for a caregiver to sleep (eg, recliner or cot)
- Accessible to emergency medical providers
- Testing bed with a mattress no smaller than a hospital bed
- One bathroom for every 3 testing rooms, including a sink and toilet

both are useful markers of chronic hypoventilation. Specifically, a forced vital capacity (FVC) less than 50% predicted or an elevated daytime serum bicarbonate greater than 27 mmol has been shown to correlate well with the presence of diurnal hypercapnia, and patients meeting either of these metrics should be considered for further evaluation with a full PSG.[5] Patients with amyotrophic lateral sclerosis (ALS) represent a notable exception to this rule of thumb and should be serially screened for respiratory insufficiency starting early in their disease course.

THE STANDARD POLYSOMNOGRAPHY AND ADDITIONAL OPTIONS

Based on the most recent practice parameters published by the AASM,[6] a minimum of the following recordings must be present to qualify a study as a full PSG: electroencephalography, electroocculography, chin electromyography (EMG), air flow (via nasal flow transducer [or via PAP machine flow sensor if the patient is receiving positive pressure during the study]), arterial oxygen saturation (SaO_2), respiratory effort (most commonly in the form of respiratory inductive plethysmography belts for measurement of thoracic and abdominal excursion), and electrocardiography or heart rate.[6] Additional EMG information obtained by placing bipolar electrodes on the anterior tibialis is often added to assess for periodic limb movements.

For patients in whom significant medical comorbidities are present or chronic alveolar hypoventilation is present, additional monitoring channels may be warranted.[6] The following sections outline several additional technologies that can be added to a traditional PSG when assessing patients with complex disease.

CARBON DIOXIDE MONITORING

In patients with suspected or documented chronic hypoventilation, accurate assessment of partial pressure of carbon dioxide ($Paco_2$) is crucial for initiating optimal therapy and ensuring persistence of clinical benefit. Direct measurement of $Paco_2$ with arterial blood gas (ABG) analysis remains the gold standard. However, when ABG is not feasible, the AASM recommends capillary blood gas testing as an acceptable alternative.[7] However, both capillary and arterial sampling are invasive and often painful enough to disrupt sleep and/or effect a change in Pco_2. Accordingly, the AASM has expanded their recommendations for CO_2 monitoring to include both end-tidal Pco_2 ($P_{ET}CO_2$) and transcutaneous CO_2 ($P_{TC}CO_2$) technologies,

---

Box 3
Causes of hypoventilation and/or respiratory instability requiring in-lab polysomnography

Decreased central respiratory drive:

- Obesity hypoventilation syndrome
- Central nervous system depressants (eg, opioids, benzodiazepines, etc.)
- Congenital alveolar hypoventilation disorders
- Brainstem disease
- Stroke

Impaired respiratory mechanics:

- Respiratory impairment due to neuromuscular disease
  - Amyotrophic lateral sclerosis
  - Multiple sclerosis
  - Muscular dystrophy
  - Cervical spine disease or injury
  - Phrenic nerve injury
- Thoracic cage disorders:
  - Kyphoscoliosis
  - Pectus excavatum
  - Ankylosing spondylitis
- Increased dead space
  - Pulmonary embolism
  - Pulmonary vascular disease
  - Dynamic hyperinflation due to obstructive lung disease (eg, COPD or asthma)
  - Advanced interstitial lung disease

Impaired respiratory stability with ataxic or Cheyne-Stokes breathing:

- Chronic narcotic or benzodiazepine use
- Heart failure (both preserved and reduced ejection fraction)
- Cardiac arrhythmias
- Stroke
- Renal failure
- Low cervical tetraplegia
- Primary mitochondrial diseases

---

of intrinsic lung disease and in cases where a mask interface is being used for administration and titration of noninvasive ventilation (NIV).[7]

When intrinsic lung disease is present, the accuracy of the $P_{ET}CO_2$ reading should be validated against an arterial or capillary P_{CO_2} level obtained during stable breathing. Differences of less than 10 mm Hg between the $P_{ET}PCO_2$ and blood gas P_{CO_2} suggest a valid $P_{ET}CO_2$ reading.[7]

If a mask interface is being used during the PSG, $P_{ET}PCO_2$ sampling should be obtained from the nares rather than the mask to avoid gas dilution in the setting of NIV-generated airflow. When using $P_{ET}CO_2$ monitoring, special attention should be paid to the expiratory plateau phase of the capnography waveform. If the plateau is lost, the $P_{ET}CO_2$ reading can no longer be trusted as valid. Alternative methods of CO_2 monitoring should be explored.

$P_{TC}CO_2$ is an alternative option for continuous, noninvasive CO_2 monitoring. The 2010 AASM guidelines for titration of NIV in patients with stable chronic alveolar hypoventilation cite a goal of transcutaneous P_{CO_2} level between 45 and 50 mm Hg.[7]

Unlike end-tidal capnography, $P_{TC}CO_2$ monitoring does not vary based on the presence of lung disease or a mask interface and thus has been recommended as a reasonable alternative to blood gas sampling, assuming optimal device calibration and documented correlation with P_{CO_2} levels obtained from a blood gas analysis (difference between $P_{TC}CO_2$ and P_{CO_2} <10 mm Hg).

RESPIRATORY MUSCLE ELECTROMYOGRAPHY

Sleep centers with significant experience performing PSG on patients with NMD often use bipolar electrodes to assess respiratory muscle activity during sleep. The methods for obtaining respiratory muscle EMG data are similar to those used for anterior tibial EMG recordings, although in the former the electrodes are placed over the diaphragm, intercostals, and sternocleidomastoid.[7] See **Fig. 1** for a detailed description of lead placement.

In healthy individuals at sea level, the accessory muscles are inactive during sleep, with the exception of brief periods of activity during arousals. Meanwhile, the intercostal muscles normally show inspiratory EMG activity during NREM sleep but become inactive during REM. The diaphragmatic electrodes normally show activity in both NREM and REM sleep, although the level of activity is intermittently decreased during bursts of rapid eye movement.[7]

of which each allows for continuous and noninvasive CO_2 assessment.[7,8]

Traditionally, the utility of $P_{ET}CO_2$ monitoring during PSG has been limited by poor correlation between $P_{ET}CO_2$ and ABG Pa_{CO_2} measurements. These issues tend to be most significant in cases

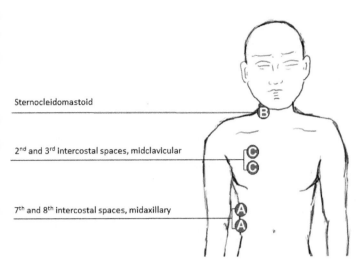

Fig. 1. Standard accessory muscle EMG electrode placement. Diaphragm (*A*), sternocleidomastoid (*B*), and intercostal (*C*) surface EMG placement for accessory muscle monitoring during polysomnography. Diaphragmatic electrodes are placed approximately 2 cm apart in the seventh and eighth intercostal spaces along the right anterior axillary line (typically only the right side is recorded in order to avoid ECG artifact). Additional electrodes are placed over the right sternocleidomastoid and within the right parasternal intercostal spaces (within the second and third right intercostal spaces along the midclavicular line).

The respiratory muscle weakness associated with NMD is thought to lead to inspiratory recruitment of accessory muscles during sleep (mostly in NREM, but occasionally throughout REM as well).[9] Because accessory muscle recruitment during sleep serves as a surrogate for increased respiratory drive/respiratory distress, cessation of accessory muscle EMG signal during the titration portion of a PSG may prove useful in determining when an effective amount of pressure support has been reached.[7]

Although not as routinely used in the COPD population, polysomnographic accessory muscle monitoring may have beneficial applications within this disease group as well. One study of 29 patients with advanced COPD found that 90% of patients had evidence of accessory muscle recruitment during sleep. Moreover, those with persistent polysomnographic accessory muscle activity were found to have more disrupted sleep and more frequent COPD exacerbations.[10] Because high-intensity pressure support works by resting respiratory muscles, cessation of accessory muscle activity on PSG suggests that optimal NIV settings have been achieved.

SUPPLEMENTAL OXYGEN

Arterial oxygen saturation (SaO_2) is another key component of the PSG that can be affected by NIV use. In situations requiring the use of supplemental oxygen during PSG, special attention should be given to the location of oxygen entrainment into the circuit. The AASM recommends using a T-shaped, 3-way connector placed between the outflow tract of the NIV device and the circuit tubing, with the side port connected to the supplemental oxygen source. Entrainment of the supplemental oxygen as close to the machine as possible allows for optimal oxygen mixing and creates a large reservoir of oxygen-enriched gas within the circuit tubing.[7]

Caution should be exercised when titrating supplemental oxygen in patients with high suspicion for chronic hypoventilation. Chronic CO_2 retention can lead to decreased central chemoreceptor sensitivity to CO_2 alterations. In this setting, hypoxemia becomes the primary driver of respiration, and this hypoxemic drive to breathe can be obliterated by the application of excessive supplemental oxygen, leading to respiratory arrest. Accordingly, the AASM recommends judicious use of supplemental oxygen during NIV titration in patients with suspected chronic hypoventilation, starting at a flow rate of 1 L/min and increasing no faster than every 5 minutes to obtain an SpO_2 level greater than 90%.[7]

MODIFIED POLYSOMNOGRAPHY TITRATION PROTOCOLS FOR NONOBSTRUCTIVE SLEEP APNEA HYPOVENTILATION

When sending patients to the sleep laboratory for evaluation, it is essential to be specific regarding what parameters and targets are to be achieved. These targets differ based on the underlying pathophysiology (NMD, COPD, OHS, etc.) and can cause provider confusion, particularly in medically complex patients who lack a straight-forward, singular diagnosis. For example, a patient with super morbid obesity (body mass index [BMI] 51 kg/m^2) with an extensive tobacco use history and evidence of obstruction on spirometry (FEV1 ~ 56% predicted) has more than one indication for in-lab PSG. In such cases, determining the most appropriate study targets will depend on figuring out which pathophysiologic process is disproportionately driving the patient's sleep-disordered breathing. This is where corroborating information is beneficial. Does the patient have evidence of daytime hypercapnia or hypoxemia on an arterial blood gas? Is there a chronically elevated serum bicarbonate? Does the patient have a history of frequent COPD exacerbations or poorly controlled symptoms? These data are important when choosing disease-specific PSG monitoring parameters and therapeutic targets.

The following sections outline important considerations to keep in mind when ordering PSG in patients with the most-commonly encountered hypoventilatory conditions.

NEUROMUSCULAR DISEASE

Chronic respiratory failure in NMD is due to progressive muscular weakness, most importantly in the diaphragm and intercostal muscles. This weakness increases respiratory work of breathing and leads to ineffective ventilation due to muscle fatigue.[11] This is most commonly seen in ALS, muscular dystrophy, spinal muscular atrophy, and myasthenia gravis.

The use of noninvasive ventilation for respiratory support in patients with NMD is well established. Specifically, all patients diagnosed with NMD-associated respiratory failure require and benefit from bilevel ventilation, with a backup rate, to support the impaired respiratory muscles. This treatment modality is also well accepted based on previous studies[12–22] that, in the United States, therapy can be initiated without sleep study or titration.[7]

Although it is not necessary to perform a PSG with NIV titration for all patients with NMD, there are certain confounding characteristics that may make in-lab titration beneficial. For example, there may be a young man with a diagnosis of Duchenne muscular dystrophy, an FVC of 45%, and concomitant morbid obesity (BMI 37 kg/m^2) due to years of immobility and systemic steroids. Such a clinical scenario creates a situation in which potentially 2disorders warrant treatment: neuromuscular respiratory weakness and suspected obstructive sleep apnea.

Although it would be possible to jump straight to therapy initiation without PSG, assessing whether OSA is present/optimally treated would be based on NIV downloads and overnight oximetry tests, which could delay confirmation of optimal settings (and in turn adequate ventilation) by up to several months. Conversely, in-lab PSG with NIV titration has the benefit of allowing for real-time EPAP and IPAP titration in order to confirm both resolution of

upper airway collapse and achievement of adequate ventilation, respectively, in a single night.

In addition, some patients with NMD may benefit from an in-lab titration PSG to evaluate issues with device synchrony and adjust comfort settings. In traditional bilevel ventilation with a back-up rate, most providers are familiar with adjusting the EPAP, IPAP, and respiratory rate. In the setting of NMD, there are other settings on the device (eg, trigger, cycle time, inspiratory time, etc.) that can have a meaningful impact on ventilation and can be effectively titrated during an in-lab PSG.

Trigger pertains to the initiation of inspiratory ventilator support. Trigger can be initiated either by the patient (spontaneous breath) or by the device (mandatory breath). The sensitivity of the trigger can be adjusted based on the patient's underlying pathophysiology. The diaphragmatic weakness associated with NMD greatly impairs a patient's ability to initiate a machine-assisted breath, so the trigger should be very sensitive (ie, low threshold) to allow for breath initiation with minimal patient effort. During a PSG, inappropriate trigger sensitivity may be suggested by an absence of patient-initiated breaths (ie, only mandatory breaths noted by the sleep technician). In such cases, increasing the trigger sensitivity would be appropriate, with the ultimate goal of making it easier for the patient to initiate an assisted breath, with the ultimate goal of having the patient initiate 10% to 25% of all delivered breaths.[23] Achieving this balance can be difficult and requires that the physician understand both the device and settings being used.

Cycle time is defined as the point at which the NIV device switches from IPAP to EPAP. Cycle time is set to limit inspiratory support and can be assessed by inspiratory airflow. When the device detects a significant reduction in the patient's inspiratory effort it will terminate the inspiratory phase of the breath (ie, the IPAP will stop) and will cycle to the expiratory phase (ie, the EPAP will start). The cycle sensitivity sets the level of inspiratory flow (generally demarcated as a percentage of peak inspiratory flow) below which the device changes from IPAP to EPAP. This is an important setting in NMD because patients may struggle when attempting to maintain the inspiratory phase of a breath due to diaphragmatic weakness, so the lower it is set, the later the inhalation support by IPAP will terminate, providing more consistent breathing, and this can be assessed on PSG via review of the inspiratory flow curve morphology and breathing pattern (ie, resolution of rapid shallow breathing with decreased longer cycle time).[23]

Inspiratory time is another important setting when titrating NIV during PSG for patients with NMD. Inspiratory time is defined as the time spent in the inspiratory phase (ie, the time during which IPAP is being supplied by the device). Aside from pressure support, inspiratory time is the important variable in providing ventilatory support to neuromuscular patients. This is because the length of the inspiratory time proportionately affects the size of tidal volume provided to the patient. Namely, the longer the time spent during inspiration, the larger the exhaled tidal volume. Patients with NMD have diaphragm dysfunction, which contributes to basilar atelectasis and leads to a ventilation-perfusion (V/Q) mismatch, hypoxia, and rapid shallow breathing. When attempting to increase a patient's exhaled tidal volume, increasing the amount of pressure support will only lead to overdistention of the low-resistance, nondependent segments of the lung, which will further impair oxygenation and V/Q mismatch. However, when the inspiratory time is prolonged, the inspiratory pressure supplied by the device will have more time to eke into atelectatic alveoli in the dependent portions of the lung, thus improving lung recruitment and oxygenation. In-lab PSG can be helpful when adjusting the inspiratory time, as a patient may start with hypoxia that gradually improves as the inspiratory time is extended over the course of the study. Over the same period, the exhaled tidal volume will also increase, leading to a decrease in CO_2 levels and an improvement in oxygenation in a real time.[23]

The rise time can also be adjusted for comfort and refers to the speed at which an NIV device transitions from EPAP to IPAP (similar to the concept of time to maximal inspiratory flow rate in traditional mechanical ventilation). Unlike the previously discussed parameters, the rise time does not directly affect the amount of ventilatory support supplied to the patient. Rather, manipulation of the rise time should be thought of as a way to improve patient-device synchrony, particularly in NMD patients with significant bulbar dysfunction, in whom oropharyngeal spasticity can contribute to glottic closures. Such events can be seen on PSG as flow limitations and tend to improve with increase in the rise time. In a patient with NMD without significant bulbar disease (often termed "limb-onset") the opposite pattern may be seen, with longer rise times leading to air hunger, which commonly manifests as a rapid respiratory rate. In this group of patients, adjusting the rise to be very quick often improves synchrony.[23]

CHRONIC OBSTRUCTIVE PULMONARY DISEASE

NIV in COPD has been controversial for decades, with some studies showing clear therapeutic benefit and others showing no benefit.[24–30] The purpose of this paper is not to readdress the question of therapeutic efficacy, but rather to take the data in the literature and practically apply it to the sleep laboratory.[24]

The goal of NIV in chronic, stable COPD is to decrease work of breathing and optimize respiratory mechanics.[31] Pathophysiologically, small airway disease and hyperinflation due to emphysema lead to increased airway resistance. This increase in resistance increases the overall mechanical work of breathing and can lead to fatigue and atrophy of the diaphragm muscle.[32,33] NIV (generally with high levels of pressure support) seeks to offload/rest the diaphragm and has also been shown in randomized controlled trials to improve ventilation by augmenting tidal volume, alveolar ventilation, and gas exchange.[24]

Two recent large randomized controlled trials[28,30] help to demonstrate the benefit of using NIV for chronic respiratory failure due to severe COPD. Both trials targeted complete control of breathing with the use of high-intensity pressure support and high backup respiratory rates and showed an improvement in both mortality and hospital readmission in patients with stable, severe COPD and chronic hypercapnia.

When referring a patient with severe COPD for an in-lab PSG, it is important to consider additional disease processes that may affect NIV titration. Specifically, with the growing epidemic of obesity in the United States, severe COPD is no longer the disease of skinny patients, with a significant portion of people living with severe COPD and comorbid obesity. Concomitant obesity confounds the treatment plan for patients with severe COPD, as it brings with it a high likelihood of upper airway/obstructive events during sleep, which, in and of themselves, have been shown to negatively affect COPD control.

As described earlier, it is crucial to understand what pathophysiology you are treating. Patients with COPD and comorbid OSA represent an overlap syndrome, which has shown improved survival and decreased COPD-associated hospitalizations with CPAP therapy, titrated to eliminate upper airway/obstructive respiratory events.

In patients with stable, chronic, severe COPD without obesity/OSA, the matter is more complicated. The first question is how to get them qualified for NIV. Under the Centers for Medicare and

Medicaid (CMS) in the United States, for the respiratory assist devices guidelines, both the presence of hypercapnia (P_{CO_2}>52 mm Hg) on arterial blood gas and the presence of hypoxia (oxygen saturation <88% for 5 minutes cumulative minutes on supplemental O_2 [2 L/min]) must be established, along with the absence of OSA. If all these criteria are met, then the patient qualifies for a bilevel device without a backup rate. The US model of starting with an NIV device without a backup rate is different from what the European literature supports (ie, an NIV device with a backup rate). This difference is primarily due to restrictions put in place by the CMS, all of which make qualifying a COPD patient for an ideal device very frustrating for providers. Perhaps not surprisingly, many providers have opted to use home mechanical ventilators (HMV) to provide high-intensity therapy to patients with COPD, as qualification criteria for an HMV have traditionally been less onerous. These devices offer the capabilities of both high-intensity pressure support and high backup rates, consistent with what has been proved to confer benefit in the European literature.[28,30]

Before beginning a titration study, both the anticipated mode of therapy and target parameters must be determined. In addition, there should be monitoring via continuous pulse oximetry to titrate supplemental oxygen therapy to the lowest level needed to keep oxygen saturation greater than 88%. Baseline CO_2 levels (either with $EtCO_2$ or transcutaneous CO_2 monitoring) should also be checked and documented before study initiation. The goal of a titration study in the setting of advanced COPD is to target high-pressure support ventilation, so sleep technicians should be adjusting NIV settings based on the following parameters:[24]

- Increase IPAP to reach pressure greater than 18 cm H2O
- Increase respiratory rate (RR) to decrease work of breathing
- Increase IPAP to reach an exhaled tidal volume of approximately 8 cc/kg (ideal body weight)
- Increase IPAP and/or RR to reach a minute ventilation of ~12 L/min

At the same time, expiratory pressure should be titrated for flow-limited events, snoring, or obstructive upper airway events. The inspiratory time should be decreased to allow for a prolonged exhalation phase, and rise time should be minimized to address air hunger. Based on overall muscle strength and deconditioning, adjustment

of the trigger and cycle sensitivities should be optimized for patient comfort.[24]

The use of NIV in COPD is Jeremy E. Orr and colleagues' article, "Management of Chronic Respiratory Failure in Chronic Obstructive Pulmonary Disease: High-Intensity and Low-Intensity Ventilation," in this issue.

NONOBSTRUCTIVE SLEEP APNEA OBESITY HYPOVENTILATION SYNDROME

Several distinct phenotypes exist among patients meeting the diagnostic criteria for OHS (obesity defined by a BMI $\geq$30 kg/m^2, daytime hypercapnia based on an awake arterial blood gas $Paco_2$ $\geq$45 mm Hg, and exclusion of other causes of hypercapnia).[34] The absence of severe obstructive sleep apnea—based on an apnea hypopnea index (AHI) less than 30 obstructive respiratory events/hour of sleep—serves as the main differentiating factor between OHS phenotypes (herein termed "low-AHI" and "high-AHI"). The daytime hypercapnia seen in OHS with severe OSA is thought to be due to inadequate time for CO_2 unloading between frequent obstructive events, whereas low-AHI OHS is thought to be predominantly centrally driven by changes in medullary chemoreceptor sensitivity that lead to daytime hypercapnia, which is exacerbated during sleep. Perhaps not surprisingly, the recommended treatment modality differs between the high- and low-AHI groups, with the former responding to CPAP therapy in most of the cases and the latter requiring NIV with a backup rate.[35]

Seeing as the workup and management of OHS with concomitant severe OSA is covered in Roop Kaw and Marta Kaminska' article, "Obesity Hypoventilation: Traditional Versus Nontraditional Populations," in this issue, for the purposes of this review the authors focus on low-AHI (ie, non-OSA) OHS.

Because non-OSA OHS is thought to be due to abnormalities in central respiratory drive, initiation of NIV with a backup rate is the recommended initial treatment modality in this patient group.[34–36] Although some practicing sleep physicians may opt to initiate NIV without a PSG, the AASM recommends an attended in-lab PSG be performed for patients with OHS initiating NIV.[7] Beyond the added benefits of being able to separately address upper airway and central respiratory events, a full PSG also provides sleep architecture data, which can be particularly helpful in assessing NIV efficacy during REM, when events are known to be more severe.[7]

Mean IPAP and EPAP levels for non-OSA OHS ranged from 16 to 18 cm H2O and 8 to 10 cm H2O, respectively in 2 major studies of this patient group. Comparatively, higher EPAP levels were generally needed in patients with high-AHI OHS, likely due to a higher critical opening pressure at the level of the upper airway in the setting of high obstructive apnea/hypopnea burden.[7]

Although the amount of pressure support is commonly considered the most important parameter when initiating NIV in patients with chronic hypoventilation, the inspiratory time can also be manipulated to recruit atelectatic lung and improve ventilation. Once adequate IPAP and EPAP levels are determined during the first portion of the PSG, those pressures are held constant, whereas the inspiratory time is gradually lengthened. By giving the breath over a longer period of time, heterogeneity in lung recruitment, and thereby abnormal air movement from dependent to nondependent areas (a phenomenon called "pendelluft") improves. Because no additional pressure is required for this recruitment maneuver, risk of barotrauma is thought to be minimal.[37]

As an added benefit, the reduction in atelectasis also improves lung compliance and ventilation by improving functional residual capacity, in turn lessening mechanical work of breathing. This point makes inspiratory time extension particularly useful in OHS, where baseline low lung volumes are thought to play a prominent role in the development of chronic hypoventilation.[38]

CONGENITAL CENTRAL HYPOVENTILATION SYNDROME AND OTHER DISORDERS OF CENTRAL RESPIRATORY CONTROL

Because of the potential for life-threatening complications if not ventilated adequately during sleep, all patients with known or suspected congenital central hypoventilation syndrome (CCHS) or other disorders of central respiratory control (eg, Chiari malformation) should undergo an attended, in-lab PSG.

Patients with CCHS often require tracheostomy and volume ventilation from birth but may be transitioned to NIV as they age, provided they only require nocturnal ventilatory support. Patients not requiring daytime ventilatory support should be assessed for transition to NIV, including evaluation

of their motivation and overall health-related adherence. Those who are thought to be reasonable candidates should then undergo an in-lab, attended PSG to document effective ventilation with NIV. The AASM strongly urges that NIV not be used in this subset of patients unless settings have been titrated during PSG and are documented to adequately ventilate the patient.[7]

Depending on the time-course of transition to NIV, potential anatomic complications involving the face and trachea exist. For patients transitioned to NIV early in life, central facial hypoplasia has been shown to occasionally develop, likely due to chronic facial pressure from the mask. Such changes in facial anatomy may create issues with mask leak and comfort.[7,39]

For patients in whom a tracheostomy tube has been in place for an extended period of time, issues relating to laryngeal injury can complicate attempts to transition to NIV. Specifically, development of subglottic stenosis following tracheostomy may delay, or even preclude, transition to NIV due to persistent central airway obstruction.[7,39]

DOCUMENTATION CONSIDERATIONS

Meticulous documentation is critical for ensuring that the results of a PSG are acceptable for both establishing a diagnosis and qualifying the patient for the most appropriate NIV device. For best practices regarding the creation and formatting of a standard PSG score report, please see the most recent AASM guidelines. For the patient groups and disease processes covered in this review, it is generally advisable to avoid standard language used for documenting OSA (eg, AHI, ODI, RDI), because such language can lead to confusion when sending test results to insurance providers and durable medical equipment companies.

Figs. 2–6 are not intended to be exhaustive. Rather, they contain the qualification criteria for NIV devices adapted from the most recent CMS policy statement regarding respiratory assist devices. The bottom of each figure also contains a

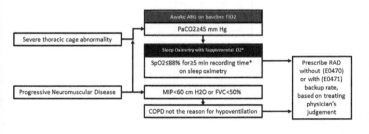

Fig. 2. Respiratory assist device (RAD) qualification criteria and PSG score report considerations for *restrictive thoracic disorders.* [a] Sleep oximetry should be performed while the patient is breathing 2 L/min supplemental oxygen or their prescribed Fio_2 (use whichever is higher). Acceptable total recording time should be greater than 2 hours.

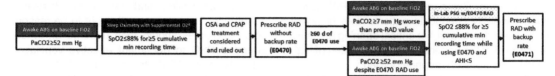

Fig. 3. Respiratory assist device (RAD) qualification criteria and PSG score report considerations for *restrictive thoracic disorders.* [a] Sleep oximetry should be performed while the patient is breathing 2 L/min supplemental oxygen or their prescribed Fio_2 (use whichever is higher). Acceptable total recording time should be greater than or equal to 2 hours. (*From* the Centers for Medicare & Medicaid Services. (2018, April). Respiratory assist device appendices A and B. (Draft R1.0b). Retrieved from: https://www.cms.gov/Research-Statistics-Data-and-Systems/Computer-Data-and-Systems/Electronic-Clinical-Templates/Downloads/Respiratory-Assist-Device-Appendices-A-and-B-Draft-20180412-R10b.pdf.)

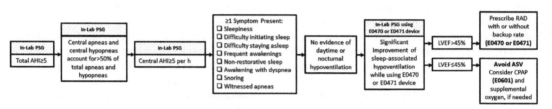

Fig. 4. Respiratory assist device (RAD) qualification criteria and PSG score report considerations for *central sleep apnea.*

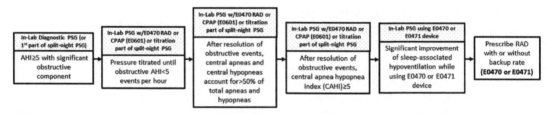

Fig. 5. Respiratory assist device (RAD) qualification criteria and PSG score report considerations for *complex sleep apnea.*

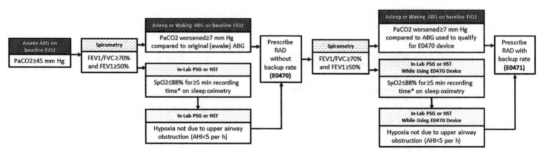

Fig. 6. Respiratory assist device (RAD) qualification criteria and PSG score report considerations for *hypoventilation syndrome.* * minimum recording time of 2 hours required

list of helpful suggestions for what to include in the final PSG score report.

DISCLOSURE

The authors have no financial disclosures to report.

REFERENCES

1. Dement W. Wake up America: a national sleep alert: executive summary and executive report, report of the national commission on sleep disorders research. Washington, DC: National Institutes of Health, US Department of Health and Human Services; 1994.
2. Quan SF, Epstein LJ. A warning shot across the bow: the changing face of sleep medicine. J Clin Sleep Med 2013;9(04):301–2.
3. Shepard JW, Buysse DJ, Chesson AL, et al. History of the development of sleep medicine in the United States. J Clin Sleep Med 2005;1(01):61–82.
4. Sleep Center Accreditation Changes: A Guide from the joint commission [press release]. Sleep Rev 2017.
5. Randerath W, Verbraecken J, Andreas S, et al. Definition, discrimination, diagnosis and treatment of central breathing disturbances during sleep. Eur Respir J 2017;49(1):1600959.
6. Kushida CA, Littner MR, Morgenthaler T, et al. Practice parameters for the indications for polysomnography and related procedures: an update for 2005. Sleep 2005;28(4):499–521.
7. Berry RB, Chediak A, Brown LK, et al. Best clinical practices for the sleep center adjustment of noninvasive positive pressure ventilation (NPPV) in stable chronic alveolar hypoventilation syndromes. J Clin Sleep Med 2010;6(5):491–509.
8. Storre JH, Steurer B, Kabitz HJ, et al. Transcutaneous PCO2 monitoring during initiation of noninvasive ventilation. Chest 2007;132(6):1810–6.
9. Arnulf I, Similowski T, Salachas F, et al. Sleep disorders and diaphragmatic function in patients with amyotrophic lateral sclerosis. Am J Respir Crit Care Med 2000;161(3 Pt 1):849–56.
10. Redolfi S, Grassion L, Rivals I, et al. Abnormal activity of neck inspiratory muscle during sleep as a prognostic indicator in COPD. Am J Respir Crit Care Med 2020;201(4):414–22.
11. Rabinstein AA. Acute neuromuscular respiratory failure. Continuum (Minneap Minn) 2015;21(5):1324–45.
12. Bourke SC, Tomlinson M, Williams TL, et al. Effects of non-invasive ventilation on survival and quality of life in patients with amyotrophic lateral sclerosis: a randomised controlled trial. Lancet Neurol 2006;5(2):140–7.
13. Gruis KL, Brown DL, Lisabeth LD, et al. Longitudinal assessment of noninvasive positive pressure ventilation adjustments in ALS patients. J Neurol Sci 2006;247(1):59–63.
14. Toussaint M, Chatwin M, Soudon P. Mechanical ventilation in Duchenne patients with chronic respiratory insufficiency: clinical implications of 20 years published experience. Chron Respir Dis 2007;4(3):167–77.
15. Benditt JO. Respiratory complications of amyotrophic lateral sclerosis. Semin Respir Crit Care Med 2002;23(3):239–47.
16. Bourke SC, Bullock RE, Williams TL, et al. Noninvasive ventilation in ALS: indications and effect on quality of life. Neurology 2003;61(2):171–7.
17. Guilleminault C, Philip P, Robinson A. Sleep and neuromuscular disease: bilevel positive airway pressure by nasal mask as a treatment for sleep disordered breathing in patients with neuromuscular disease. J Neurol Neurosurg Psychiatry 1998;65(2):225–32.
18. Lechtzin N, Wiener CM, Clawson L, et al. Use of noninvasive ventilation in patients with amyotrophic lateral sclerosis. Amyotroph Lateral Scler Other Motor Neuron Disord 2004;5(1):9–15.
19. Mellies U, Ragette R, Dohna Schwake C, et al. Long-term noninvasive ventilation in children and adolescents with neuromuscular disorders. Eur Respir J 2003;22(4):631–6.
20. Vianello A, Bevilacqua M, Salvador V, et al. Long-term nasal intermittent positive pressure ventilation in advanced Duchenne's muscular dystrophy. Chest 1994;105(2):445–8.
21. Jackson CE, Lovitt S, Gowda N, et al. Factors correlated with NPPV use in ALS. Amyotroph Lateral Scler 2006;7(2):80–5.
22. Berlowitz DJ, Detering K, Schachter L. A retrospective analysis of sleep quality and survival with domiciliary ventilatory support in motor neuron disease. Amyotroph Lateral Scler 2006;7(2):100–6.
23. Selim BJ, Wolfe L, Coleman JM III, et al. Initiation of noninvasive ventilation for sleep related hypoventilation disorders: advanced modes and devices. Chest 2018;153(1):251–65.
24. Coleman JM III, Wolfe LF, Kalhan R. Noninvasive ventilation in chronic obstructive pulmonary disease. Ann Am Thorac Soc 2019;16(9):1091–8.
25. Casanova C, Celli BR, Tost L, et al. Long-term controlled trial of nocturnal nasal positive pressure ventilation in patients with severe COPD. Chest 2000;118(6):1582–90.
26. Clini E, Sturani C, Rossi A, et al. Rehabilitation and Chronic Care Study Group-Italian Association of Hospital Pulmonologists (AIPO). The Italian multicentre study on noninvasive ventilation in chronic obstructive pulmonary disease patients. Eur Respir J 2002;20(3):529–38.

27. McEvoy RD, Pierce RJ, Hillman D, et al. Nocturnal non-invasive nasal ventilation in stable hypercapnic COPD: a randomised controlled trial. Thorax 2009; 64(7):561–6.

28. Köhnlein T, Windisch W, Köhler D, et al. Non-invasive positive pressure ventilation for the treatment of severe stable chronic obstructive pulmonary disease: a prospective, multicentre, randomised, controlled clinical trial. Lancet Respir Med 2014; 2(9):698–705.

29. Struik F, Sprooten R, Kerstjens H, et al. Nocturnal non-invasive ventilation in COPD patients with prolonged hypercapnia after ventilatory support for acute respiratory failure: a randomised, controlled, parallel-group study. Thorax 2014;69(9):826–34.

30. Murphy PB, Rehal S, Arbane G, et al. Effect of home noninvasive ventilation with oxygen therapy vs oxygen therapy alone on hospital readmission or death after an acute COPD exacerbation: a randomized clinical trial. JAMA 2017;317(21):2177–86.

31. Ferguson GT. Why does the lung hyperinflate? Proc Am Thorac Soc 2006;3(2):176–9.

32. Ottenheijm CA, Heunks LM, Dekhuijzen PN. Diaphragm muscle fiber dysfunction in chronic obstructive pulmonary disease: toward a pathophysiological concept. Am J Respir Crit Care Med 2007;175(12):1233–40.

33. Similowski T, Yan S, Gauthier AP, et al. Contractile properties of the human diaphragm during chronic hyperinflation. N Engl J Med 1991; 325(13):917–23.

34. Lopez-Jimenez M, Masa J, Corral J, et al. Mid- and long-term efficacy of non-invasive ventilation in obesity hypoventilation syndrome: the Pickwick's study. Arch Bronconeumol 2016;52(3):158–65.

35. Masa J, Corral J, Caballero C, et al. Non-invasive ventilation in obesity hypoventilation syndrome without severe obstructive sleep apnoea. Thorax 2016;71(10):899–906.

36. Noda J, Masa J, Mokhlesi B. CPAP or non-invasive ventilation in obesity hypoventilation syndrome: does it matter which one you start with? Thorax 2017;72(5):398–9.

37. Teggia Droghi M, De Santis Santiago RR, Pinciroli R, et al. High positive end-expiratory pressure allows extubation of an obese patient. Am J Respir Crit Care Med 2018;198(4):524–5.

38. Kallet R, Diaz J. The physiologic effects of noninvasive ventilation. Respir Care 2009;54(1):102–15.

39. Ramesh P, Boit P, Samuels M. Mask ventilation in the early management of congenital central hypoventilation syndrome. Arch Dis Child Fetal Neonatal Ed 2008;93(6):F400–3.

Noninvasive Ventilation Downloads and Monitoring

Philip Choi, MD[a], Veronique Adam, RRT[b], David Zielinski, MD, FRCPC, FCCP[c],*

KEYWORDS

- Noninvasive ventilation • Downloads • Adherence • Exhaled tidal volume • Leak • Oximetry
- Transcutaneous CO_2

KEY POINTS

- Patients on chronic NIV therapy require close monitoring through interpretation of data downloads.
- Proper mask interface should be chosen to minimize leak and maximize patient adherence.
- Several factors impact exhaled tidal volume including leak, set pressures, mode of ventilation, and inspiratory time.
- Overnight oximetry and transcutaneous CO_2 are used to help interpret challenging data downloads.
- Clinicians should take a stepwise approach to download interpretation.

INTRODUCTION

Noninvasive ventilation (NIV) is becoming increasingly prescribed for nonobstructive sleep apnea–related conditions[1–3] including neuromuscular disease,[4] thoracic cage disorders,[5] chronic obstructive pulmonary disease,[6] and hypoventilation syndromes.[7] Although understanding the indications for NIV therapy can be challenging in and of itself, once patients are started on NIV, management over time is particularly challenging. Structures put in place to manage home NIV may differ based on institution, region, and even insurance plans. However, regardless of the health care system in place, effective management and monitoring of NIV relies on the close interactions between pulmonary clinicians, respiratory therapists, and patients. This article discusses various parameters found within the data downloads and provides suggestions based on clinical experience to help provide high-quality care for patients on home NIV. Although there are multiple manufacturers, for the purpose of this article we focus on practical aspects of Philips Respironics and ResMed devices because they are the predominant manufacturers in North America. An extensive discussion of NIV devices and modes is provided in Gaurav Singh and Michelle Cao's article, "Noninvasive Ventilator Devices and Modes," in this issue.

PARAMETERS

One of the first steps in interpreting NIV downloads is to understand what the parameters are and how they are determined. NIV at home is typically delivered through a single-limb passive circuit (Fig. 1). This means that during inhalation, the device delivers a flow toward the patient to reach its target pressure. Certain parameters during this phase are directly measured by the device. Adherence data are measured in hours used, and is often reported as percentage of days used and percentage of days used greater than 4 hours, given

[a] University of Michigan, 3916 Taubman Center/1500 East Medical Center Drive, SPC 5360, Ann Arbor, MI 48109, USA; [b] Programme National d'assistance Ventilatoire à Domicile, McGill University Health Center, Building V - Division of Clinical Epidemiology, 1025 Pine Ave W, Montreal, Quebec H3A 1A1, Canada; [c] Montreal Children's Hospital, Research Institute of McGill University Health Centre, McGill University, 1001 Decarie Boulevard, Montreal, Quebec H4A 3J1, Canada
* Corresponding author.
E-mail address: david.zielinski@muhc.mcgill.ca

Sleep Med Clin 15 (2020) 569–579
https://doi.org/10.1016/j.jsmc.2020.08.012
1556-407X/20/© 2020 Elsevier Inc. All rights reserved.

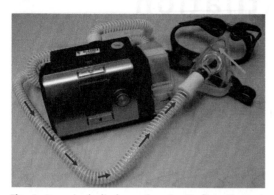

Fig. 1. In a single limb passive circuit, flow through the tubing is always in the direction of the patient as indicated by the *red arrows*. The *blue arrow* identifies the leak valve on the mask where excess flow and exhalation leave the circuit.

current insurance guidelines for adherence. Inspiratory and expiratory pressures are set in standard bilevel modes, but with more advanced volume-targeted algorithms, inspiratory and expiratory pressures are measured and reported as averages, medians, and 95th percentiles depending on the specific device. Several aspects of the respiratory cycle are reported from direct measurements including the delivered breath rate, patient triggering (percent of breaths initiated by the patient), and inspiratory time (Ti).

Tidal volume and leak, however, are calculated by the devices.[8] The volume that leaves the ventilator is not exclusively the inspired tidal volume, because a significant portion is lost to leak. Furthermore, during exhalation, air escapes via a leak valve in the mask to ensure that expired CO_2 does not reenter the tubing and cause CO_2 rebreathing with the next inhalation. Therefore, it is important to acknowledge that reported tidal volumes are not actually measured and are dependent on the calculations of device-specific algorithms. Studies have shown that leak estimations may vary by device, and with increasing expiratory leak, calculated tidal volume accuracy decreases.[9,10] Therefore, clinicians must be cognizant of these potential limitations of calculated versus measured data included in each individual device download.

The apnea-hypopnea index (AHI) is another important parameter calculated on NIV devices. The AHI does not replicate an AHI determined by polysomnography (PSG), so should not be used for diagnostic purposes. However, there is evidence that there is good correlation with PSG particularly at higher AHI.[11] Although each individual manufacturer has different proprietary algorithms, the key concept is that devices measure obstructive events as they sense changes in flow

or impedance.[12–14] For example, newer generations of Philips Respironics devices use a system called AHI_{flow}, which score a hypopnea as a 10-second decrease in flow of 40% to 80% and an apnea as a 10-second decrease of flow greater than 80%. This correlates well with PSG, especially when the AHI is less than 10 per hour.[15] New NIV devices with autotitrating expiratory positive airway pressure (EPAP) use a forced oscillation technique to adjust EPAP to minimize obstructive events.[14,16]

ADHERENCE

When obtaining data downloads, a clinician must first look at adherence. This is particularly important in the United States where the Centers for Medicare and Medicaid Services have set guidelines for NIV adherence within the first 30 to 90 days after device initiation. Patients are required to show adherence of greater than 4 hours per night for 70% of the nights during a consecutive 30-day period to receive continued coverage of the device. However, beyond using it solely for insurance coverage issues, adherence data can also guide clinicians in their history taking to help determine what specific issues may be limiting patient tolerance. Clinicians should first determine whether patients have received the appropriate interface.[17–19] Interfaces range from nasal to various forms of oronasal units. Comfort of these various interfaces is often determined by objective factors, such a facial size and features, and subjective factors, such as feelings of claustrophobia. Finding the appropriately sized and designed interface for each individual patient may be the only step necessary to improve adherence for many patients. Logistical factors can sometimes be to blame. For example, patients with neuromuscular disease with limited arm movement may have difficult putting on certain interfaces without assistance. In this case, some newer interfaces have such features as magnetic clasps that make putting the headgear on easier for those with limited movement and strength.

For those patients who state that the interface is comfortable, but still find positive pressure difficult to tolerate, clinicians must explore other factors that may impede tolerance. Even with a comfortable interface, high leaks may make treatment uncomfortable and lead to asynchrony, thereby leading to poor adherence. If patients are not synchronous with the device, then clinicians must determine whether the Ti, rise time, and trigger are set appropriately. Patients with various pathologies may have different physiologic needs that may aid in patient-device synchrony. In the rest of this article, we discuss approaches to these parameters that ultimately help with patient adherence.

Aerophagia is another common side effect of NIV use. Mild symptoms are treated with medication, such as simethicone. However, some patients may have severe symptoms that limit their use of NIV. If patient adherence does not improve with reassurance and conservative measures, considerations can include increasing rise time and Ti. As a further step inspiratory pressure or target volume settings may need to be decreased to minimize the amount of aerophagia.

Another common side effect with NIV is excessive dry mouth. Most patients use active heated humidification systems. Furthermore, proper hydration with adequate fluid intake should be assessed and recommended. For patients using NIV during the day, heat and moisture exchanger filters may be used. However, this may add resistance into the circuit and may have limited benefit because exhalation occurs via the leak valve and this is assessed on a case-by-case basis. Despite taking these measures, some patients may still find dry mouth to be a side effect that limits adherence. If a patient has this complaint, clinicians must first determine whether there is excessive leak that is exacerbating dry mouth. If the leak is minimal, the level of heated humidity should be increased if that has not yet been maximized. Finally, if dry mouth is still a problem, over-the-counter oral moisturizing products may be used for symptomatic relief.

To maximize patient adherence, clinicians should take measures to educate patients on potential side effects. This allows patients to understand the most common issues that may arise in the initial setup period. In addition, close follow-up should be scheduled to troubleshoot any problems that can easily improve patient adherence. **Table 1** lists some common problems that affect patient adherence and potential solutions.

LEAK

Before interpreting the multitude of data from an NIV download, one must first examine the leak within the system. Total leak is made up of intentional and unintentional leak. Intentional leak is built into all NIV interfaces, to prevent the recycling of CO_2 rich air, and depends on the inspiratory pressure flow and the type of mask used. Unintentional leak refers to any leak in excess of this that may include leak around the mask and leak from the mouth.

With excessive leak, ventilation may ultimately become ineffective. The reliability of autotitrating volume-assured pressure support (VAPS)

Table 1
Problems that may affect patient adherence to NIV with potential solutions

Problem	Potential Solutions
Pressure sores	Switch mask interface
High leak	Properly size mask Switch mask interface
Dry mouth	Check leak Increase heated humidification Ensure adequate hydration Oral moisturizer rinses for symptomatic relief
Aerophagia	Simethicone for symptomatic relief Increase rise time, inspiratory time Decrease inspiratory pressure Decrease target tidal volume if in volume-assured pressure support
Asynchrony	Adjust inspiratory time, rise time, trigger

algorithms, such as average VAPS (AVAPS) and intelligent VAPS (iVAPS), rely on a reasonable leak, so it is imperative that leak is controlled so that information from the download is being interpreted appropriately.

The total amount of unintentional leak that is tolerated is patient dependent and should factor in symptomatic complaints (discomfort, dry mouth, tolerance) and effectiveness of ventilation. Similar leaks in different patients may lead to important clinical differences. However, there are certain levels that should alert the clinician that further adjustments should be made. When analyzing the leak data from a device download, clinicians must first understand whether they are looking at total leak or unintentional leak. ResMed devices provide the unintentional leak only. The intentional leak is subtracted out based on the expected leak of the mask being used. Interpreting these data correctly is contingent on having the appropriate interface entered into the device. Assuming that the correct mask is entered into the device, we recommend looking at two values to determine whether the leak is appropriate. Ideally the median leak should be less than 10 L/min and the 95th percentile leak less than 24 L/min (**Fig. 2**). Philips Respironics devices, however, report the total leak. Ideally clinicians should have easy access to charts with expected leaks for the different masks used in their practice at different pressure settings. Whereas most masks with

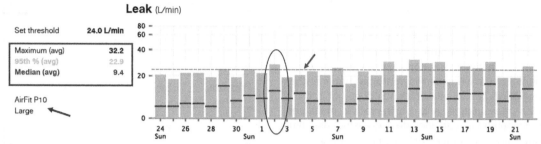

Fig. 2. Unintentional leak data as presented from a ResMed device. The *blue circle* outlines a 24-hour period with the top of the *yellow bar* representing the 95th percentile leak and the *solid black line* in the bar representing the median leak for that day. The *dotted line* across the graph identified by the *blue arrow* represents the set threshold for elevated unintentional leak of 24.0 L/min. The *red box* indicates the average daily median, maximum, and 95th percentile leaks for the 30-day period. Because ResMed downloads provide the unintentional leak only, it is important to ensure that the selected mask interface as indicated by the *red arrow* is the same interface the patient is using. In this example the patient's average median are less than 10 L/min and most nights the 95th percentile leak is less than 24 L/min. However, careful assessment of the daily graphs reveals that the leaks are elevated on many nights and further assessment to correct this should be considered.

mean pressures of 10 cm H_2O have an expected total leak ranging from 25 to 35 L/min, at pressures of 20 cm H_2O the expected total leaks are more typically at the 40 to 55 L/min range. As with ResMed devices, aiming for median leaks less than 10 L/min higher than the expected is reasonable. In the absence of easy access to expected leak charts, the clinician may choose to use as a general rule that once total leaks are in excess of 60 L/min, titrating algorithms may not be accurate. If greater than 5% of the night is spent in a high leak state, Philips Respironics recommends that

the leak needs to be addressed. **Fig. 3** provides an example of high leak.

When encountering a high and persistent leak, one must first consider the mask interface and ensure that patients are installing and adjusting them appropriately and whether it is the right interface for them. Nasal mask or nasal pillow interfaces are often preferred by patients who suffer from an element of claustrophobia, or who require daytime ventilation, because they facilitate better speech and vision as a result of less facial obstruction. There is also smaller surface area contacting

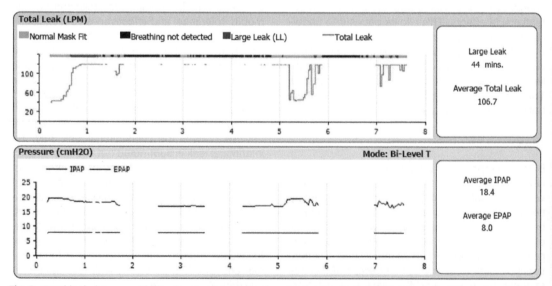

Fig. 3. Total leak data on a Philips Respironics device showing a large leak. In this example, although only 44 minutes are indicated for a large leak, in fact it is almost 50% of the night without breathing detected because of the leak being too high. Furthermore, the impact of the leak does not allow the delivered pressure. The patient's IPAP and EPAP settings are 20 cm H_2O and 8 cm H_2O, respectively; however, the attained average IPAP is only 18/8 cm H_2O. IPAP, inspiratory positive airway pressure.

the skin, making them easier to adjust to minimize leaks. However, for those who have some degree of mouth breathing and/or facial muscle weakness, the leak may be too large to maintain adequate ventilation. Chin straps are used, but patient tolerance may vary greatly. Nasal masks, as opposed to nasal pillows, can cause excess pressure at the bridge of the nose, which can lead to skin breakdown. For those patients unable to use nasal masks because of high leaks, full facemask interfaces may minimize the leak in the system. Standard oronasal masks must be sized appropriately to ensure a tight seal. Facial shape differs between patients and must therefore be considered when choosing the mask. Some of the challenges of full facemasks include pressure at the bridge of the nose, more surface area covered by the mask leading to potential high leaks, and more adjustments needed to obtain proper fit. For those patients predisposed to developing sores at the bridge of the nose with prolonged NIV usage, newer oronasal masks that fit just below the nares may be more comfortable for some patients. They also allow for eyewear to be worn to improve quality of life for some patients. Regardless of which interface is chosen, the best interface for each individual patient balances quality of life with adequate ventilation and safety. Clinicians must remember that patients with neuromuscular disease, quadriplegia, or decreased mental status may not be able to remove full face masks on their own. This must be considered when the interface is chosen.

In situations where median leaks are appropriate but 95th percentile is high, this may be indicative of variable mouth and/or positional leaks. Efforts should be taken to adjust the interface to have the 95th percentile leak closer to the median leak. **Table 2** lists some suggestions for interface and circuit assessment to help prevent leak.

EXHALED TIDAL VOLUME

For patients who are using NIV for ventilation purposes (as opposed to pure sleep apnea), maintaining adequate minute ventilation is of vital importance. Current NIV is based on positive pressure technology. The difference between inspiratory and expiratory pressure, along with chest wall and lung compliance, determine the delivered tidal volume. Given that current NIV technology are pressure modes of ventilation with built in leak, the delivered volume is estimated by a calculated exhaled tidal volume. We generally aim for 8 mL/kg ideal body weight estimated by height as a target volume.[14] For patients with neuromuscular disease, chest wall compliance decreases as the

Table 2 **Suggestions for interface and circuit assessment to help prevent leak**	
Type of mask	Nasal mask has a smaller surface to cover, may limit leaks Facial mask may limit leak from the mouth
Headgears	Use the minimum tension required to keep in place the mask When adjustment is needed, always detach both sides and place them equally on both sides of the head
Position	Always adjust the mask in the position in which it will be used
Machine	Start the machine before readjusting the mask
Silicone air cushion[a]	Lift the mask to inflate the air cushion to optimize the comfort and decrease leaks
Cleaning silicone	Clean the mask daily to remove the greasy film left by the sebum of the skin
Chin strap	Could help to decreased mouth leaks Could be tried before considering to change for a full face mask
Circuit	Check: Circuit parts are well connected Check that each part of the circuit is in good condition (no cracks or other signs of wear and tear) Ensure that the circuit is adequately positioned so that there is no pulling or tension on the circuit
Humidity chamber	Make sure it is correctly installed in the device No cracks or holes

[a] Air cushion: All types of masks have an air cushion, sometimes they have a double wall or other times created only by the bulge of the silicone bubble. The role of the air cushion is to maintain a good seal and to avoid high pressure points on the patient's face. To be effective, it must be able to inflate when positive pressure is started. If the headgears are too tight, the air cushion is not able to inflate and does not function appropriately.

disease progresses. For standard modes, such as spontaneous (S), spontaneous/timed (S/T), and pressure control, if the exhaled tidal volume declines between visits, then the inspiratory pressure must be increased to maintain the same exhaled volume. With VAPS modes, target tidal volumes (AVAPS) or alveolar ventilations (iVAPS) are set to maintain an adequate minute ventilation.[16] However, exhaled tidal volumes must still be evaluated on the data downloads to ensure that these volumes are being delivered. If the exhaled volumes do not match the target tidal volumes, then one must troubleshoot the underlying problem. First, the leak must be assessed to make sure that the delivered pressure is primarily being delivered to the respiratory system. Furthermore, if the leak is excessive, increasing the inspiratory pressure may further worsen the leak. If the leak is appropriate, then there are several reasons the exhaled volume may not match the target volume. First, the volume may be limited by the maximum inspiratory pressure. When the VAPS feature is being used, a range of inspiratory pressures (since one can set pressure support in AVAPS AE) is set. If the maximum inspiratory pressure is set too low in patients with poor lung or chest wall compliance, the delivered pressure may consistently reach that inspiratory pressure maximum. In this case, the average inspiratory pressure would equal the maximum inspiratory pressure. If the maximum pressure is being reached and target volume has not yet been attained, this is remedied by increasing the maximum inspiratory pressure or pressure support. The data downloads will provide the inspired pressure ranges and the clinician can also examine the nightly graphic summaries to observe this. Most standard bilevel devices with VAPS can deliver a maximum inspiratory pressure of 30 cm H_2O and ventilators (eg, ResMed Astral and Philips Respironics Trilogy) can deliver pressures up to 50 cm H_2O.

If the target volume is not being reached, one must also consider whether airway obstruction is adequately being treated. If persistent obstruction is suspected based on history or the presence of an elevated AHI, even with an adequate inspiratory positive airway pressure (IPAP) or IPAP range, target volumes may remain low. In this case, the EPAP should be increased to minimize obstructive events. VAPS with autoadjusting EPAP (AVAPS-AE, iVAPS-AE) is used for patients with ventilation needs who may also have variable obstruction through the night. These algorithms maintain airway patency with an adjustable EPAP, while maintaining adequate minute ventilation based on the volume-targeted algorithms.

Another reason the exhaled volume may be suboptimal is an inadequate Ti being delivered. This is especially relevant to patients with underlying neuromuscular disease because they are predisposed to developing rapid shallow breathing patterns as their respiratory muscles weaken. At high respiratory rates with short Ti, there may not be adequate time during inspiration to achieve the set inspiratory pressure and/or deliver the target tidal volume.[20] In examining the download, the clinician should first look at the data addressing the respiratory cycle. This information may be reported differently based on device manufacturer. For ResMed devices, depending on the platform, either a Ti or an inspiratory/expiratory (I/E) ratio is reported as median, 95th percentile, and maximum values. For Philips Respironics devices, an average Ti/total duration of the respiratory cycle value is reported. In neuromuscular disease, if I/E ratios are close to 1:1 and respiratory rates remain high, then it is unlikely that the device will be able to deliver the desired volume of air for each breath.[20] In this case the clinician needs to look at whether the Ti is inadequate, the set respiratory rate needs to be adjusted, or the mode should be reconsidered. As such, the clinician must also understand the various modes of NIV and the differences between manufacturers.

With Philips Respironics devices, in spontaneous mode (S), the set inspiratory pressure is provided with each patient-triggered breath and the Ti is determined by the duration of the patient's effort. Patients with extreme neuromuscular weakness may continue with rapid shallow breathing because of a naturally short Ti. In S/T, a backup rate and Ti are added. However, if the patient is breathing higher than the ventilator set rate, the breaths will remain spontaneous and may not achieve an adequate Ti. Only machine-triggered breaths will deliver the set Ti.[16] Therefore, if the Ti is low, one should examine the percentage of patient-triggered breaths and if most breaths are patient triggered, adjusting the Ti will have minimal impact. The clinician may choose to increase the set respiratory rate to closer match the patient's rate or preferably the mode is changed to a pressure control mode where a fixed Ti is delivered with each breath, whether patient or machine triggered (**Fig. 4**).[20]

With ResMed devices with S and S/T modes, the clinician sets a minimum and maximum Ti and can therefore ensure that an adequate Ti is allowed. The default settings for Ti minimum and maximum are 0.3 and 2.5 seconds, respectively. These extremes allow for patients to essentially breathe spontaneously, which may provide more

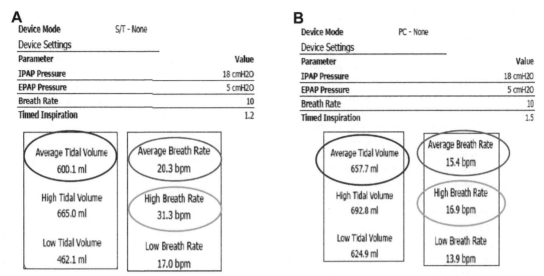

A

Device Mode	S/T - None

Device Settings

Parameter	Value
IPAP Pressure	18 cmH2O
EPAP Pressure	5 cmH2O
Breath Rate	10
Timed Inspiration	1.2

Average Tidal Volume
600.1 ml

Average Breath Rate
20.3 bpm

High Tidal Volume
665.0 ml

High Breath Rate
31.3 bpm

Low Tidal Volume
462.1 ml

Low Breath Rate
17.0 bpm

B

Device Mode	PC - None

Device Settings

Parameter	Value
IPAP Pressure	18 cmH2O
EPAP Pressure	5 cmH2O
Breath Rate	10
Timed Inspiration	1.5

Average Tidal Volume
657.7 ml

Average Breath Rate
15.4 bpm

High Tidal Volume
692.8 ml

High Breath Rate
16.9 bpm

Low Tidal Volume
624.9 ml

Low Breath Rate
13.9 bpm

Fig. 4. Summary of two downloads in a 23 year old with diaphragmatic paralysis indicating the impact in change of two parameters as indicated by *blue circles*. Changes in mode from S/T (*A*) to pressure control (*B*) and an increase in inspiratory time from 1.2 to 1.5 seconds led to a significant increase in tidal volume (*red circle*) and decreases in average breath rate (*blue circle*) and high breath rate (*green circle*) to more physiologic levels. PC, pressure control.

comfort. However, this may not be appropriate for certain pathologies including neuromuscular disease, thoracic cage abnormalities, or obesity.[16] To provide more consistent controlled breaths, the minimum Ti should be increased to a time well higher than the default settings. This ensures that enough time is allowed for the target tidal volume to be delivered. With that increased amount of support, the respiratory rate will likely decrease as the patient experiences less air hunger. It should be noted that the newest version of the Philips Respironics Trilogy, the Trilogy Evo, also allows the user to set a minimum and maximum Ti in S and S/T modes.

In chronic obstructive pulmonary disease, because of airway obstruction and decreased elastic recoil, patients are predisposed to developing air trapping and hyperinflation, which may lead to worsening hypercapnia. In this situation, careful attention should be paid to the Ti. Too long of a Ti may lead to worsening of air trapping. Therefore, the Ti should be adjusted appropriately based on the percentage of time spent in the inspiratory cycle. A prolonged I/E ratio is preferred in patients with obstructive physiology.

PERCENT TRIGGERED BREATHS

Clinicians should also look at the percentage of breaths that are triggered by the patient. The interpretation of this depends on the patient's underlying conditions and the clinical settings. A low

percentage of patient-triggered breaths may indicate that the trigger sensitivity setting is not set sensitive enough and not able to sense the patient's spontaneous efforts. In these circumstances the clinician may need to increase the trigger sensitivity. With ResMed devices this entails going to a "higher" sensitivity (eg, from medium to high) and with Philips Respironics devices, this entails changing from autotrak to autotrak sensitive or to a flow trigger with a lower flow setting (eg, from 5 L/min to 3 L/min).

Alternatively, a low-percent triggered breath may indicate the backup rate is set at or greater than the patient's own physiologic respiratory rate and the device may be delivering a breath before the patient initiates their own breath. In neuromuscular disease this may be desirable and some clinicians aim to provide "respiratory muscle rest" overnight and have the device initiate and deliver most breaths. In this circumstance downloads are used to increase the respiratory rate until less than 10% to 20% patient-triggered breaths at their baseline.[21] The clinician, however, may require clinical assessments over time to ensure that as the patient's neuromuscular disease progresses, the trigger sensitivity remains adequate because the patient will still need to trigger the device intermittently and during times of illness.

High leaks may also interfere with patient triggering and cause autotriggering. This is more difficult to ascertain from a download.

OVERNIGHT OXIMETRY

Although a significant amount of information is interpreted from the data download alone, these data have limitations in terms of physiologic changes through the night. Although PSG is the gold standard to monitor overnight physiologic changes during sleep, repeat PSG may be undesirable given the burden to patients, particularly those with neuromuscular weakness, and cost and resource limitations.[22] Overnight oximetry is a cost-effective alternative for physiologic monitoring for patients already initiated on NIV. It has several advantages including simplicity of use, easy installation, and relative affordable cost.[9,23]

Overnight oximetry alone, however, has several limitations. There may be artifact depending on position or movement, and moments of poor perfusion at the site of monitoring. Also, desaturation events cannot be interpreted in isolation because there may be various reasons for low oxygen saturations, including obstructive events, hypoventilation, or changes in ventilation/perfusion matching. Another challenge is the lack of standardized criteria for oximetry assessment of NIV. The most specific criteria for suspected hypoventilation include Sao_2 less than 88% for 5 consecutive minutes and/or a mean Sao_2 less than 90% or Sao_2 less than 90% for greater than 10% of the night.[24] However, there would need to be significant impairment before those are met. Other groups have used a 4% desaturation index (ODI4%) to monitor NIV outcomes.[25] The ODI4% is useful in long-term monitoring and if it

is increasing may be a sign that ventilator or mask adjustments may be required.

The most informative way to interpret the oximetry is in conjunction with a data download. If periods of desaturation coincide with periods of large leak, then efforts should be focused on the mask interface to attempt to minimize the periods of leak (**Fig. 5**). If mask leaks seem to be well controlled, the clinician must consider whether there are residual obstructive events present. If the AHI on the download is elevated, one should consider increasing the EPAP.

If leaks and obstructive events are controlled, and desaturations are suspected to be caused by periods of nocturnal hypoventilation, then adjustments are made to various settings including backup rate, tidal volume, or inspiratory pressures to increase minute ventilation. However, given the limitations of overnight oximetry, appropriate follow-up with repeat oximetry should be scheduled. If desaturations persist, PSG should be considered.

One must remember that hypoventilation may be masked when supplemental oxygen alone used to treat desaturations; therefore, oxygen therapy alone is not recommended without a clear understanding of the underlying physiology causing the desaturation.

TRANSCUTANEOUS CO_2 MONITORING

Although arterial blood gas (ABG) remains the gold standard for measurement of $Paco_2$ levels and acid/base status, regular monitoring using ABG

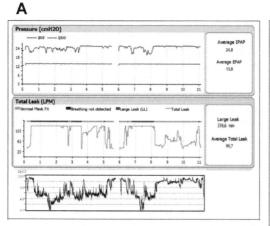
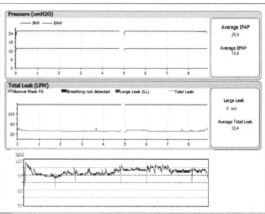

Fig. 5. (*A*) The oximetry in 65 year old with chronic obstructive pulmonary disease and obesity hypoventilation reveals frequent and prolonged desaturations to <80% documented throughout the night with the largest desaturations related to the large leaks on the download. Furthermore, during these periods the set IPAP of 25 cm H_2O is not being reached because of the excessive leak. (*B*) After appropriate teaching for mask adjustment the leak improved with associated improvement in oxygenation.

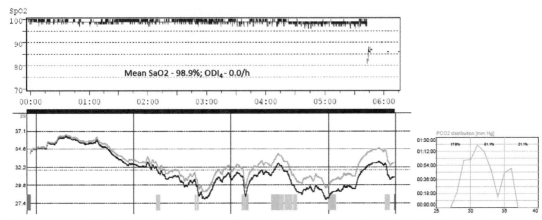

Fig. 6. A 9 year old with spinal muscular atrophy type 2 on NIV. The patient's download (not shown) revealed 100% nightly adherence, normal leaks, exhaled tidal volume of 9 mL/kg, and AHI of 0.2/h. (*Top*) The oximetry is normal with a normal mean saturation and no desaturations of 4% or more as indicated by a 4% desaturation index (ODI4%) of 0.0/h. (*Bottom*) However, the TCO$_2$ tracing reveals most of the night TCO$_2$ less than 35 mm Hg indicating they are overventilated on the current settings. On the TCO$_2$ tracing, the *green line* indicates the measured TCO$_2$ and the *blue line* is the drift corrected TCO$_2$ and is the tracing that should be used. To the right is a distribution graph of the cumulative times spent at different TCO$_2$ during the night.

is limited by several factors including patient body habitus, patient discomfort, and practicalities of obtaining real-time ABGs during periods of hypoventilation. Newer transcutaneous CO$_2$ (TCO$_2$) devices have been shown to be reliable in estimation of Pa$_{CO_2}$ levels.[26] Combined with overnight oximetry and data downloads, clinicians can more reliably detect periods of hypoventilation before patients developing daytime hypercapnia. Appropriate adjustments are made to NIV settings to

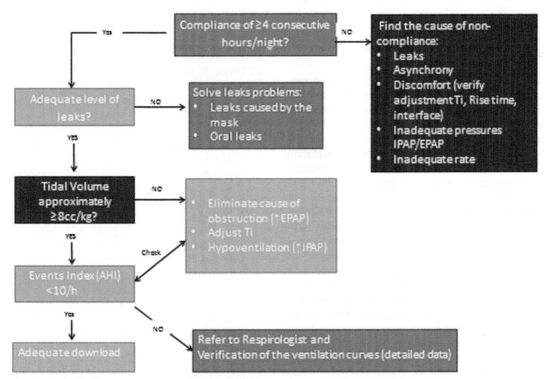

Fig. 7. Approach to evaluating NIV data download. (*Courtesy of* Veronique Adam and Programme National d'Assistance Ventilatoire à Domicile (PNAVD), Montreal, Quebec, Canada.)

minimize these periods of hypoventilation. Furthermore, if a patient is overventilated, then all indices on download and oximetry may be normal and this would not be detected without CO_2 measurements (**Fig. 6**).

As with overnight oximetry, TCO_2 monitoring may be limited by artifact and poor perfusion. In addition, TCO_2 monitors are expensive, fragile, and not widely used by many home care companies. Therefore, widespread use in the home environment remains limited. However, if TCO_2 monitoring is available, then clinicians should consider it as an additional tool to ensure adequate ventilation for patients on NIV.

PROTOCOLS

Given the complexities involved in monitoring home mechanical ventilation, we recommend instituting respiratory therapy–based protocols for effective longitudinal follow-up. A systematic approach involving a home-based respiratory therapist is vital to ensure most effective adherence to the therapy and appropriate management of settings. In **Fig. 7**, we outline a systematic approach that can be followed by a home-based respiratory therapist to manage most of the problems that may be encountered when a patient is initiated on home mechanical ventilation. If these parameters are not able to be controlled, then further diagnostic testing, such as PSG, may be warranted.

SUMMARY

Long-term monitoring of patients on home mechanical ventilation is aimed at treating the patient's underlying problem in a cost-effective and efficient manner. Routine PSG and ABG monitoring is not practical, cost-effective, or comfortable for patients. Therefore, proper interpretation of data downloads, in conjunction with noninvasive testing, such as overnight oximetry and TCO_2 monitoring, should be used to optimize NIV settings. Efforts should be made to minimize mask leaks, achieve adequate tidal volumes, and limit obstructive events. Clinicians must also take detailed histories to elicit any symptoms of nocturnal hypoventilation. When performed in a systematic way, home-based respiratory therapists partnered with pulmonary clinicians can provide effective NIV monitoring that can lead to increased adherence to therapy and appropriate ventilation.

DISCLOSURE

No financial disclosures.

REFERENCES

1. MacIntyre EJ, Asadi L, McKim DA, et al. Clinical outcomes associated with home mechanical ventilation: a systematic review. Can Respir J 2016;2016: 6547180.
2. Rose L, McKim DA, Katz SL, et al. Home mechanical ventilation in Canada: a national survey. Respir Care 2015;60(5):695–704.
3. King AC. Long-term home mechanical ventilation in the United States. Respir Care 2012;57(6):921–30 [discussion: 30–2].
4. Bourke SC, Bullock RE, Williams TL, et al. Noninvasive ventilation in ALS: indications and effect on quality of life. Neurology 2003;61(2):171–7.
5. Annane D, Orlikowski D, Chevret S. Nocturnal mechanical ventilation for chronic hypoventilation in patients with neuromuscular and chest wall disorders. Cochrane Database Syst Rev 2014;(12):CD001941.
6. Ergan B, Oczkowski S, Rochwerg B, et al. European Respiratory Society guidelines on long-term home non-invasive ventilation for management of COPD. Eur Respir J 2019;54(3):1901003.
7. Couillard A, Pepin JL, Rabec C, et al. Noninvasive ventilation: efficacy of a new ventilatory mode in patients with obesity-hypoventilation syndrome. Rev Mal Respir 2015;32(3):283–90 [in French].
8. Lujan M, Sogo A, Monso E. Home mechanical ventilation monitoring software: measure more or measure better? Arch Bronconeumol 2012;48(5):170–8.
9. Rabec C, Georges M, Kabeya NK, et al. Evaluating noninvasive ventilation using a monitoring system coupled to a ventilator: a bench-to-bedside study. Eur Respir J 2009;34(4):902–13.
10. Contal O, Vignaux L, Combescure C, et al. Monitoring of noninvasive ventilation by built-in software of home bilevel ventilators: a bench study. Chest 2012;141(2):469–76.
11. Georges M, Adler D, Contal O, et al. Reliability of apnea-hypopnea index measured by a home bilevel pressure support ventilator versus a polysomnographic assessment. Respir Care 2015;60(7): 1051–6.
12. Pevernagie DA, Proot PM, Hertegonne KB, et al. Efficacy of flow- vs impedance-guided autoadjustable continuous positive airway pressure: a randomized cross-over trial. Chest 2004;126(1):25–30.
13. Morgenthaler TI, Aurora RN, Brown T, et al. Practice parameters for the use of autotitrating continuous positive airway pressure devices for titrating pressures and treating adult patients with obstructive sleep apnea syndrome: an update for 2007. An American Academy of Sleep Medicine report. Sleep 2008;31(1):141–7.
14. Berry RB, Parish JM, Hartse KM. The use of autotitrating continuous positive airway pressure for treatment of adult obstructive sleep apnea. An

American Academy of Sleep Medicine review. Sleep 2002;25(2):148–73.

15. Li QY, Berry RB, Goetting MG, et al. Detection of upper airway status and respiratory events by a current generation positive airway pressure device. Sleep 2015;38(4):597–605.

16. Selim BJ, Wolfe L, Coleman JM 3rd, et al. Initiation of noninvasive ventilation for sleep related hypoventilation disorders: advanced modes and devices. Chest 2018;153(1):251–65.

17. Schonhofer B, Sortor-Leger S. Equipment needs for noninvasive mechanical ventilation. Eur Respir J 2002;20(4):1029–36.

18. Elliott MW. The interface: crucial for successful noninvasive ventilation. Eur Respir J 2004;23(1):7–8.

19. Fernandez R, Cabrera C, Rubinos G, et al. Nasal versus oronasal mask in home mechanical ventilation: the preference of patients as a strategy for choosing the interface. Respir Care 2012;57(9):1413–7.

20. Rimmer KP, Kaminska M, Nonoyama M, et al. Home mechanical ventilation for patients with amyotrophic lateral sclerosis: a Canadian Thoracic Society clinical practice guideline. Canadian Journal of Respiratory, Critical Care, and Sleep Medicine 2019;3(1):9–27.

21. Perrem L, Mehta K, Syed F, et al. How to use noninvasive positive airway pressure device data reports to guide clinical care. Pediatr Pulmonol 2020;55(1):58–67.

22. Katz SL, Witmans M, Barrowman N, et al. Paediatric sleep resources in Canada: the scope of the problem. Paediatr Child Health 2014;19(7):367–72.

23. Janssens JP, Borel JC, Pepin JL. [Nocturnal monitoring of home non-invasive ventilation: contribution of simple tools such as pulse-oximetry, capnography, built-in ventilator software and autonomic markers of sleep fragmentation]. Rev Mal Respir 2014;31(2):107–18.

24. Ogna A, Quera Salva MA, Prigent H, et al. Nocturnal hypoventilation in neuromuscular disease: prevalence according to different definitions issued from the literature. Sleep Breath 2016;20(2):575–81.

25. Orr JE, Coleman J, Criner GJ, et al. Automatic EPAP intelligent volume-assured pressure support is effective in patients with chronic respiratory failure: a randomized trial. Respirology 2019;24(12):1204–11.

26. Aarrestad S, Tollefsen E, Kleiven AL, et al. Validity of transcutaneous PCO_2 in monitoring chronic hypoventilation treated with non-invasive ventilation. Respir Med 2016;112:112–8.

Extubating to Noninvasive Ventilation
Noninvasive Ventilation from Intensive Care Unit to Home

Ashima S. Sahni, MD[a],*, Lien-Khuong Tran, MD[b], Lisa F. Wolfe, MD[c]

KEYWORDS

- Weaning • Home respiratory care • Noninvasive ventilation • Acute respiratory failure
- Hypercapnia

KEY POINTS

- Determining persistent hypercapnic state after chronic obstructive pulmonary disease (COPD) exacerbation before initiation of home noninvasive ventilation (NIV) is important.
- High-intensity pressure support is better than low-intensity pressure support for adequate ventilation especially in patients with COPD.
- COPD plus patients (COPD + decompensated heart failure, acute myocardial infarction, or pneumonia) do not need NIV at the time of the discharge.
- In a patient with hypercapnic respiratory failure with obesity in which obesity hypoventilation syndrome cannot be ruled out, discharging them on NIV has shown to have mortality benefit.
- Closely following the bedside respiratory muscle strength is important to determine the timing of weaning of patients with primary neuromuscular disorder prompting respiratory failure.

INTRODUCTION

Weaning in intensive care unit (ICU) setting is the process of gradual reduction in the ventilator support or immediate withdrawal of full ventilator support, thus forcing the patient to resume a period of breathing without assistance from the ventilator. Because of improved technology and better interfaces, noninvasive ventilation (NIV) use is evolving in the weaning process. The use of NIV in weaning from mechanical ventilation is associated with decreased incidence of ventilator-associated pneumonia, decreased hospital mortality, and decreased ICU length of stay. Once the patients are liberated from the mechanical ventilator to NIV, a clinician must sort the subgroup of patients who would benefit from prolonged NIV support in a home care setting. In this article the authors strive to help guide the clinician in determining which patients would benefit from NIV, the timing of initiation of chronic NIV, the optimal settings, and the criteria needed for insurance approval for setting up NIV for home care use.

Chronic Obstructive Pulmonary Disease

Brief introduction

NIV in chronic obstructive pulmonary disease (COPD) is also Jeremy E. Orr and colleagues' article, "Management of Chronic Respiratory Failure in Chronic Obstructive Pulmonary Disease: High-Intensity and Low-Intensity Ventilation," in this issue. In patients with COPD

a Pulmonary, Critical Care, Sleep, and Allergy, University of Illinois at Chicago, 909 S Wolcott Ave, Room 3135 (MC 719), Chicago, IL 60612, USA; b Pulmonary, Critical Care and Sleep, Texas Pulmonary & Critical Care Consultants, 1201 Fairmount Avenue, Fort Worth, TX 76104, USA; c Department of Pulmonary and Critical Care, Northwestern University, 675 North Saint Clair Street, 14 th floor Pulmonary Medicine, Chicago, Illinois 60611, USA
* Corresponding author.
E-mail address: asahni@uic.edu

Sleep Med Clin 15 (2020) 581–592
https://doi.org/10.1016/j.jsmc.2020.08.010

NIV helps to offload the work of respiratory muscles (including the diaphragm), improve alveolar ventilation, and stent open airways allowing for improvement in gas exchange and reduction of air trapping. In an inpatient setting, physicians will likely see 3 different phenotype of patients with COPD (**Fig. 1**)[1]:

1. COPD with predominant obstructive sleep apnea (OSA)
2. Acute COPD exacerbation
3. COPD plus patients (COPD + heart failure/pneumonia/myocardial infarction [MI])

An intensivist will likely see the latter 2 categories in an ICU setting presenting with acute hypercapnic respiratory failure prompting the following questions once the acute episode resolves, which are addressed later in this article:

1. How to wean these patients to NIV if intubated previously?
2. How to determine which patients need to be discharged home with NIV?
3. How to qualify them for this device?

Extubation to noninvasive ventilation

Based on several randomized control trials (RCTs),[2–5] European Respiratory Society/American Thoracic Society (ATS) guidelines recommend extubating patients to NIV who are considered high risk for reintubation. However, this recommendation is applicable for a select group of patients with the following risk factors: age greater than 65 years, presentation with acute cardiogenic pulmonary edema/decompensated heart failure as their reason for initial respiratory failure, or presence of hypercapnic respiratory failure due to COPD. In unselected patients, there was no difference in reintubation rates when extubating to conventional oxygen therapy compared with extubating to NIV.[6]

Acute chronic obstructive pulmonary disease exacerbation

Once the acute episode of COPD exacerbation has resolved and the patient is ready for extubation, weaning to NIV is ideal. However, the dilemma arises in how to determine the optimal settings to benefit the patient.

How are the settings determined for noninvasive ventilation in these patients?

Previous studies have shown that NIV in patients with severe COPD with conventional settings (ie, lower inspiratory positive airway pressure [PAP]) did not clearly work to improve survival, quality of life, or lower $Paco_2$ levels.[7–9] However, it was postulated that perhaps minimal benefits were seen with NIV in patients with severe COPD due to inadequate inspiratory PAP (IPAP) settings

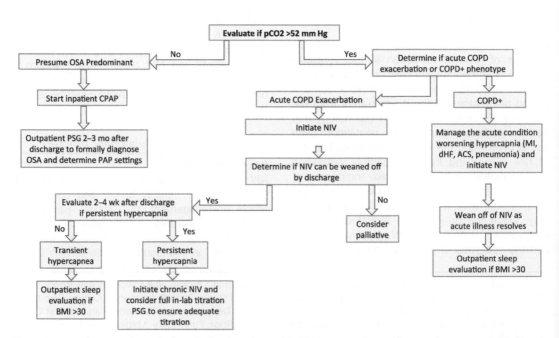

Fig. 1. Proposed approach to the hospitalized patient with COPD presenting with acute hypercapnic respiratory failure and suggested posthospitalization approach to NIV. [a] COPD+: patients with COPD and other comorbid conditions that can increase risk of developing acute hypercapnic respiratory failure (eg, decompensated heart failure, acute MI, or pneumonia).

used. It was thought that higher IPAP would allow for improvement in diaphragmatic muscle weakness, increase in tidal volume while reducing respiratory rate, and improvement in respiratory muscle oxygen consumption.[10]

Subsequent studies[11,12] tested this hypothesis and demonstrated that higher IPAP settings (mean 28 mm Hg) led to a reduction of nocturnal hypercapnia and improvement in daytime hypoxia. This is postulated to be due to muscle unloading that occurs with higher intensity IPAP settings.[11,12] Another larger RCT was able to notably demonstrate that using high-intensity IPAP (mean 21.6 mm Hg) along with high mandatory backup rate improved not only $PaCO_2$, PaO_2, and serum bicarbonate levels but also 1-year survival.[13] A mandatory and higher backup rate is thought to help offload and rest the diaphragm. Therefore, based on existing data it is recommended that for patients with COPD who are planned for initiation of chronic nocturnal NIV to start with high IPAP settings of 16 to 18 cmH2O, which can be titrated upward to the following goal points—maximum IPAP tolerable by the patient, normocapnia, or a predetermined reduction from baseline $PaCO_2$ level[14]—and to consider a high backup respiratory rate.[15] The expiratory PAP (EPAP) should be kept to a minimum if possible or, in the presence of concomitant OSA, titrated to resolve OSA.

A summary of the comparison of high-intensity and low-intensity NIV is discussed in **Table 1**.

Once the patients are successfully extubated and weaned to NIV in the acute care setting, the physician is tasked with an important question of determining which subgroup of patients will benefit from long-term NIV.

Who benefits from noninvasive ventilation and what is the timeline as to when to start noninvasive ventilation for chronic obstructive pulmonary disease?

Over time 2 important phenotypes have arisen:

1. Patients with severe COPD with hypercapnia who were evaluated within 48 hours after acute exacerbation—RESCUE study patients.[16] In this study, those patients who started on chronic NIV during hospitalization demonstrated an improvement in nocturnal hypercapnia; however, there was no significant

Table 1
Comparison of effects of high-intensity and low-intensity noninvasive ventilation on various outcomes

	High-Intensity NIV Settings	Low-Intensity NIV Settings
Daytime $PaCO_2$	↓[13, 11], no change [12]	No change [12, 7, 9], ↓[8]
Nocturnal $PaCO_2$	↓[12]	↓[12]
Change in serum bicarbonate	↓[13], ↓[12]	↓[12]
pH	↓[13]	No change [7]
Change in FEV1	↑[13, 11]	↑[12]. No change [7, 8, 9]
Work of breathing	↓[12]	-
6MWT	↑[13[a], 12]	No change [8]
Hospital readmissions	↓[11]	No change [7, 8, 9]
Intubations	-	No change [7]
Survival	↑[13,11]	No change [7, 8]

Abbreviations: FEV1, forced expiratory volume in the first second; 6MWT, 6-minute walking test.
  [13] = Kohnlein. Lancet. 2014. Mean IPAP 21.6, EPAP 4.8, BUR 16, 1-year survival.
  [12] = Dreher. Thorax.2010. HI-NIV: Mean IPAP 28.6, EPAP 4.5, LI-NIV: 14.6, EPAP 4.0.
  [7] = Casanova. Chest 2000. LI-NIV with mean IPAP 12, 1-year survival.
  [8] = Clini. ERJ 2002. LI-NIV with mean IPAP 14, EPAP 2, 1-year survival.
  [9] = Mcevoy. Thorax 2009. LI-NIV with mean IPAP 13.
  [11] = Windisch. Int J Med Sci 2009. HI-NIV: mean IPAP 28, mean EPAP 5 (2 and 5-year survival).
  [a] Not statistically significant.

difference in overall survival, quality of life, frequency of exacerbations, or time to readmission as compared with those who did not start NIV during hospitalization and before discharge.[16]

2. Patients with severe COPD with persistent hypercapnia who were evaluated at 2 to 4 weeks after acute exacerbation—HOT-HMV study patients.[17] The patients who received home mechanical ventilation with backup rate had longer time to readmission or death compared with those receiving home oxygen therapy alone (4.3 vs 1.4 months) and also had reduction in number of COPD exacerbations (3.8 vs 5.1/y)[17]

3. A third multicenter RCT trial to come from Europe regarding timing of initiation of chronic NIV for patients with COPD randomized stable COPD stage GOLD IV patients who were chronically hypercapnic.[13] These patients were given either chronic NIV for more than 6 hours usage versus conventional therapy (standard COPD therapy without NIV) and followed-up for a year. The results of the study noted that the NIV group had statistically significant improvement in 1-year survival (12% mortality in NIV group vs 33% mortality in control), along with improvements in levels of $Paco_2$, pH, and serum bicarbonate, and improvements with forced expiratory volume in the first second and quality of life.[13]

Therefore, it is suggested that patients with acute COPD exacerbation be reassessed at 2 to 4 weeks after their exacerbation and if hypercapnia persists, the patient should be considered for NIV, as stable and chronically hypercapnic patients with COPD seem to benefit most from NIV.[18]

In addition, patients who are initiated on chronic NIV have been demonstrated to have reduction in hospital readmissions and improvement in 1-year survival if their posthospital care is also accompanied by a multidisciplinary bundled care intervention, which includes regular home visits by the respiratory therapist, COPD and NIV education, and pharmacist assistance with medication reconciliation.[19]

These 2 phenotypes highlight the fact that timing of NIV initiation and patient selection is of utmost importance in determining who successfully benefits from NIV in the long term.

How to qualify a hospitalized patient with chronic obstructive pulmonary disease exacerbation for noninvasive ventilation?

Once a patient has been identified as possibly benefiting from a bi-level device, the US Medicare Respiratory Assist Device (RAD) guidelines (a set of Medicare-created criteria established for coverage of noninvasive ventilatory devices) have outlined an algorithm in order to qualify the patient for a bilevel device on discharge. In the United States, to qualify for a bilevel device based on chronic COPD

- A diagnosis of OSA should be ruled out based on clinical judgment; sleep study is not mandatory.
- Patients should have an awake arterial blood gas (ABG) analysis performed on the prescribed Fio_2 demonstrating a $Paco_2$ level greater than or equal to 52 mm Hg.
- Overnight pulse oximetry equipped with downloadable data should be used to demonstrate that the patient desaturated to $SpO_2 <$ 88% for > 5 minutes (cumulatively). The pulse oximetry can be performed on 2 L/min of O_2 or on the patient's prescribed Fio_2, whichever flow rate is higher.

If these aforementioned criteria are met, then based on the RAD guidelines the patient is eligible for a bilevel device albeit without a backup rate.[20]

Qualifying patients for a bilevel with a backup rate is significantly more difficult to do and involves documenting that the patient has failed bilevel therapy without a backup rate. After 3 months, the provider has to document an ABG showing a $Paco_2$ worsening of greater than or equal to 7 mm Hg as compared with the patient's original ABG, along with an in-laboratory polysomnography (PSG) to rule out OSA as the cause to the patient's chronic, nocturnal hypoxia. The second way to qualify for a bilevel with backup rate in the United States is, after a period of 2 months, to again document that despite bilevel use, the patient's $Paco_2$ remains greater than or equal to 52 mm Hg and overnight pulse oximeter again confirms O_2 less than or equal to 88% for a cumulative total of greater than or equal to 5 minutes (performed on 2 L/min of O_2 or on the patient's prescribed Fio_2, whichever is higher). Despite studies demonstrating that a high backup respiratory rate in these patients with chronic COPD confers benefit from reducing diaphragmatic fatigue, these patients often are not able to easily receive a bilevel with a backup rate from insurance companies in a timely manner.

In other patients in United States—especially in institutions that do not have the capacity to perform printable pulse oximetry—one can qualify a patient for home mechanical ventilation by documentation of the following:

1. Diagnosis of chronic respiratory failure
2. ICU admission requiring noninvasive ventilation
3. ABG demonstrating $Paco_2$ greater than 52 mm Hg

This should be followed-up by an outpatient PAP titration to determine the ideal settings.

COPD Plus Patients

Brief introduction

Patients with COPD may also have other comorbid conditions that can increase their risk of developing acute hypercapnic respiratory failure, including decompensated heart failure, acute MI, or pneumonia. The authors refer to this subset of patients as COPD plus patients and strive to outline the NIV management for patients with COPD with each of these concomitant conditions. Although there is a preponderance of data regarding the benefits of positive pressure ventilation in patients with decompensated heart failure, MI, and a select subset with pneumonia, there is a paucity of studies examining the role of NIV in these patients with concomitant COPD and lack of data in how to wean NIV in these patients. However, it is the authors' opinion that the robust pre-extubation NIV data can be extrapolated to postextubation as well.

Once the physician determines that the patient is ready to be extubated, either CPAP or NIV may be used. Sometimes the addition of backup rate may be helpful.[1]

Noninvasive Ventilation in Patients with Chronic Obstructive Pulmonary Disease and Concurrent Acute Cardiogenic Pulmonary Edema /Heart Failure Decompensation

Patients with COPD who develop acute cardiogenic pulmonary edema can often present in acute hypercapnic respiratory failure. It has been well shown that PAP (delivered via either NIV or CPAP[21,22]) improves hypercapnic respiratory failure in these patients by means of reducing left ventricular afterload, reducing respiratory muscle fatigue and work of breathing, and increasing oxygenation by improving alveolar ventilation and lung compliance, and often times obviating invasive mechanical ventilation.[23]

Either way, as the focus of the article is weaning to NIV and home discharge, once the precipitating condition that triggered acute hypercapnia resolves and the underlying pulmonary edema improves, these patients should not require NIV at the time of the discharge.

Patients with Chronic Obstructive Pulmonary Disease on Noninvasive Ventilation—Risk of Acute Coronary Syndrome/Myocardial Infarction?

Previously, there was a concern that patients experiencing acute coronary syndrome who also received NIV were at increased incidence of acute MI,[24] but this has since been disproved and subsequent studies have demonstrated that patients with acute hypercapnic respiratory failure receiving NIV are not at increased risk of acute MI.[25]

What About Patients with Chronic Obstructive Pulmonary Disease Who Develop Pneumonia? Can These Patients Be Managed with Noninvasive Ventilation?

Again, this subgroup of patients should not need NIV at the time of the discharge, as resolution of pneumonia should treat hypercapnia as well.

Obesity Hypoventilation Syndrome

Brief introduction and definition

NIV in obesity hypoventilation syndrome (OHS) is also Roop Kaw and Marta Kaminska' article, "Obesity Hypoventilation: Traditional Versus Nontraditional Populations," in this issue. The prevalence of OHS has been steadily increasing in recent decades due to increasing rates of obesity in both developed and developing countries.[26] The conventional criteria for defining OHS includes presence of sleep-disordered breathing and awake hypoventilation ($Paco_2 \geq 45$ mm Hg) in the setting of body mass index (BMI) greater than or equal to 30 kg/m^2, along with exclusion of other primary causes of daytime hypoventilation.[27]

Obstructive sleep apnea and obesity hypoventilation syndrome in the intensive care unit patient

OHS Roop Kaw and Marta Kaminska' article, "Obesity Hypoventilation: Traditional Versus Nontraditional Populations," in this issue. It is estimated that approximately 90% of patients with OHS have concomitant OSA and approximately 70% of patients with OHS qualify as having severe OSA.[28]

A common scenario that pulmonologists and intensivists face is the patient with suspected OHS who has been admitted to the ICU with acute on chronic hypercapnic respiratory failure. Recognizing patients who may have OHS in the acute care setting has important implications, as patients with OHS face increased mortality during or after hospitalization as compared with their counterparts with the same BMI but who are eucapnic.[29,30] In addition, observational studies have shown that patients with suspected or known OHS who are discharged with PAP therapy have improved outcomes and mortality as compared with those discharged without PAP therapy. However, initiation of noninvasive ventilation in the above situation should not be a substitute for outpatient sleep study and PAP titration, which should be done ideally within 3 months of hospital discharge.[31]

In an ambulatory setting, serum bicarbonate, Paco2, pulse oximetry, and nocturnal capnometry can be used as tools to screen for OHS, but in the hospital setting, one can only suspect OHS based on BMI and presence of hypercapnic respiratory failure.

Several ventilator modalities are available for management of patients with suspected OHS with acute or chronic hypercapnic respiratory failure in the ICU—these include NIV, endotracheal intubation with mechanical ventilation, and trach ± mechanical ventilation.[32] Inpatient CPAP is only recommended for those patients with stable OHS, but oftentimes, patients with OHS in the ICU are battling acute on chronic hypercapnic respiratory failure, and CPAP is therefore not the modality of choice owing to its lack of ability to optimally ventilate these hypercapnic patients. It is not always clear once their respiratory status has stabilized whether these patients with suspected OHS and/or OSA would benefit more from CPAP or NIV therapy on discharge. Multiple RCTs have shown that in patients with OHS and stable respiratory status, both CPAP and NIV yield similar benefits in improvement of daytime Paco2 level, daytime sleepiness, and quality-of-life measures, while also demonstrating similar treatment failure rates.[33,34]

In the Pickwick Project, 2 parallel multicenter RCTs were performed in Spain evaluating the efficacy of CPAP versus NIV in patients with OHS and OSA. A notable finding in these studies is that for patients with OHS and severe OSA with an AHI of greater than or equal to 30/hr, CPAP and NIV were found to confer similar benefits including reduction of daytime hypercapnia.[28] However, for patients with OHS but with nonsevere OSA (AHI <30/hr), NIV was shown to be beneficial in improving Paco2 and serum bicarbonate levels.[35]

Recent guidelines have emerged recommending that all patients with suspected OHS admitted in the critical care setting be subsequently discharged with NIV therapy, as NIV has been demonstrated to improve survival in this population.[36] This recommendation is based on a meta-analysis of 10 observational studies, which showed an increased 3-month mortality in patients with confirmed or suspected OHS who were not discharged on PAP therapy (16.8%) as compared with those who were discharged with PAP (2.3%, PAP included both CPAP and NIV).[31] Therefore, when stable for discharge, arrangements should be made for these patients to receive an NIV device or a RAD device. The ATS panel did remark that in situations where NIV is not available due to limited resources, auto-PAP is preferable to no PAP therapy.

What noninvasive ventilation settings to use?

NIV provides benefit for patients with OHS ± OSA presenting with acute on chronic hypercapnic respiratory failure, as IPAP allows for ventilation and EPAP allows for maintaining airway patency for OSA treatment. Multiple studies have suggested that in the OHS population, high inspiratory pressure and high backup rates improve outcomes for these patients. In these studies, IPAP pressures were titrated upward to obtain optimal levels based on various strategies, including maintaining goal Paco2 less than 65 mm Hg with pH greater than 7.35, achieving SpO2 greater than or equal to 88%,[29] or achieving a TV of at least 800 mL, and to resolve sensation of "air hunger" in the patients, with goal minimum peak inspiratory pressure of greater than 20 cmH2O. With these strategies, high inspiratory pressures of 17 to 18 cmH2O were attained and shown to significantly reduce daytime Paco2. Optimal EPAP settings were obtained by increasing PEEP until "unhindered and comfortable inhalation triggering" was possible for the patient[37] or titrating until apneas and desaturations were no longer observed during sleep in the acute care setting[38] with average EPAP of 3 to 7 cmH2O used in these studies.

Algorithm to achieve optimal noninvasive ventilation settings for the patient with obesity hypoventilation syndrome

A proposed algorithm for in hospital titration of NIV settings includes inspiratory positive airway pressure (IPAP) titration which should be initiated around 16 cm H2O and increased by 2 cm of H2O to achieve a) resolution of hypoxemia - (SpO2> 90% consistently) b) improvement in acidosis - (ph > 7.3) c) target TV of 8 cc/kg of IBW - (ideally) d) chest wall expansion on physical exam and e) resolution of respiratory distress with improvement in tachypnea. Expiratory positive airway pressure (EPAP) should be initiated at EPAP of 4-6 cm H2O and increased by 2 cm of H2O to obtain a final pressure which eliminates a)snoring b) apneas, c) Oxygen desaturations and d) Paradoxical breathing. Lastly addition of supplemental oxygen may be needed if the SpO_2 < 88% despite high IPAP pressures. It should be slowly initiated at 1 L/min and increased by 1L/min to achieve SpO_2> 88% consistently.[38,39]

Another novel ventilator strategy that may be used to determine optimal settings involves use of volume-assured pressure support (VAPS) ventilators. These are noninvasive ventilators that, using an algorithm, automatically adjust inspiratory pressure support settings to reach a predetermined tidal volume, thereby maintaining adequate ventilation for the OHS patient. These devices can have the added capability of automatically titrating EPAP to maintain upper airway patency. One RCT compared fixed bilevel PAP therapy with AVAPS therapy with auto-EPAP (AVAPS-AE) capability and suggested that AVAPS-AE is noninferior in the treatment of OHS, and both methods of NIV showed similar improvements in daytime $Paco_2$ and Epworth sleepiness scale scores.[40]

The above-proposed NIV titration process can be done at the bedside or auto-EPAP can be used in VAPS mode to assist with the process. No matter which initial NIV device (CPAP, bilevel, VAPS) the OHS patient is discharged with, as mentioned previously, an in-laboratory PSG within 3 months of discharge should be performed to determine if the patient can be downgraded to a CPAP or for further titration of optimal NIV or VAPS settings. For a full discussion on NIV devices and modes, Gaurav Singh and Michelle Cao' article, "Noninvasive Ventilator Devices and Modes," in this issue.

How to qualify patients for noninvasive ventilation on discharge from intensive care unit?

Once optimal NIV settings have been established, how do, in the United States, we qualify these patients for an NIV device on discharge?

The first method is outlined as follows:

- Document diagnosis of chronic respiratory failure and its associated ICD-10 code.
- Document ABG during admission demonstrating awake hypercapnia ($Paco_2$ >45 mm Hg).

This will allow the patient to receive a mechanical ventilator bilevel device.

A second method for qualifying a patient with OHS to receive an RAD on hospital discharge is based on the RAD guidelines and is outlined as follows:

- Document an awake ABG performed on prescribed Fio_2 demonstrating $Paco_2$ level greater than or equal to 52 mm Hg.

- Obtain printable nocturnal pulse oximetry data showing desaturation less than 88% for more than 5 mins on 2L of oxygen.
- Pulmonary function tests are not needed.

Following this second method, the patient will fall in the category of chronic lung disease category A. This will allow the patient with suspected OHS to receive either a bilevel without a backup rate (E0470) or a bilevel with a backup rate (E0471). RAD criteria for OHS exist but are laborious and thus rarely used.

Role of oxygen in patients with obesity hypoventilation syndrome on discharge

Oftentimes, these patients present with hypoxic respiratory failure and are placed on supplemental oxygen during their hospital course and subsequent discharge. The mechanisms by which hypoxia occurs in patients with OHS may be due to alveolar hypoventilation and ventilation/perfusion mismatch due to basilar atelectasis.[36] It has been demonstrated that Pao_2 levels less than 50 mm Hg in patients with OHS is an independent predictor of mortality.[41] However, providing supplemental oxygen therapy has also been found to be a contributing factor for mortality in these patients with OHS.[36] The increase in mortality may be attributed to the fact that more hypoxic patients had a higher rate of cardiovascular disease in this study population also also that chronic hypoxia increases the risk for development or worsening of pulmonary hypertension, which may be contributing to mortality in patients with OHS.

Fig. 2 illustrates the algorithm for obtaining NIV following an acute hypercapnic respiratory failure.

Neuromuscular disorder

Respiratory failure caused by Guillain-Barré syndrome (GBS) and that caused by myasthenia gravis crisis are the 2 most common primary neurologic diseases encountered in an ICU setting. Other causes of neuromuscular respiratory failure, including botulism, tick paralysis, porphyria, and critical exacerbations of chronic inflammatory demyelinating polyradiculoneuropathy, are fortunately rare, and little research has been published in regard to their specific ventilator management.[42] As we all know, this subgroup of patients has unique challenges including the readiness of weaning and deciding appropriate NIV settings postextubation.

Weaning in Patients with Myasthenia Gravis and Guillain-Barre Syndrome

Once the patient has been intubated due to respiratory failure, determination of readiness to

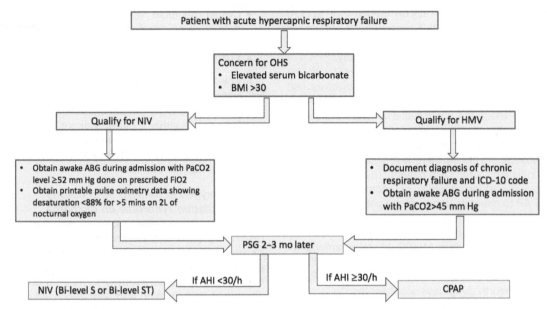

Fig. 2. Proposed algorithm for approach to the ICU patient with acute hypercapnic respiratory failure.

extubation is crucial. Prolonged intubation in such patients contributes to various medical complications, especially respiratory and infectious complications. Independent risk factors for prolonged intubation are age greater than 50 years, vital capacity less than 25 mL/kg on postintubation day 1 to 6, and serum bicarbonate level greater than 30 mmol/L.[43]

Recovery of the neurologic function is crucial in considering extubation. Along with aggressive medical management with steroids, plasmapheresis, intravenous immunoglobulin, or immunosuppressants, efforts are needed for appropriate respiratory care. Respiratory care is essential to achieving good recovery in patients with critical neurologic conditions. Intensive respiratory care protocols aimed at reducing the risk of pneumonia and atelectasis must be instituted as soon as a myasthenic patient is intubated. Extubation of these patients may be associated with considerable risks of need for reintubation. Thus, use of bilevel ventilation after extubation may be a useful strategy to prevent this complication.[42]

When to Consider Weaning?

Physical examination findings—appropriate neurologic examination showing some neurologic recovery is crucial in determining the readiness to weaning. Increased strength in the neck flexor has been associated with some improvement in the respiratory and bulbar muscle strength.[44]

Respiratory Function Tests

These tests may be useful but are less dependable in myasthenia patients than in GBS. More so, these testing are more unpredictable in patients with bulbar weakness who can perform better on the test but are at higher risk of upper airway collapse after extubation versus patients with facial weakness who may perform poorly on the test but are otherwise ready for a trial of extubation.[42,45] Nonetheless, weaning trials should be considered[46] once the patient shows

1. Maximal inspiratory pressure (MIP) > −20 cm H2O
2. Maximal expiratory pressure (MEP) > 40 cm
3. Forced vital capacity (FVC) > 10 mL/kg

Extubation should be attempted when the patient is breathing comfortably, not fatigued,[47] and FVC remains greater than 15 mL/kg, MIP greater than −20 cm, and patient has near normal blood gas.

Some investigators have recommended to consider weaning once the patient demonstrates some clinical improvement (vital capacity > 15 mL/kg).[48,49]

Another study looking at patients with GBS ventilated for longer than 3 weeks showed that a drop in vital capacity, MIP, and MEP between measures at baseline and day 12 predicted the need for prolonged intubation. The investigators proposed the use of an integrated measurement, the pulmonary function (PF) score, calculated by

PF score = VC + MIP + MEP; PF ratio = PF score on day 1/PF score on day 12. A PF ratio of less than 1 (indicating worsening strength of inspiratory and expiratory muscles compared with the time of intubation) was uniformly associated with ventilatory requirement longer than 3 weeks.[50]

Invasive Testing

Koyama and colleagues[51] described monitoring diaphragm function by its electrical activity (E-di) using nasogastric probes. They reported tidal volume/ΔE-di (calculated as the maximum minus the minimum E-di during inspiration) to be a more reliable tool to monitor weaning in myasthenia gravis on mechanical ventilator based on one case report.

Diaphragm Ultrasound

In recent years, diaphragmatic ultrasonography has emerged as a safe, bed-side tool for assessment of diaphragm function.[52] It provides both morphologic and functional information in real time. Several ultrasound techniques, such as B-mode and M-mode, have been used to assess diaphragm sonographic predictors.

- Diaphragm inspiratory excursion (DE)—distance that the diaphragm is able to move during the respiratory cycle; correlates to MIP[53]
- Time to peak inspiratory amplitude of the diaphragm (TPIA dia)
- Diaphragm thickness
- Diaphragm thickness difference (DTD)
- Diaphragm thickening fraction—ratio between the difference in thickness from inspiration and expiration divided by the thickness on expiration (Tinsp−Texp)/Texp—correlates to lung volume[54]

A prospective study looked at 68 adult patients needing mechanical ventilation and found that TPIA dia had a good performance in predicting the success of weaning from mechanical ventilation. The TPIA dia greater than 0.8 had a sensitivity of 92%, specificity of 46%, positive predictive value of 89%, and negative predictive value of 56%.[55]

A recent meta-analysis looking at diaphragm ultrasonography for prediction of ventilator weaning found that the pooled sensitivity and specificity of DE was 0.786 and 0.711. The pooled sensitivity and specificity of DTD were 0.893 and 0.796, making it a promising tool although there is a need for large scale studies.[56]

The summary of the abovementioned parameters is outlined in **Fig. 3**.

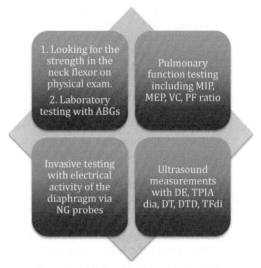

Fig. 3. Weaning parameters. ABG, arterial blood gas; DE, diaphragm inspiratory excursion; DT, diaphragm thickness; DTD, diaphragm thickness difference; MEP, maximal expiratory pressure; MIP, maximal inspiratory pressure; NG probes, nasogastric probes; PF ratio, pulmonary function score; TFdi, diaphragm thickening fraction; TPIA dia, time to peak inspiratory amplitude of the diaphragm; VC, vital capacity.

How to Perform Weaning?

There is a debate on the correct mode for weaning. Most investigators suggest pressure support ventilation but T-piece trial can also be done.[48] In a single-center experience of 5 patients, the investigators report failure to wean with the help of T-piece, and weaning attempts were made on low level of pressure support ventilation with IPAP less than or equal to 10 mm Hg and EPAP less than or equal to 8 mm Hg at the time of the extubation to bilevel support. Once weaned to the bilevel, the patients were kept on IPAP ranging from 18 to 8 mm Hg and EPAP from 8 to 4 mm Hg. They concluded that weaning to bilevel is feasible and may shorten the time of intubation.[57]

Spinal Cord Injury

Asil Daoud and colleagues' article, "Noninvasive Ventilation and Spinal Cord Injury," in this issue also discusses spinal cord injury in depth. In regard to weaning, the most crucial aspect in these patients is recovery of the muscle strength. In patients with cervical or high thoracic spinal cord injury this may take weeks to months as the patient comes out of the spinal shock or as inflammation resolves.[58] Prolonged weaning is common but slowly increasing the ventilator free time helps. Prevention of atelectasis is a key for weaning success alongside accurate neurologic assessment. In one study, the investigators used ventilator-free breathing according to vital capacity, followed by rest periods with controlled ventilation. When the vital capacity reduced two-thirds of the starting value or the patient appeared in distress, patients were placed back on controlled ventilation ensuring a tidal volume of 10 to 15 mLl/kg. Overall based on this, the vital capacity of the patients improved from 525 to 1415 mL.[59]

How to Qualify the Patients for a Noninvasive Ventilation at the Time of Discharge?

Patients will qualify for NIV based on the diagnosis of a neuromuscular disorder with clear documentation of FVC less than 50% or printable overnight pulse oximetry showing SpO2 less than 88% for 5 minutes (only possible in institutes with capability of printable spirometry) or ABG showing $Paco_2$ greater than 45 mm Hg.[60]

Empirical settings can be given to these patients but adding a backup rate or initiating them on VAPS with assured tidal volume is crucial to ensure adequate minute ventilation.

How to Qualify the Challenging Neuromuscular Patient?

If there is debate about the correct neuromuscular disorder, one may request the neurologist a tentative diagnosis of motor neuron disease–based physical examination provided the nerve conduction or electromyography studies are not feasible while hospitalized.

In the case of patients with transverse myelitis and cerebral palsy who need NIV support, a diagnosis of scoliosis based on the examination will qualify them under RAD guidelines.

DISCLOSURE

The authors have no disclosures related to any relationship with a commercial company that has a direct financial interest in subject matter or materials discussed in article or with a company making a competing product.

REFERENCES

1. Selim B, Wolfe L, Coleman JM, Dewan NA. Initiation of noninvasive ventilation for sleep related hypoventilation disorders: advanced modes and devices. Chest 2018;153(1):251–65.
2. Nava S, Gregoretti C, Fanfulla F, et al. Noninvasive ventilation to prevent respiratory failure after extubation in high-risk patients. Crit Care Med 2005;33:2465–70.
3. Ferrer M, Valencia M, Nicolas JM, et al. Early noninvasive ventilation averts extubation failure in patients at risk: a randomized trial. Am J Respir Crit Care Med 2006;173:164–70.
4. Ferrer M, Sellares J, Valencia M, et al. Non-invasive ventilation after extubation in hypercapnic patients with chronic respiratory disorders: randomised controlled trial. Lancet 2009;374:1082–8.
5. Ornico SR, Lobo SM, Sanches HS, et al. Noninvasive ventilation immediately after extubation improves weaning outcome after acute respiratory failure: a randomized controlled trial. Crit Care 2013;17:R39.
6. Su CL, Chiang LL, Yang SH, et al. Preventive use of noninvasive ventilation after extubation: a prospective, multicenter randomized controlled trial. Respir Care 2012;57:204–10.
7. Casanova C, Celli BR, Tost L, et al. Long- term controlled trial of nocturnal nasal positive pressure ventilation in patients with severe COPD. Chest 2000;118:1582–90.
8. Clini E, Sturani C, Rossi A, et al. Rehabilitation and Chronic Care Study Group, Italian Association of Hospital Pulmonologists (AIPO). The Italian multicentre study on noninvasive ventilation in chronic obstructive pulmonary disease patients. Eur Respir J 2002;20:529–38.
9. McEvoy RD, Pierce RJ, Hillman D, et al. Australian trial of non-invasive Ventilation in Chronic Airflow Limitation (AVCAL) Study Group. Nocturnal non-invasive nasal ventilation in stable hypercapnic COPD: a randomised controlled trial. Thorax 2009; 64:561–6.
10. Field S, Sanci S, Grassino A. Respiratory muscle oxygen consumption estimated by the diaphragm pressure-time index. J Appl Physiol 1984;57:44–51.
11. Windisch W, Haenel M, Storre JH, et al. High-intensity non-invasive positive pressure ventilation for stable hypercapnic COPD. Int J Med Sci 2009;6: 72–6.
12. Dreher M, Storre JH, Schmoor C, et al. High-intensity versus low-intensity non-invasive ventilation in patients with stable hypercapnic COPD: a randomised crossover trial. Thorax 2010;65:303–8.
13. Köhnlein T, Windisch W, Köhler D, et al. Non-invasive positive pressure ventilation for the treatment of severe stable chronic obstructive pulmonary disease: a prospective, multicentre, randomised, controlled clinical trial. Lancet Respir Med 2014;2(9):698–705.
14. Wiles SP, Aboussouan LS, Mireles-cabodevila E. Noninvasive positive pressure ventilation in stable patients with COPD. Curr Opin Pulm Med 2020; 26(2):175–85.
15. Murphy PB, Brignall K, Moxham J, et al. High pressure versus high intensity noninvasive ventilation in

stable hypercapnic chronic obstructive pulmonary disease: a randomized crossover trial. Int J Chron Obstruct Pulmon Dis 2012;7:811–8.

16. Struik FM, Sprooten RT, Kerstjens HA, et al. Nocturnal non-invasive ventilation in COPD patients with prolonged hypercapnia after ventilatory support for acute respiratory failure: a randomised, controlled, parallel-group study. Thorax 2014;69:826–34.

17. Murphy PB, Rehal S, Arbane G, et al. Effect of home noninvasive ventilation with oxygen therapy vs oxygen therapy alone on hospital readmission or death after an acute COPD exacerbation: a randomized clinical trial. JAMA 2017;317(21):2177–86.

18. Murphy PB, Hart N. Home non-invasive ventilation for COPD: how, who and when? Arch Bronconeumol 2018;54(3):149–54.

19. Coughlin S, Liang WE, Parthasarathy S. Retrospective assessment of home ventilation to reduce rehospitalization in chronic obstructive pulmonary disease. J Clin Sleep Med 2015;11(6):663–70.

20. Available at:https://www.resmed.com/us/dam/documents/articles/1010293_RAD_Guidelines.pdf. Accessed September 25, 2020.

21. Winck JC, Azevedo LF, Costa-pereira A, et al. Efficacy and safety of non-invasive ventilation in the treatment of acute cardiogenic pulmonary edema– a systematic review and meta-analysis. Crit Care 2006;10(2):R69.

22. Pisani L, Corcione N, Nava S. Management of acute hypercapnic respiratory failure. Curr Opin Crit Care 2016;22:45–52.

23. Bersten AD, Holt AW, Vedig AE, et al. Treatment of severe cardiogenic pulmonary edema with continuous positive airway pressure delivered by face mask. N Engl J Med 1991;325:1825–30.

24. Mehta S, Jay GD, Woolard RH, et al. Randomised, prospective trial of bilevel versus continuous positive airway pressure in acute pulmonary edema. Crit Care Med 1997;25:620–8.

25. Yamamoto T, Takeda S, Sato N, et al. Noninvasive ventilation in pulmonary edema complicating acute myocardial infarction. Circ J 2012;76:2586–91.

26. Ng M, Fleming T, Robinson M, et al. Global, regional, and national prevalence of overweight and obesity in children and adults during 1980-2013: a systematic analysis for the Global Burden of Disease Study 2013. Lancet 2014;384(9945):766–81.

27. Mokhlesi B. Obesity hypoventilation syndrome: a state-of-the-art review. Respir Care 2010;55(10):1347–62.

28. Masa JF, Corral J, Alonso ML, et al. Efficacy of different treatment alternatives for obesity hypoventilation syndrome. Pickwick study. Am J Respir Crit Care Med 2015;192(1):86–95.

29. Perez de Llano LA, Golpe R, Ortiz Piquer M, et al. Short-term and long-term effects of nasal intermittent positive pressure ventilation in patients with obesity-hypoventilation syndrome. Chest 2005;128:587–94.

30. Nowbar S, Burkart KM, Gonzales R, et al. Obesity-associated hypoventilation in hospitalized patients: prevalence, effects, and outcome. Am J Med 2004;116(1):1–7.

31. Mokhlesi B, Masa JF, Brozek JL, et al. Evaluation and management of obesity hypoventilation syndrome. Am J Respir Crit Care Med 2019;200(3):e6–24.

32. Lee WY, Mokhlesi B. Diagnosis and management of obesity hypoventilation syndrome in the ICU. Crit Care Clin 2008;24(3):533–49, vii.

33. Piper AJ, Wang D, Yee BJ, et al. Randomised trial of CPAP vs bilevel support in the treatment of obesity hypoventilation syndrome without severe nocturnal desaturation. Thorax 2008;63:395–401.

34. Howard ME, Piper AJ, Stevens B, et al. A randomized controlled trial of CPAP versus non-invasive ventilation for initial treatment of obesity hypoventilation syndrome. Thorax 2017;72:437–44.

35. Masa JF, Corral J, Caballero C, et al. Non-invasive ventilation in obesity hypoventilation syndrome without severe obstructive sleep apnoea. Thorax 2016;71(10):899–906.

36. Priou P, Hamel JF, Person C, et al. Long-term outcome of noninvasive positive pressure ventilation for obesity hypoventilation syndrome. Chest 2010;138(1):84–90.

37. Blankenburg T, Benthin C, Pohl S, et al. Survival of hypercapnic patients with COPD and obesity hypoventilation syndrome treated with high intensity non invasive ventilation in the Daily routine care. Open Respir Med J 2017;11:31–40.

38. Sequeira TCA, Bahammam AS, Esquinas AM. Noninvasive ventilation in the critically ill patient with obesity hypoventilation syndrome: a review. J Intensive Care Med 2017;32(7):421–8.

39. Masa JF, Pepin J-L, Borel J-C, et al. Obesity hypoventilation syndrome. Eur Respir Rev 2019;28:180097.

40. Patout M, Gagnadoux F, Rabec C, et al. AVAPS-AE vs. ST mode: a randomised controlled trial in patients with obesity hypoventilation syndrome. Eur Respir J 2018;52(Suppl. 62):PA1674.

41. Budweiser S, Riedl SG, Jörres RA, et al. Mortality and prognostic factors in patients with obesity-hypoventilation syndrome undergoing noninvasive ventilation. J Intern Med 2007;261(4):375–83.

42. Rabinstein AA. Update on respiratory management of critically ill neurologic patients. Curr Neurol Neurosci Rep 2005;5:476–82.

43. Thomas CE, Mayer SA, Gungor Y, et al. Myasthenic crisis: clinical features, mortality, complications, and risk factors for prolonged intubation. Neurology 1997;48:1253–60.

44. Meriggioli MN. Myasthenia gravis: immunopathogenesis, diagnosis, and management. Continuum (Minneap Minn) 2009;15:35–62.

45. Multz AS, Aldrich TK, Prezant DJ, et al. Maximal inspiratory pressure is not a reliable test of inspiratory muscle strength in mechanically ventilated patients. Am Rev Respir Dis 1990;142(3):529–32.

46. Mayer SA. Intensive care if myasthenia patient. Neurology 1997;48:s7–75.

47. Varelas PN, Chua HC, Natterman J, et al. Ventilatory care in myasthenia gravis crisis : assessing the baseline adverse event rate. Crit Care Med 2002; 30(12):2663–8.

48. Kirmani JF, Yahia AM, Qureshi AI. Myasthenic crisis. Curr Treat Options Neurol 2004;6:3–15.

49. Wendell LC, Joshua L. Myasthenic crisis. Neurohospitalist 2011;1(1):16–22.

50. Lawn ND, Wijdicks EF. Post-intubation pulmonary function test in Guillain-Barre syndrome. Muscle Nerve 2000;23:613–6.

51. Koyama Y, Yoshida T, Uchiyama A, et al. Monitoring diaphragm function in a patient with myasthenia gravis: electrical activity of the diaphragm vs maximal inspiratory pressure. J Intensive Care 2017;5:66.

52. Matamis D, Soilemezi E, Tsagourias M, et al. Sonographic evaluation of the diaphragm in critically ill patients. Technique and clinical applications. Intensive Care Med 2013;39:801–10.

53. Mccool FD, Conomos P, Benditt JO, et al. Maximal inspiratory pressures and dimensions of the diaphragm. Am J Respir Crit Care Med 1997;155: 1329–34.

54. Cohn D, Benditt JO, Eveloff S, et al. Diaphragm thickening during inspiration. J Appl Physiol 1997; 83:291–6.

55. Theerawit P, Eksombatchai D, Sutherasan Y, et al. Diaphragmatic parameters by ultrasonography for predicting weaning outcomes. BMC Pulm Med 2018;18:175.

56. Li C, Li X, Han H, et al. Diaphragmatic ultrasonography for predicting ventilator weaning: a meta-analysis. Medicine 2018;97(22):e10968.

57. Rabinstein AA, Wijdicks EF. Weaning from the ventilator using BiPAP in myasthenia gravis. Muscle Nerve 2003;27:252–3.

58. Hassid VJ, Schinco MA, Tepas JJ, et al. Definitive establishment of airway control is critical for optimal outcome in lower cervical spinal cord injury. J Trauma 2008;65:1328–32.

59. Atito-Narh E, et al. Slow ventilator weaning in spinal cord injury. Br J Intensive Care 2008;95–102.

60. Sahni A, Wolfe L. Respiratory care in neuromuscular diseases. Respir Care 2018;63(5):601–8.

Tracheostomy to Noninvasive Ventilation
From Acute Care to Home

Jeanette Brown, MD, PhD

KEYWORDS

- Acute care • Care transitions • Long-term acute care (LTAC)
- Noninvasive positive pressure ventilation (NIPPV) • Rehabilitation • Tracheostomy

KEY POINTS

- Patients who undergo tracheostomy in the intensive care unit, especially ones with neuromuscular disorders, will undergo several care transitions.
- There are several aspects of transition that can be problematic if not proactively addressed. Potential solutions are detailed in this article.
- The trajectory for these patients are diverse and some patients will require long-term tracheostomy, transitioned to noninvasive positive pressure ventilation, or able to be decannulated.

INTRODUCTION

The number of patients experiencing prolonged mechanical ventilation is increasing over time[1,2] and is expected to increase further. The timing of tracheostomy placement varies considerably.[3] There is uncertainty as to the optimal time for tracheostomy placement, leading to considerable variation in placement practice in the US. Patients who have a tracheostomy placed in a critical care setting have been described as having an average of 4 separate transitions between the acute care setting, long-term acute care (LTAC), and home.[2] These transitions are points where variable practices can also come into play. We describe the transition between acute care to home for patients with tracheostomy and the transition to noninvasive positive pressure ventilation (NIPPV).

SCOPE OF PROBLEM

One of the major challenges with evaluating patients who require prolonged mechanical ventilation is that it is a heterogeneous population with many different origins and varying prognosis. These can be from primary respiratory failure, septic shock with critical illness myopathy, neurologic

origin, including spinal cord injury, trauma, postoperative, and cardiac causes. The expected clinical course would be shorter for a younger trauma patient but could be very prolonged for a patient with a primary neurologic injury with comorbidities but each case can have complications requiring transitions of care.

Patients with chronic neuromuscular respiratory failure that use NIPPV for support are at high risk for requiring intubation due to an exacerbating factor, such as a pneumonia or viral infection. These patients are at high risk for failing extubation, leading to reintubation and then subsequent tracheostomy placement. Liberation from ventilators has been assisted by extubation to directly to noninvasive ventilation and heated high flow also,[4] but some patients will still fail this due to weakness of the diaphragm and other respiratory muscles. Other coexisting conditions that may complicate extubation include obesity hypoventilation (discussed further in Roop Kaw and Marta Kaminska's article, "Obesity Hypoventilation: Traditional Versus Nontraditional Populations"; and Asil Daoud and colleagues' article, "Noninvasive Ventilation and Spinal Cord Injury," in this issue) and obstructive sleep apnea (OSA).

Division of Pulmonary Medicine, University of Utah, 26 North 1900 East, Salt Lake City, UT 84132, USA
E-mail address: Jeanette.Brown@hsc.utah.edu

Sleep Med Clin 15 (2020) 593–598
https://doi.org/10.1016/j.jsmc.2020.08.003
1556-407X/20/© 2020 Elsevier Inc. All rights reserved.

Acute high-level spinal cord injury with or without traumatic brain injury is another population that will frequently be ventilator dependent. These patients will often also have tracheostomies placed. Incomplete injuries of the spinal cord may have improvement over time. Some may elect for early placement of phrenic nerve stimulators to facilitate weaning off ventilation.

Critical illness myopathy after a prolonged intensive care unit (ICU) stay has been linked to prolonged mechanical ventilation. Diaphragm atrophy has been confirmed by biopsy after as little as 7 days of ventilator support.[5] This population is a significant portion of patients with prolonged mechanical ventilation requiring care after the ICU. This is a heterogeneous population with a variety of preexisting and acquired comorbidities that can further prolong ventilator dependency.

The timing of tracheostomy placement early (at 4 days) versus late (at 14 days) has been debated.[6] Early placement has been advocated to improve mobility and for patients with low likelihood of weaning due to underlying condition. Early tracheostomy placement did not show any improvement in days on the ventilator or length of ICU stay. The practice pattern has therefore been variable between practitioners and regions. Placement of a tracheostomy can be done by interventional pulmonary, general surgery, otolaryngology, or oral and maxillofacial surgery in the operating room or can be done bedside in the ICU with percutaneous tracheostomy placement. Placement of tracheostomy has significant impact on where patients then receive their care going forward.

Some patients will be transferred to an LTAC facility. These facilities became more common in the 1990s due to changes in incentives for these patients.[7] From an ICU perspective, this could free up beds for more acutely ill patients although some data suggest that up to one-third of patients could have completed weaning in an ICU.[8] In patients who are transferred to an LTAC the acute issues should have been resolved and should be stable on ventilator settings prescribed at the time of transfer. Typically, these patients have a secure tracheostomy and means for providing nutrition, such as a Dobhoff tube or gastrostomy tube. The focus of LTAC facilities is liberation of mechanical ventilation and physical rehabilitation. Care will typically include physicians who specialize in this population, nurses, and respiratory therapists. Weaning protocols vary depending on the facility as there is no standard of care for ventilator weaning protocols. Tracheostomy care can be completed also, including downsizing of the tracheostomy tube to facilitate speech and swallowing. Downsizing may be limited if patients need frequent suctioning for secretion removal.

Alternatively, some patients can be transferred to an acute rehabilitation center. Patients sent to these centers have to be able to complete at least 3 hours per day of physical therapy. These patients typically are stronger than those who go to LTACs and the cost of acute rehabilitation centers is less than LTACs.[1] Weaning from mechanical ventilation can take place at these facilities also.

Depending on location around the US or availability of insurance coverage, patients who require ventilatory support long term may or may not have access to an LTAC or acute rehabilitation facility. This can be an even greater issue if the patient requires chronic dialysis and continued ventilation. These patients may end up undergoing ventilator weaning in the ICU of the acute hospital or a step-down ICU unit, if available.

FROM THE INTENSIVE CARE UNIT TO LONG-TERM ACUTE CARE OR ACUTE REHABILITATION CENTER

Care transitions can be a major challenge when patients going from the ICU to either an LTAC or acute rehabilitation center. Handoff of care between providers presents an opportunity for errors[9] especially when transitioning neuromuscular patients (eg, those with Duchenne muscular dystrophy, amyotrophic lateral sclerosis [ALS], spinal cord injury) to a facility that does not routinely care for these patients. A discussion between the medical practitioners is recommended for a better handoff. This can be especially important after a prolonged hospitalization. In addition, a discharge summary should be sent to the new facility detailing the hospital stay with specific discharge instructions and scheduled follow-ups with applicable subspecialists.

There are continued risks of nosocomial infections in these facilities. Proper care protocols and personal protective equipment are essential to decrease the risk of disease transmission.

VENTILATOR ASYNCHRONY ON NEW VENTILATOR

The acute care hospital and the receiving facility may use different ventilators, and it is a common misconception that the devices will perform in equivalent fashion as long as comparable modes and setting are used. If possible, the patient will be given a trial on the ventilator that will be used at the new facility before transport, with ample opportunity to make adjustments to ensure stability and comfort. Neuromuscular patients may benefit from using volume assured pressure support modes (called AVAPS and iVAPS depending on manufacturer of the device) for comfort. Adjusting trigger sensitivity and inspiratory time may also be needed (Gaurav Singh and Michelle Cao's article, "Noninvasive Ventilator Devices and Modes," in this issue discusses in detail various modes and devices.)

TRACHEOSTOMY PLACEMENT WITH PLAN FOR DOWNSIZING AND DECANNULATION

The transferring facility should provide information as to when the tracheostomy was placed, the type and size of the tracheostomy tube, and method for placement (eg, percutaneous placement). Recently placed tracheostomy tubes should typically have sutures removed after 10 to 14 days. Tracheostomy size is important for secretion removal and can also be patient dependent. Tracheostomy tubes can be downsized to facilitate speaking and swallowing and this is typically done at provider discretion as there are no formal guidelines.[10] The summary of discussions with the patient and family/caregivers about goals and expectations regarding weaning and decannulation are also important to provide to the transferring facility.

ADVANCING FROM TRACHEOSTOMY TO NONINVASIVE POSITIVE PRESSURE VENTILATION

Patients with underlying chronic neuromuscular respiratory failure may be able to be decannulated to NIPPV. Bach and Saporito[11] found that patients with a peak cough flow greater than 160 L/min were able to be decannulated or extubated. These patients are extubated to NIPPV with frequent cough clearance therapy (mechanical insufflator/exsufflator). These protocols typically require significant patient monitoring and respiratory therapy support and could be done in the ICU or in the LTAC environment. Monitoring oxygen saturation and Pco_2 is important to manage these patients through this transition.

Some patients may be able to wean off the ventilator for part of the day and still require ventilator support at night. These patients would have their tracheostomy tube capped during the daytime. If they are able to tolerate this, then it is also possible to try NIPPV support at night instead of ventilation by tracheostomy. If NIPPV support is tolerated, then it is possible to consider decannulation also.

Some spinal cord injury patients have been started on phrenic nerve pacers in combination with nocturnal NIPPV support while the tracheostomy tube is capped. Monitoring pulse oximetry and arterial or venous Pco_2 are useful in guiding adjustment of these therapies.

When considering a patient's needs for ventilator support and weaning off this support it is important to consider whether patients have underlying sleep disordered breathing that is contributing to the requirement for ventilatory support. Patients with spinal cord injuries have a much higher rate of OSA than typical estimations from the general population.[12] Unfortunately, these patients may not have had a formal polysomnography (PSG) before acute ventilation. If a patient has a capped tracheostomy and looking toward decannulation, a formal PSG can be done to evaluate for sleep disordered breathing. Performing full PSGs in a sleep lab can be prohibitively challenging for some of these patients due to the need for specialized beds, equipment, and patient care. Continuous transcutaneous CO_2 monitoring can be used to evaluate for central hypoventilation. Settings for NIPPV can be titrated based on overnight oximetry and arterial or venous Pco_2 monitoring if a formal PSG is not available at the patient's location.

Another way to titrate settings without a formal PSG is to evaluate data downloads from ventilators, which is discussed in depth in Philip Choi and colleagues' article, "Noninvasive Ventilation Downloads and Monitoring," in this issue. Evaluation of respiratory rate, pressure required to achieve set tidal volume, mask leak, and apnea hypopnea index flow[13] can be helpful, depending on the settings and patient's specific device.

CHOOSING A DEVICE FOR LONG-TERM VENTILATION: INVASIVE OR NONINVASIVE

Before the late 1990s, there were few ventilatory support devices that a patient could use in the home. They had limited modes, typically SIMV and AC, and were large and bulky. New devices, such as the Trilogy (Phillips), Astral (ResMed), and recently the VOCSN (Ventec Life Systems) have made delivery of care easier for patients. The devices are smaller, quieter, and battery operated making them more portable. The alarm settings are improved and the devices have multiple modes with capacity for varied settings such as day or night. Newer modes, such as VAPS, allow for a set tidal volume with a set pressure range to achieve that tidal volume. This can be used for invasive and noninvasive ventilation. They have touch screen options for setting up the device, which can be helpful if adjustments are necessary. They also allow for detailed data downloads via

Bluetooth so that providers can monitor use and data parameters. The new VOCSN is a multifunction device that combines a ventilator, oxygen concentrator to 6 L, cough clearance function, suction machine, and nebulizer all in 1 unit. When deciding which device a patient will need in the LTAC and at home, it is important to consider what devices and settings they are using currently. If a patient uses the Trilogy or Astral and needs cough clearance therapy, they will need a separate device. Cough clearance devices have also improved, including the CoughAssist device (Phillips) and the VitalCough (Hill-Rom). These have both an inspiratory phase and expiratory phase to rerecruit lung and pull up secretions to the larger airways. These devices have been shown to reduce mucus plugging, respiratory events, and the incidence of pneumonia[14] for neuromuscular patients. Cough clearance devices can be used in patients with a diagnosis of functional quadriplegia and other neuromuscular disorders using mask and or a mouthpiece or if they have a tracheostomy, it is directly attached to their tube.

Patients who are expected to remain on the ventilator who need oxygen, suctioning, and other devices may be better suited to a VOCSN device for ease of training caregivers and for avoiding the expense of multiple pieces of equipment. Another option for high-level spinal cord injured patients would be a phrenic pacer system. After gaining diaphragm strength, some patients can wean off NIPPV completely and use just the pacing system. Pacing systems in the US are made by Avery and Synapse. The Avery system in completely contained within the body and the Synapse system has a wire that comes through the abdominal wall to connect to the system for stimulation. There has been hesitation to use these systems outside of patients with spinal cord injury or congenital central hypoventilation syndrome because of the negative outcomes reported for patients with ALS in European studies.[15] There are current clinical trials for temporary pacers in the ICU setting to see if they will help shorten the duration of ventilatory support.[16] Overall, the choice of device should be tailored to the patients' individual needs and desires.

FROM LONG-TERM ACUTE CARE OR ACUTE REHABILITATION CENTER TO HOME

Many patients would prefer to be in their own homes instead of any form of medical institution. Cost of care at home is typically less expensive and there is considerably less concern about nosocomial infection.[17] With transition to home, there are many factors to consider, including whether the acute care issues are resolved, whether the patient maintains stable vital signs, and the overall goal of the patient. Issues that we have encountered in the past include patients having enough caregivers available, as we recommend at least 2 fully trained caregivers.

Patients who are discharged home with full-time caregivers (both family and private duty) will need follow-up in the clinic with a pulmonologist and other subspecialists depending on the complexity of the patient's medical care.[1] A primary care provider should be the central hub of the care but often a subspecialist, such as a physiatrist will assume that role. It is important that, as patients are transitioned home, they have easy access to a point person if they have needs or concerns at home. This helps reduce anxiety. Before going home, our patient's caregivers are required to demonstrate competency in care tasks for 24 hours or longer so that they can feel comfortable going home. They also should be comfortable in responding to emergencies, such as mucus plugs or ventilator alarms. Despite this training, questions and problems often arise and going home with a loved one can have a lot of unknowns. Phone numbers should be provided for these support staff at the time of discharge. Close follow-up is necessary soon after discharge to ease the stress and allow for questions. Consider telehealth as a simpler and more efficient follow-up. Arranging prompt follow-up with social work and palliative care support is also important. **Table 1** summarized our recommendations to improve outcomes with transitioning to home based on experiences at the University of Michigan and the University of Utah.

TO DECANNULATE OR NOT TO DECANNULATE

Often the issue is brought up about the possibility of decannulation, in LTAC, acute rehabilitation or after discharge to home. Decannulation can aid with speech and swallowing, but if a patient develops respiratory failure in the future that may require repeat tracheostomy placement, which can be more complicated. The patient's underlying medical conditions must be considered heavily when pondering decannulation. Consider a patient with ALS who develops pneumonia and who failed extubation attempts and had a percutaneous tracheostomy placed in the ICU. After months of rehabilitation, he was able to cap his tracheostomy during the daytime and use the ventilator at night. He wanted to be decannulated but his bulbar symptoms had the team concerned that he would

Table 1
Summary of recommendations to improve outcomes with transitioning to home based on experiences at the University of Michigan and the University of Utah

Problems Transitioning to Home	Recommended Solutions
Education for caregivers for managing the patient at home	24 h of care provided by selected home caregivers while still at facility using the equipment they plan to be using at home
Hospital ventilator to home ventilator transition	Transition from hospital ventilator to home ventilator in the facility to adjust settings if needed before transition
Identification of all those to be called with questions on discharge summaries (nursing, respiratory therapy, other providers)	Discharge paperwork with clear discharge instructions and clinic contact numbers
Emergencies at home or out of the house	"To go" bag/emergency bag content: • Portable suction machine • Suction catheters • Gloves • Hand sanitizer • Saline bullets • Trach tube (same size and size smaller) • Obturator for current trach • Scissors • Hemostats • Extra tracheostomy ties • Syringe for cuffed tracheostomy tube • Contact numbers for the clinic
Emotional support going home	Social work and palliative care consultation

have another pneumonia. In the end, he elected for a tracheal button that would preserve the stoma for future tracheostomy placement, but he could use NIPPV via mask for nocturnal support. Months later, he did develop pneumonia and had to go back to using his tracheostomy for ventilation and secretion clearance with the cough assist device.

As in the example, the question of whether to remove the tracheostomy tube is a complex one. The patient's clinical trajectory and underlying condition should factor heavily making these decisions, in concert with the patient and family/caregivers. It also depends on the underlying condition that led to the need for intubation and failure of extubation. If it was due to critical illness myopathy, then more likely the patient will be able to be decannulated once their strength improves. If there is an underlying neuromuscular disorder, then this is more difficult and the likelihood of recurrent respiratory failure is an issue to be considered. One option, as in the example above, is to place a tracheal button that preserves the stoma but does not protrude out of the skin much or into the airway. This way, if the patient needs to be ventilated again the button can be replaced by a standard tracheostomy tube without

the need for repeat tracheostomy placement, which is typically more complicated.

SUMMARY

In summary, patients who undergo tracheostomy in the ICU, especially ones with neuromuscular disorders, will undergo several care transitions that have many areas that need to be addressed proactively. The trajectory for these patients are diverse. Some may be able to have their tracheostomy removed and some may need to have it for long term. This again will be based on underlying conditions and shared decision making with patient, caregiver, and care team. Some may be able to transition to NIPPV and will need long-term follow-up for this going forward. It is essential to discuss all these issues in detail with patients and caregivers during each transition.

DISCLOSURE

serves on the Advisory Board for Biogen for SMA.

REFERENCES

1. Unroe M, Kahn JM, Carson SS, et al. One-year trajectories of care and resource utilization for

recipients of prolonged mechanical ventilation: a cohort study. Ann Intern Med 2010;153(3):167–75.

2. Zilberberg MD, Luippold RS, Sulsky S, et al. Prolonged acute mechanical ventilation, hospital resource utilization, and mortality in the United States. Crit Care Med 2008;36(3):724–30.

3. Nathens AB, Rivara FP, Mack CD, et al. Variations in rates of tracheostomy in the critically ill trauma patient. Crit Care Med 2006;34(12):2919–24.

4. Thille AW, Muller G, Gacouin A, et al. Effect of post-extubation high-flow nasal oxygen with noninvasive ventilation vs high-flow nasal oxygen alone on reintubation among patients at high risk of extubation failure: a randomized clinical trial. JAMA 2019;322(15): 1465–75.

5. Schepens T, Verbrugghe W, Dams K, et al. The course of diaphragm atrophy in ventilated patients assessed with ultrasound: a longitudinal cohort study. Crit Care 2015;19:422.

6. Khammas AH, Dawood MR. Timing of tracheostomy in intensive care unit patients. Int Arch Otorhinolaryngol 2018;22(4):437–42.

7. Kahn JM, Benson NM, Appleby D, et al. Long-term acute care hospital utilization after critical illness. JAMA 2010;303(22):2253–9.

8. Jubran A, Grant BJB, Duffner LA, et al. Long-term outcome after prolonged mechanical ventilation. A long-term acute-care hospital study. Am J Respir Crit Care Med 2019;199(12):1508–16.

9. The Joint Commission Patient Safety Topics: sentinel event. Available at: https://www.jointcommission.org/resources/patient-safety-topics/sentinel-event.

10. White AC, Kher S, O'Connor HH. When to change a tracheostomy tube. Respir Care 2010;55(8): 1069–75.

11. Bach JR, Saporito LR. Criteria for extubation and tracheostomy tube removal for patients with ventilatory failure. A different approach to weaning. Chest 1996;110(6):1566–71.

12. Brown JP, Bauman KA, Kurili A, et al. Positive airway pressure therapy for sleep-disordered breathing confers short-term benefits to patients with spinal cord injury despite widely ranging patterns of use. Spinal Cord 2018;56(8):777–89.

13. Li QY, Berry RB, Goetting MG, et al. Detection of upper airway status and respiratory events by a current generation positive airway pressure device. Sleep 2015;38(4):597–605.

14. Bach JR. Noninvasive respiratory management of patients with neuromuscular disease. Ann Rehabil Med 2017;41(4):519–38.

15. Jackson CE, McVey AL, Rudnicki S, et al. Symptom management and end-of-life care in amyotrophic lateral sclerosis. Neurol Clin 2015;33(4):889–908.

16. A protocol comparing temporary transvenous diaphragm pacing to standard of care for weaning from mechanical ventilation (RESCUE3). Available at: https://clinicaltrials.gov/ct2/show/NCT03783884.

17. Bach JR, Intintola P, Alba AS, et al. The ventilator-assisted individual. Cost analysis of institutionalization vs rehabilitation and in-home management. Chest 1992;101(1):26–30.

1. Publication Title	2. Publication Number	3. Filing Date
SLEEP MEDICINE CLINICS	025 – 0X3	9/18/2020

4. Issue Frequency	5. Number of Issues Published Annually	6. Annual Subscription Price
MAR, JUN, SEP, DEC	4	$218.00

7. Complete Mailing Address of Known Office of Publication (Not printer) (Street, city, county, state, and ZIP+4®)

ELSEVIER INC.
230 Park Avenue, Suite 800
New York, NY 10169

Contact Person
Malathi Samayan

Telephone (Include area code)
91-44-4299-4507

8. Complete Mailing Address of Headquarters or General Business Office of Publisher (Not printer)

ELSEVIER INC.
230 Park Avenue, Suite 800
New York, NY 10169

9. Full Names and Complete Mailing Addresses of Publisher, Editor, and Managing Editor (Do not leave blank)

Publisher (Name and complete mailing address)

DOLORES MELONI, ELSEVIER INC.
1600 JHON F KENNEDY BLVD. SUITE 1800
PHILADELPHIA, PA 19103-2899

Editor (Name and complete mailing address)

JOANNA COLLETT, ELSEVIER INC.
1600 JOHN F KENNEDY BLVD. SUITE 1800
PHILADELPHIA, PA 19103-2899

Managing Editor (Name and complete mailing address)

PATRICK MANLEY, ELSEVIER INC.
1600 JOHN F KENNEDY BLVD. SUITE 1800
PHILADELPHIA, PA 19103-2899

10. Owner (Do not leave blank. If the publication is owned by a corporation, give the name and address of the corporation immediately followed by the names and addresses of all stockholders owning or holding 1 percent or more of the total amount of stock. If not owned by a corporation, give the names and addresses of the individual owners. If owned by a partnership or other unincorporated firm, give its name and address as well as those of each individual owner. If the publication is published by a nonprofit organization, give its name and address.)

Full Name	Complete Mailing Address
WHOLLY OWNED SUBSIDIARY OF REED/ELSEVIER, US HOLDINGS	1600 JOHN F KENNEDY® BLVD. SUITE 1800 PHILADELPHIA, PA 19103-2899

11. Known Bondholders, Mortgagees, and Other Security Holders Owning or Holding 1 Percent or More of Total Amount of Bonds, Mortgages, or Other Securities. If none, check box ▶ ☐ None

Full Name	Complete Mailing Address
N/A	

12. Tax Status (For completion by nonprofit organizations authorized to mail at nonprofit rates) (Check one)
The purpose, function, and nonprofit status of this organization and the exempt status for federal income tax purposes:
☒ Has Not Changed During Preceding 12 Months
☐ Has Changed During Preceding 12 Months (Publisher must submit explanation of change with this statement)

PS Form 3526, July 2014 (Page 1 of 4 (see instructions page 4)) PSN: 7530-01-000-9931   PRIVACY NOTICE: See our privacy policy on www.usps.com.

13. Publication Title	14. Issue Date for Circulation Data Below
SLEEP MEDICINE CLINICS	JUNE 2020

15. Extent and Nature of Circulation			Average No. Copies Each Issue During Preceding 12 Months	No. Copies of Single Issue Published Nearest to Filing Date
a. Total Number of Copies (Net press run)			238	190
b. Paid Circulation (By Mail and Outside the Mail)	(1)	Mailed Outside-County Paid Subscriptions Stated on PS Form 3541 (Include paid distribution above nominal rate, advertiser's proof copies, and exchange copies)	168	137
	(2)	Mailed In-County Paid Subscriptions Stated on PS Form 3541 (Include paid distribution above nominal rate, advertiser's proof copies, and exchange copies)	0	0
	(3)	Paid Distribution Outside the Mails Including Sales Through Dealers and Carriers, Street Vendors, Counter Sales, and Other Paid Distribution Outside USPS®	34	27
	(4)	Paid Distribution by Other Classes of Mail Through the USPS (e.g., First-Class Mail®)	0	0
c. Total Paid Distribution [Sum of 15b (1), (2), (3), and (4)]			202	164
d. Free or Nominal Rate Distribution (By Mail and Outside the Mail)	(1)	Free or Nominal Rate Outside-County Copies included on PS Form 3541	21	13
	(2)	Free or Nominal Rate In-County Copies Included on PS Form 3541	0	0
	(3)	Free or Nominal Rate Copies Mailed at Other Classes Through the USPS (e.g., First-Class Mail)	0	0
	(4)	Free or Nominal Rate Distribution Outside the Mail (Carriers or other means)	0	0
e. Total Free or Nominal Rate Distribution (Sum of 15d (1), (2), (3) and (4))			21	13
f. Total Distribution (Sum of 15c and 15e)			223	177
g. Copies not Distributed (See Instructions to Publishers #4 (page #3))			15	13
h. Total (Sum of 15f and g)			238	190
i. Percent Paid (15c divided by 15f times 100)			90.58%	92.65%

* If you are claiming electronic copies, go to line 16 on page 3. If you are not claiming electronic copies, skip to line 17 on page 3.

16. Electronic Copy Circulation	Average No. Copies Each Issue During Preceding 12 Months	No. Copies of Single Issue Published Nearest to Filing Date
a. Paid Electronic Copies ▶		
b. Total Paid Print Copies (Line 15c) + Paid Electronic Copies (Line 16a) ▶		
c. Total Print Distribution (Line 15f) + Paid Electronic Copies (Line 16a) ▶		
d. Percent Paid (Both Print & Electronic Copies) (16b divided by 16c × 100) ▶		

☒ I certify that 50% of all my distributed copies (electronic and print) are paid above a nominal price.

17. Publication of Statement of Ownership

☒ If the publication is a general publication, publication of this statement is required. Will be printed in the DECEMBER 2020 issue of this publication.   ☐ Publication not required.

18. Signature and Title of Editor, Publisher, Business Manager, or Owner

Malathi Samayan   Date 9/18/2020

Malathi Samayan - Distribution Controller

I certify that all information furnished on this form is true and complete. I understand that anyone who furnishes false or misleading information on this form or who omits material or information requested on the form may be subject to criminal sanctions (including fines and imprisonment) and/or civil sanctions (including civil penalties).

PS Form 3526, July 2014 (Page 3 of 4)   PRIVACY NOTICE: See our privacy policy on www.usps.com

Moving?

Make sure your subscription moves with you!

To notify us of your new address, find your **Clinics Account Number** (located on your mailing label above your name), and contact customer service at:

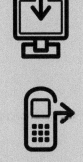

Email: journalscustomerservice-usa@elsevier.com

800-654-2452 (subscribers in the U.S. & Canada)
314-447-8871 (subscribers outside of the U.S. & Canada)

Fax number: 314-447-8029

Elsevier Health Sciences Division
Subscription Customer Service
3251 Riverport Lane
Maryland Heights, MO 63043

*To ensure uninterrupted delivery of your subscription, please notify us at least 4 weeks in advance of move.

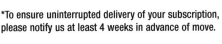